Proceedings of the 9th International Cancer Congress

UICC Monograph Series · Volume 10

Proceedings of the 9th International Cancer Congress

Tokyo October 1966
Panel Discussions

Edited by
R. J. C. Harris

With 111 figures

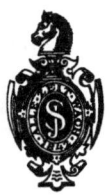

Springer-Verlag Berlin Heidelberg GmbH 1967

R. J. C. Harris, Imperial Cancer Research Fund, Burtonhole Lane,
London N. W. 7, Great Britain

ISBN 978-3-662-12798-8   ISBN 978-3-662-12796-4 (eBook)
DOI 10.1007/978-3-662-12796-4

Library of Congress Catalog Card Number 67-27724

Title-No. 7521

Contents

Panel Chairmen

1
M. Kuru, National Cancer Center Hospital, Tokyo, Japan

2
L. C. Robbins, Division of Chronic Diseases, U.S., Public Health Service, Washington D.C., U.S.A.

11
K. Shanmugaratnam, 29 Yarwood Avenue, Singapore 21, India

13
S. Watanabe, Research Institute for Nuclear Medicine and Biology, Kasumi-cho, Hiroshima, Japan

14
J. Wakefield, Christie Hospital and Holt Radium Institute, Manchester 20, England

15
G. H. Fletcher, M. D. Anderson Hospital and Tumor Institute, Houston, Texas 77025, U.S.A.

H. Imanaga, Hazama-cho, Showa-ku, Nagoya, Aichi-ken, Japan

17
R. Doll, Medical Research Council, Statistical Research Unit, 115, Gower Street, London, W.C. 1., England

20
J. H. Burchenal, Sloan-Kettering Institute for Cancer Research, 5701, N. Park Avenue, Philadelphia, Pa. 19141, U.S.A.

21
D. A. Karnofsky, Division of Chemotherapy Research, Sloan-Kettering Institute, New York, N.Y., U.S.A.

22
R. N. Grant, American Cancer Society, 219 East 42nd. St., New York, N.Y. 10017, U.S.A.

Contributors

ALEXANDR CHAKLIN, Department of Epidemiology, Institute for Experimental Clinical Oncology of Academy of Medical Science, Moscow, USSR

JOHANNES CLEMMESEN, Finsen Institute, Copenhagen, Denmark

W. M. COURT BROWN, Medical Research Council, Clinical Effects of Radiation Research Unit, Western General Hospital, Edinburgh, Scotland

R. DOLL, Medical Research Council, Statistical Research Unit, 115 Gower Sreet, London, W. C. 1, England

VASILE DRAGON, Oncological Institute of Bucharest, Bucharest, Rumania

G. H. FLETCHER, M. D. Anderson Hospital and Tumor Institute, Houston, Texas 77025, U. S. A.

EMIL FREI, III, The University of Texas, M. D. Anderson Hospital and Tumor Institute, Houston, Texas 77025, U. S. A.

WILLIAM HAENSZEL National Cancer Institute, National Institutes of Health, Bethesda, Maryland 20014, U. S. A.

M. HAKAMA, Finnish Cancer Register, Helsinki, Finland

JOHN L. HAYWARD, Department of Surgery, Guy's Hospital, London, S. E. 1, England

L. H. HEMPELMANN, Division of Experimental Radiology, University of Rochester, Rochester, N. Y., U. S. A.

JOHN HIGGINSON, International Agency for Research on Cancer, Lyon, France

TAKESHI HIRAYAMA, Epidemiology Division, National Cancer Center, Research Institute, Tokyo, Japan

ABRAHAM HOCHMAN, Department of Oncology, Hadassah Medical Organization, Jerusalem, Israel

DANIEL HORN, National Clearinghouse for Smoking and Health, U. S. Public Health Service, Arlington, Virginia, U. S. A.

C. D. HOWE, M. D. Anderson Hospital and Tumor Institute, Houston, Texas 77025, U. S. A.

W. C. HUEPER, National Cancer Institute, Bethesda, Md. 20014, U. S. A.

ANTONIO C. C. JUNQUEIRA, Central Institute of Cancer, São Paulo, Brazil

DALI J. JUSSAWALLA, Indian Cancer Society, Parel-Bombay 12, India

K. KARRER, Institut für experimentelle Krebsforschung, Universität Wien, Vienna, Austria

HANNA KOLODZIEJSKA, Institute of Oncology, Garncarska 11, Kraków, Poland

YOSHIYUKI KOYAMA, The First National Hospital of Tokyo, Tokyo, Japan

M. KURU, National Cancer Center Hospital, Tokyo, Japan

R. D. LINDBERG, M. D. Anderson Hospital and Tumor Institute, Houston, Texas 77025, U.S.A.

A. C. McKENNELL, Social Survey Division, Central Office of Information, London, England

MASASUMI MIYAKAWA, Nagoya University, School of Medicine, Nagoya, Japan

RODOLFO MORAN, Cancer Clinic, City Hospital of Guadalajara, Guadalajara, Mexico

V. ANOMAH NGU, Department of Surgery, University of Ibadan, Nigeria

ROAR NISSEN-MEYER, Norwegian Radium Hospital, Oslo 3, Norway

MICHAEL E. PALKO, Department of National Health and Welfare, Ottawa, Canada

MARIO PAREDES, Cancer Clinic, City Hospital of Guadalajara, Guadalajara, Mexico

A. J. PHILLIPS, National Cancer Institute of Canada, Toronto, Canada

J. W. PIFER, Division of Experimental Radiology, University of Rochester, Rochester, N. Y., U.S.A.

EVA J. SALBER, Department of Epidemiology, Harvard University, School of of Public Health, One Shattuck Street, Boston, Mass., U.S.A.

M. L. SAMUELS, M. D. Anderson Hospital and Tumor Institute, Houston, Texas, 77025, U.S.A.

RYOZO SANO, National Cancer Center Hospital, Tokyo, Japan

E. A. SAXÉN, Finnish Cancer Register, Helsinki, Finland

MARVIN SCHNEIDERMANN, National Cancer Institute, Bethesda, Maryland 20014, U.S.A.

MITSUO SEGI, Department of Public Health, Tohoku University School of Medicine, Sendai, Japan

J. P. SMITH, M. D. Anderson Hospital and Tumor Institute, Houston, Texas, 77025, U.S.A.

P. SMITH, Medical Research Council, Statistical Research Unit, 115, Gower Street, London, W. C. 1., England

G. N. STEMMERMAN, Kuakini Hospital, Department of Pathology, University of Hawaii, School of Medicine, Honolulu, Hawaii, U. S. A.

HAROLD L. STEWART, National Cancer Institute, Bethesda, Maryland 20014, U.S.A.

H. D. SUIT, M. D. Anderson Hospital and Tumor Institute, Houston, Texas 77025, U.S.A.

HENRI J. TAGNON, Institut Jules Bordet, Brussels, Belgium

SHINJI TAKAHASHI, Department of Radiology, Nagoya University, School of Medicine, Nagoya, Japan

KEMPO TSUKAMOTO, National Institute of Radiobiological Sciences, Chiba, Japan

J. WAKEFIELD, Christie Hospital and Holt Radium Institute, Manchester 20, England

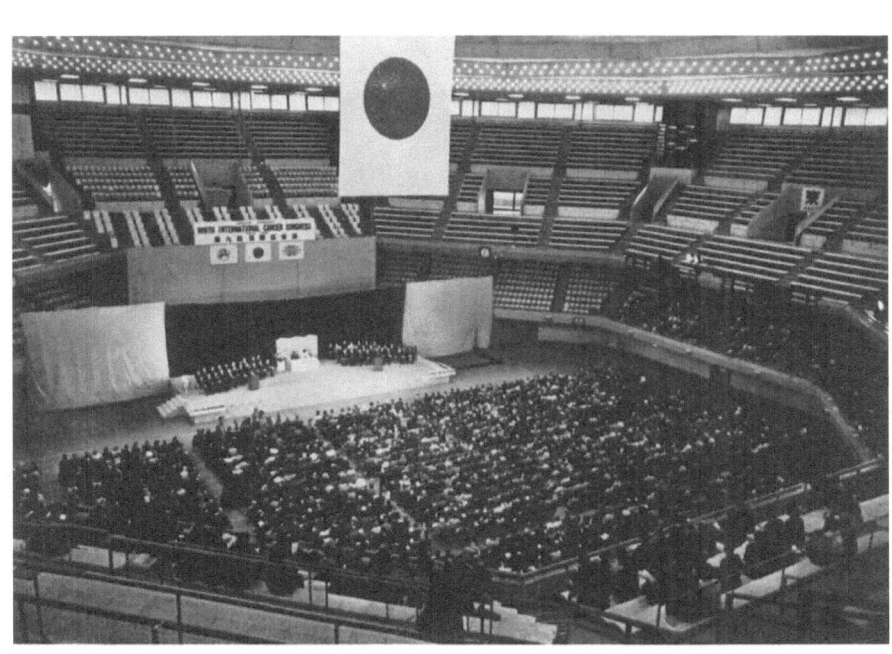

Panel 1

Pathogenesis and Epidemiology of Cancer of the Stomach

Chairman:

M. KURU (Japan)

Co-Chairman:

T. HIRAYAMA (Japan)

Members:

A. CHAKLIN (U.S.S.R.), W. HAENSZEL (U.S.A.), J. F. HIGGINSON (U.S.A.),
E. SAXÉN (Finland), M. SEGI (Japan), G. N. STEMMERMAN (U.S.A.),
H. L. STEWART (U.S.A.)

Histogenetical Study of Gastric Carcinomas in the Japanese. Analysis of 150 Cases Treated in Relatively Early Stages

MASARU KURU and RYOZO SANO

National Cancer Center Hospital, Tokyo, Japan

Introduction

From the viewpoint of early diagnosis, as well as of prophylaxis, the problem of precursors in human gastric carcinomas is a matter of paramount importance. The remarkable progress in gastric diagnostics during the last 10 years has enabled us to examine a number of gastric carcinomas in relatively early stages. In such early preparations the problem of precursors can be discussed much more easily and accurately. The present report is on a histogenetical investigation of one hundred and fifty gastric carcinomas in which cancerous invasion was restricted either to the mucous membrane or to the muco-submucous layer.

Material and Methods

Since the establishment of National Cancer Center Hospital in May 1961 till April 1966 1,050 gastrectomies were performed for carcinoma of the stomach. All the material underwent precise histological examination. Of these 1,050, in 150 there was no invasion into the muscular coat and the cancerous focus was restricted to the mucosa or the muco-submucous layer. These 150 cases were used for the histogenetical investigation. Clinical data, X-ray and gastro-camera findings of representative cases are shown in the monograph recently published by one of us (KURU, 1966b). After fixation, the part of the stomach including the whole lesion was divided into 5–20 longitudinal strips from the cardiac to the pyloric stump along or parallel to the lesser curvature. Not only the cancerous focus, but also the surrounding mucous membrane were examined in detail, paying special attention to co-existing ulcerative lesion(s). Beside the haematoxylin-eosin stain, VAN GIESON, MALLORY and PAS stains were routinely used. Silver impregnation technic was employed to trace the attitude of basal membrane in necessary cases.

Results

From their gross appearance these 150 gastric carcinomas in relatively early stages can be classified into five groups:
1. polypous or polypoid cancer,
2. ulcer-cancer,
3. superficial spreading cancer with ulcer,
4. *in situ* carcinoma of the mucosa, and
5. submucous carcinoma.

The first group differs from the other four in that the cancer has a polypous or polypoid appearance. In this group, the cancerous focus protrudes from the surroundings and its boundary is quite distinct. In 7 cases it was markedly pedunculate, while in 9 it was more sessile and in 6 more flattened (Fig. 1). In all these 22 cases the existence of adenomatous tissue beneath or in the cancerous focus could be easily demonstrated, so that a cancerous transformation of an adenoma was reasonably postulated. An example of the pedunculate form is demonstrated in Fig. 2 and that of a more sessile form is shown in Fig. 3. In the lower half of these figures both carcinomatous and adenomatous foci are shown in high magnification. However in 13 other cases of this group, adenomatous tissue could no longer be recognized despite the polypoid appearance (Fig. 4). These polypoid cancers can be interpreted as being a later stage of the polypous cancers demonstrated above or of the *in situ* carcinomas to be discussed below. Histologically papillo-tubular structure was common and in the surrounding mucosa marked atrophic or atrophic-hyperplastic gastritis with intestinal metaplasia was observed (Fig. 5). Correspondingly gastric anacidity prevailed in the majority of cases (Fig. 6).

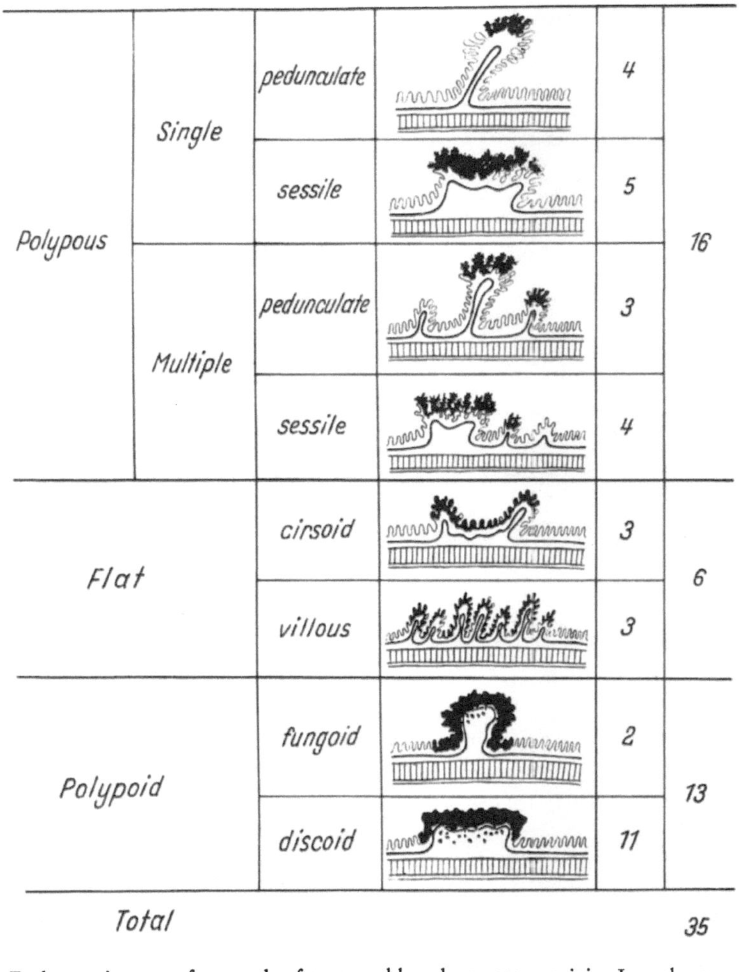

Polypous	Single	pedunculate		4
		sessile		5
	Multiple	pedunculate		3
		sessile		4
Flat		cirsoid		3
		villous		3
Polypoid		fungoid		2
		discoid		11
Total				35

(group totals: Polypous 16, Flat 6, Polypoid 13)

Fig. 1. Early carcinomas of stomach of presumably adenomatous origin. In polypous and flat groups co-existence of adenomas was confirmed

In the second and third groups the cancer is characteristic in being accompanied by an ulcer (Fig. 7). The depth of the ulcer differs from case to case. In 49 cases the muscularis mucosae was destroyed, leaving the muscular coat completely intact, whereas the defect of the muscular coat was partial in 29 cases and complete in 23 cases.

On the other hand, the extent of the mucosal invasion also varied considerably. In 15 cases it was especially localized, in 8 cases of which it was in the shape of a crescent confined to one side of the margin, whereas it was annular and encircled the ulcer-margin in 7 other cases (Fig. 8). However, in

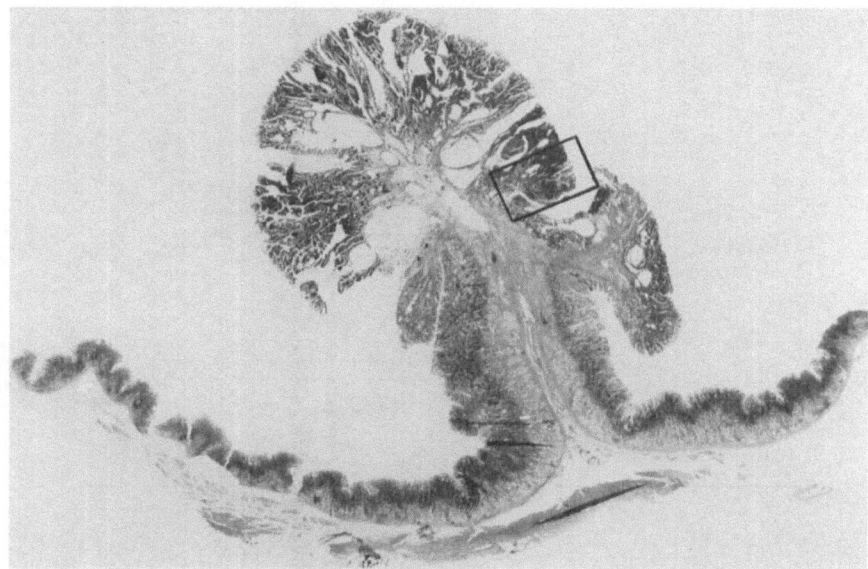

A

B   C

Fig. 2 A—C. Carcinomatous degeneration of pedunculate adenomatous polyp. A. General view.
B. High magnification of the part indicated with a rectangle in A. C. High magnification of
the part indicated with an arrow in B. 57 years old, male. Gastric hypoacidity

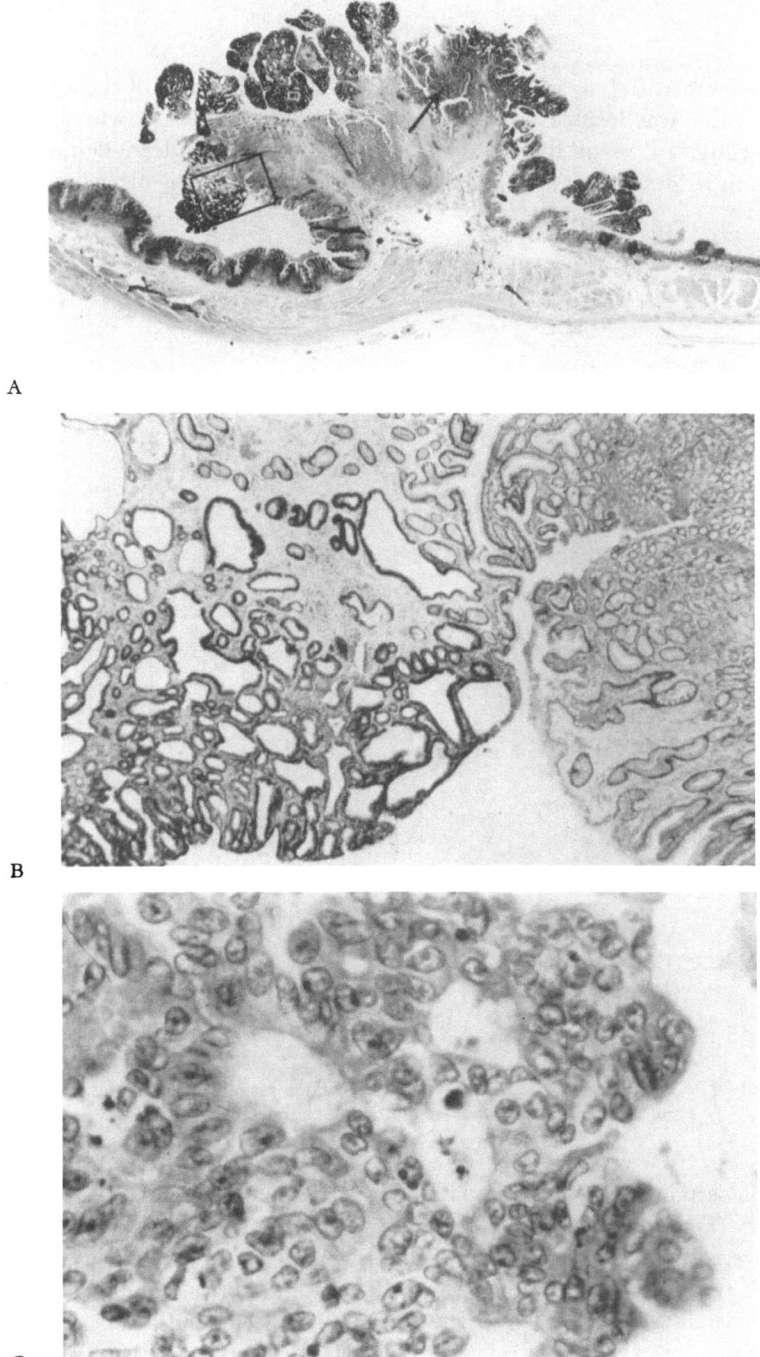

Fig. 3 A—C. Carcinomatous degeneration of sessile adenomatous polyp. A General view.
B. High magnification of the part inside the rectangle in A. C. High magnification of the part
indicated with an arrow in A. 57 years old, male. Gastric anacidity

86 cases the superficial invasion was more or less extensive. In 30 of these spread cases the ulcer was located eccentrically, whereas in 56 cases it was situated concentrically. In 64 of these 101 cases, the floor of the ulcer, despite the variation in its depth, was free from cancerous infiltration. The ulcer-floor was

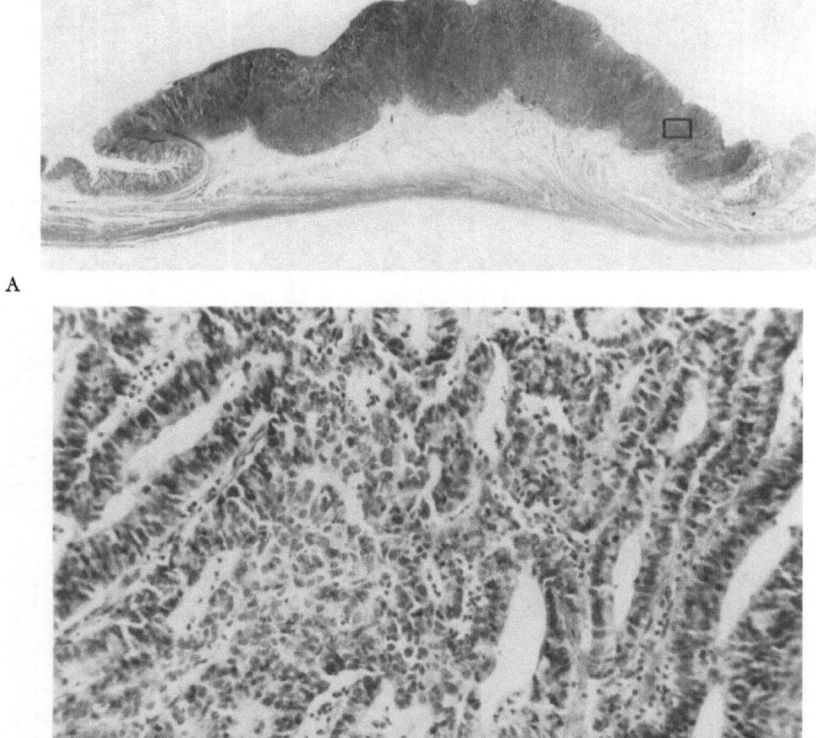

A

B

Fig. 4 A and B. Polypoid carcinoma. A. General view. B. High magnification of the part inside the rectangle in A. 60 years old, male. Gastric anacidity

covered in certain cases with granulation tissue and in others with regenerating epithelium (Figs. 9 and 10). In 37 cases, however, the regenerating epithelium which covered the ulcer-floor was partially or completely invaded by cancerous cells (Fig. 9). Even in such cases, in view of the thickness of the connective tissue in the deeper layer of the floor (Figs. 9 and 10), it seems more reasonable to postulate the pre-existence of an ulcer, than to consider, as MALLORY (1940) once did, that secondary ulceration of an *in situ* carcinoma of the gastric mucosa had occurred. Also the conspicuous convergence of rugae toward the ulcer center implies the chronicity of the ulcer (Fig. 11). On the other hand the distribution of 258 benign ulcers operated on in the same period coincides fairly well with that of carcinomas in this group, if the benign ulcers, too, are classified into three subgroups and comparison is done in each corresponding

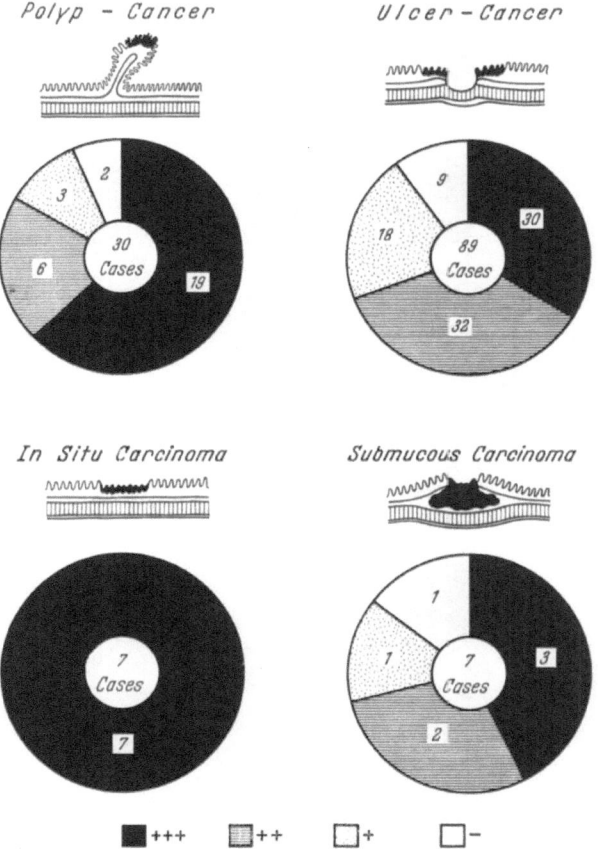

Fig. 5. Intestinal metaplasia found in surrounding mucosa of early gastric carcinomas. Superficial spreading carcinomas with ulcers are included in ulcer-cancer group. +++, conspicuous intestinalization all over the specimen. ++, intermediate between + and +++. +, intestinalization restricted to the antrum

subgroup (Fig. 12). This fact also supports the above view. Summarizing the findings in these groups, it can be concluded, that the initial cancerization took place at the mucous margin bordering the ulcer and expanded gradually into the surrounding mucosa. These types of gastric carcinoma, therefore, have the appearance of the superficial spreading type with ulcer in their later stages (Fig. 13).

It should be noted that the second and third groups contain two-thirds of the total cases. In younger patients, these types of carcinoma mostly appear histologically as a highly anaplastic carcinoma with signet ring cell formation (Fig. 9). In old patients, however, tubular adenocarcinoma was more frequently

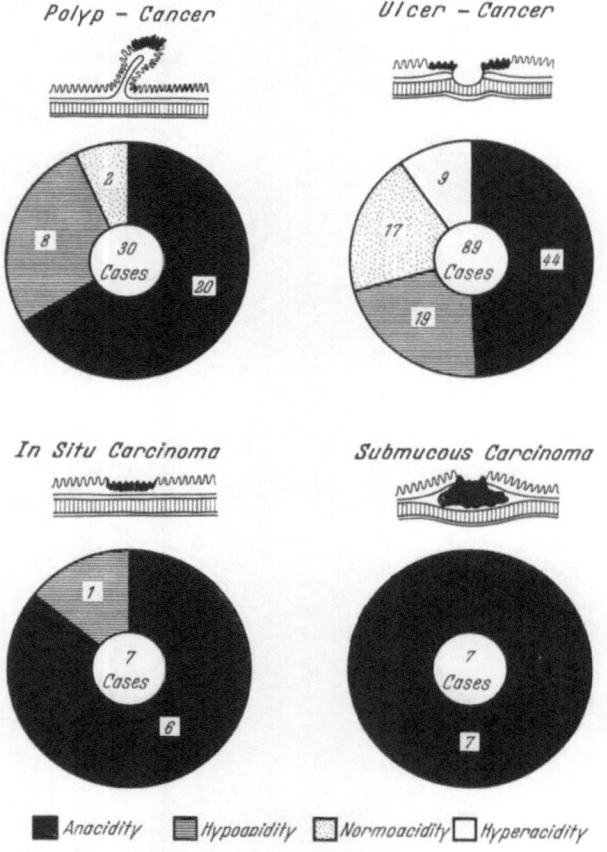

Fig. 6. Gastric acidity (Katsch-Kalk method) in cases of early gastric carcinomas. Superficial spreading carcinomas with ulcers are included in ulcer-cancer group

encountered (Figs. 8 and 10). The intestinal metaplasia in the surrounding mucosa was observed less frequently and less conspicuously than in case of polypous cancer (Fig. 5 B). However, anacidity was much more frequently observed than had been expected and hyperacidity could be confirmed only in a small number of cases (Fig. 6 B).

The cancer in the fourth group is non-polypoid pre-invasive form without ulceration and corresponds to the so-called *in situ* cancerization of the gastric mucosa. In this group the muscularis mucosae was neither markedly elevated nor deficient but was well preserved in its normal position almost parallel to the muscular coat which was similarly quite intact. The cancerous focus was confined to the mucous membrane and macroscopically slightly protruded, almost flat, or slightly depressed. Only 7 cases could be classified in this group

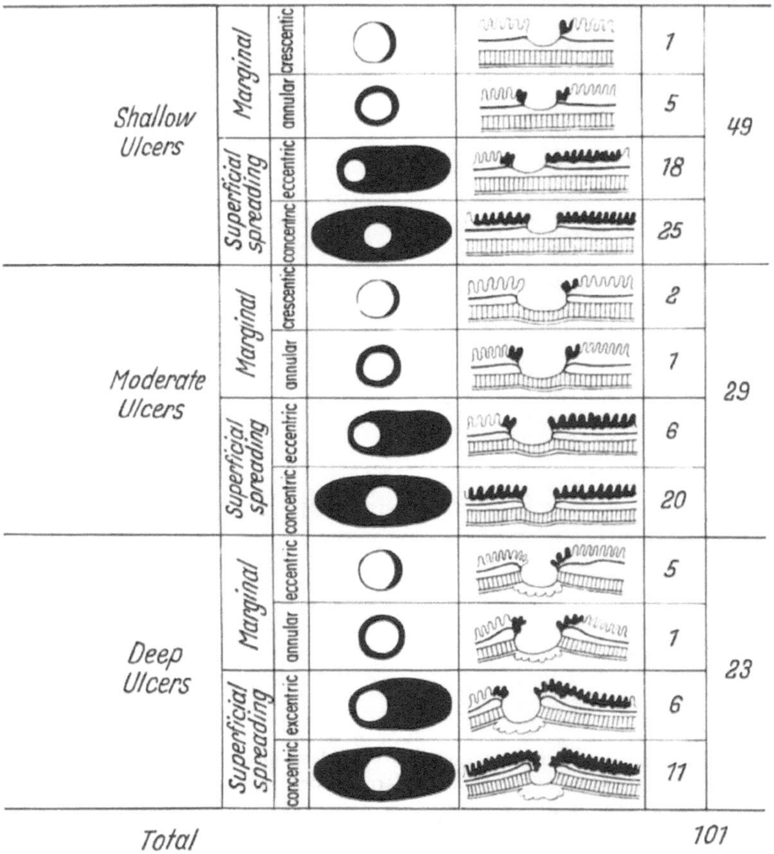

Shallow Ulcers	Marginal	crescentic			1	49
		annular			5	
	Superficial spreading	eccentric			18	
		concentric			25	
Moderate Ulcers	Marginal	crescentic			2	29
		annular			7	
	Superficial spreading	eccentric			6	
		concentric			20	
Deep Ulcers	Marginal	annular	eccentric		5	23
		annular			1	
	Superficial spreading	concentric	excentric		6	
		concentric	excentric		11	
Total						101

Fig. 7. Classification of early gastric carcinomas with ulcer. Superficial spreading carcinomas with ulcer are included in this group

(Fig. 14). In Fig. 15 is demonstrated an example of *in situ* carcinoma. This was the smallest carcinoma of the stomach we ever diagnosed. The diameter of the lesion did not surpass 7 mm. In Fig. 15 A readers might scarcely recognize the cancerous focus as a wedge-like lesion restricted completely in the mucous membrane. This last is enlarged in B of the same figure. The cancerous focus reveals itself a papillary adenocarcinoma and is just on the brink of penetrating the muscularis mucosae. In the surrounding tissue atrophic gastritis is marked.

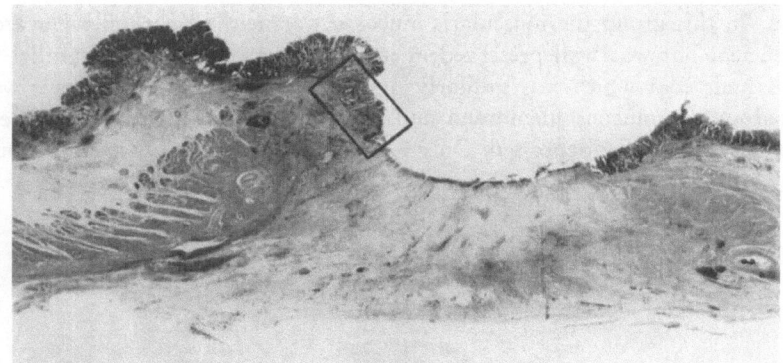

A

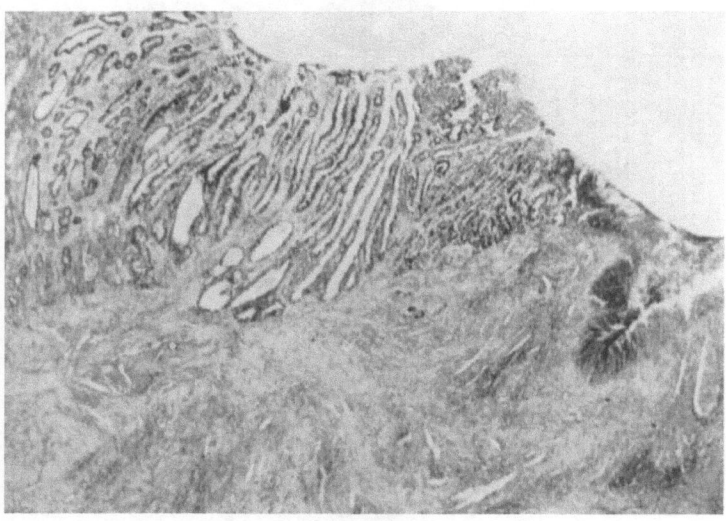

B

Fig. 8 A and B. Cancerous focus at the margin of a deep ulcer. Floor of ulcer is completely free from carcinoma. Note the gap of muscularis propria and fusion of muscularis mucosae with it. A. General view. B. Enlargement of the part inside the rectangle. 74 years old, male. Gastric anacidity

Transformation of cancers of this group into the flat form of the polypous cancers might be possible, since in some cases as shown in Fig. 16, slight elevation of muscularis mucosae can be recognized. However, transformation of these into the ulcer-cancers due to ulceration seems, as mentioned above, to be less likely at least in the earlier stages.

It should be noted that most of the cancers of this group belong to papillary or tubular adenocarcinoma (Figs. 15 and 16) similar to the polypous carcinoma and unlike the ulcer-cancers which are more frequently anaplastic carcinomas with signet ring cells formation.

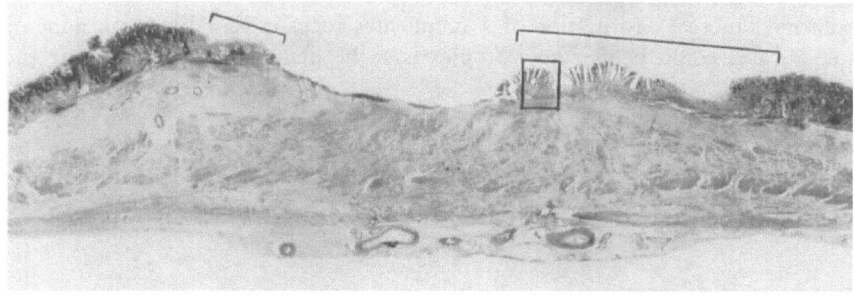

A

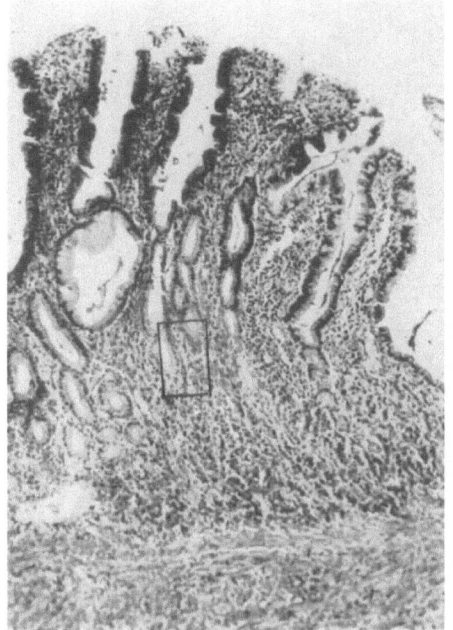

B

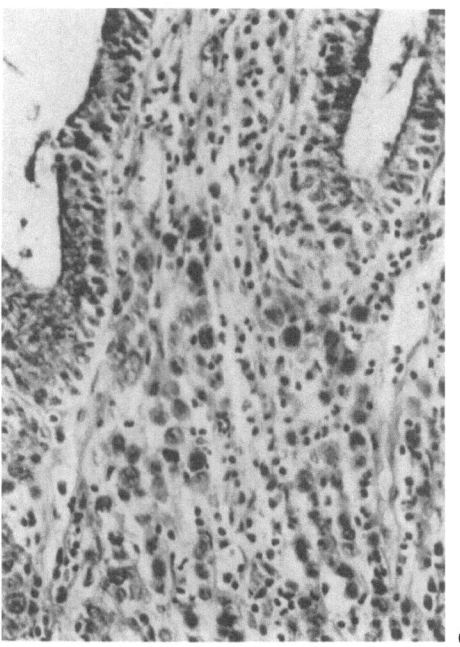

C

Fig. 9 A—C. Cancerous focus at the margin of a shallow ulcer, which is partially covered with regenerating epithelium. Muscularis propria is almost completely preserved. Note endoarteritis obliterans and increased connective tissue corresponding to ulcer floor. Parts indicated with lines are infiltrated with cancerous cells. A. General view. B. Enlargement of the part inside the rectangle in A. C. Enlargement of the part inside the rectangle in B. Note signet ring cells with deeply stained cytoplasm and excentric nucleus. 56 years old, male. Gastric anacidity

In the fifth group, the main lesion exists in the submucous layer. Seven cases could be classified in this group. Histologically, all were adenocarcinoma tubulare and in one mucoid degeneration was marked (Fig. 17). Although in cases of cancerous transformation of the submucous heterotopic tissue (especially accessory pancreas), formation of a submucous focus is very likely, in none of these 7 cases could benign heterotopic tissue be demonstrated in or near the lesion.

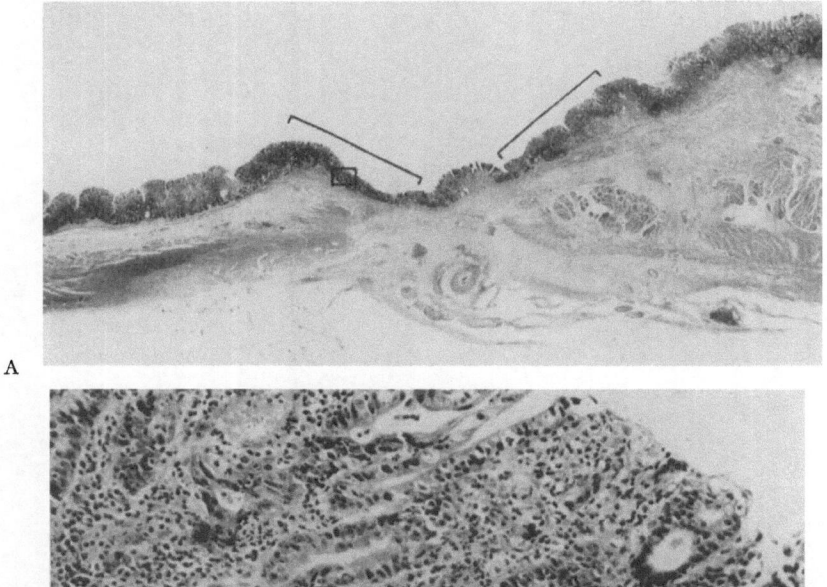

Fig. 10 A and B. Cancerous focus at the margin of a healed ulcer. A deep ulcer with gap of muscularis propria is covered completely with regenerating epithelium. Cancerous infiltration is restricted to areas indicated with lines, leaving in the center uninvaded regenerating epithelium. Note the endoarteritis and the scar forming ulcer floor. A. General view. B. Enlargement of the part inside the rectangle in A. 59 years old, male. Gastric anacidity

Discussion

1. On Polypous and Polypoid Cancers

The cancerous transformation of adenomatous polyp of the gastrointestinal tract was first discussed histologically by MÉNÉTRIER (1888). Further detailed study was done by VERSÉ (1908), whose material involved 3 cases of polyposis adenomatosa intestini, in which hundreds of polyps of histologically different features coexist, so that transformation of a benign adenoma into a malignant adenoma and that of a malignant adenoma into a carcinoma can be deduced in specimens derived from a single case. Further precise investigations concerning the polyposis adenomatosa intestini were done by LOCKHART-MUMMERY and DUKES (1928), who concluded the rectal and colonic polyps to be one of the most important precancers. Relationship of rectal and colonic polyps to carcinomas were subjected to detailed discussion also by SCHMIEDEN and WEST-HUES (1927) and WESTHUES (1934). They also emphasized the precancerous role of some kinds of adenomatous polyps.

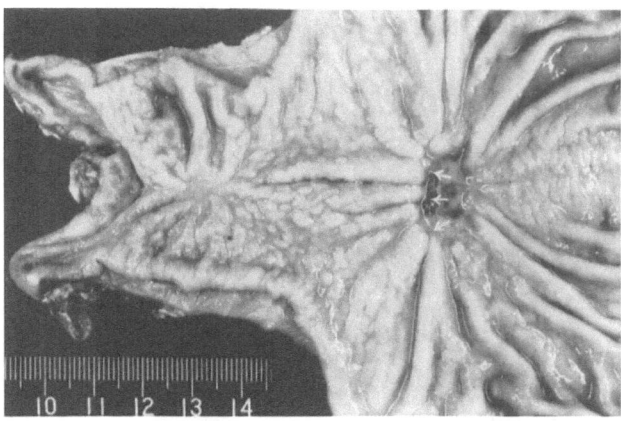

Fig. 11. Cancerous focus at the margin of a deep callous ulcer. Crescentic focus is found at the part indicated with an arrow. Note marked convergence of rugae towards the ulcer. Another healed ulcer is visible near pyloric ring. 60 years old, male. Gastric acidity 70/54. Histology: Signet ring cell carcinoma

In view of the difficulties connected with biopsy, the histological analysis of the gastric polyps based on a sufficient personal experience had been reported less frequently. However, review of cases (BRUNN and PEARL, 1926; MILLER et al., 1930; PEARL and BRUNN, 1943; YARNIS et al., 1952; PLACHTA and SPEER, 1957; MONACO et al., 1962), case reports of gastric polyps as well as polyposis (DOUGLAS, 1923; GLEAVE, 1923; MILLS, 1922–23; NIEMETZ and WHARTON, 1955) and gastric polyps or polyposis co-existing with carcinomas (STEWART, 1913–14; GLEAVE, 1923; RIGLER and ERICKSEN, 1938) gradually increased. Most authors are unanimous in regarding the gastric polyps, similar to intestinal polyps, as precancerous (STEWART, 1929; MILLS, 1922–23; MILLER et al., 1930; MALLORY, 1940; KONJETZNY, 1938; PEARL and BRUNN, 1943; SPRIGGS, 1948; RÖSSLE, 1944–45, EDWARDS and BROWN, 1950; HAY, 1953, 1956; BERG, 1958; OCHSNER and JANETOS, 1965). However, MONACO et al., (1962), inspite of the histological recognition of focal atypicality in certain cases of pedunculated polyps, hesitated to ascribe malignancy because of the

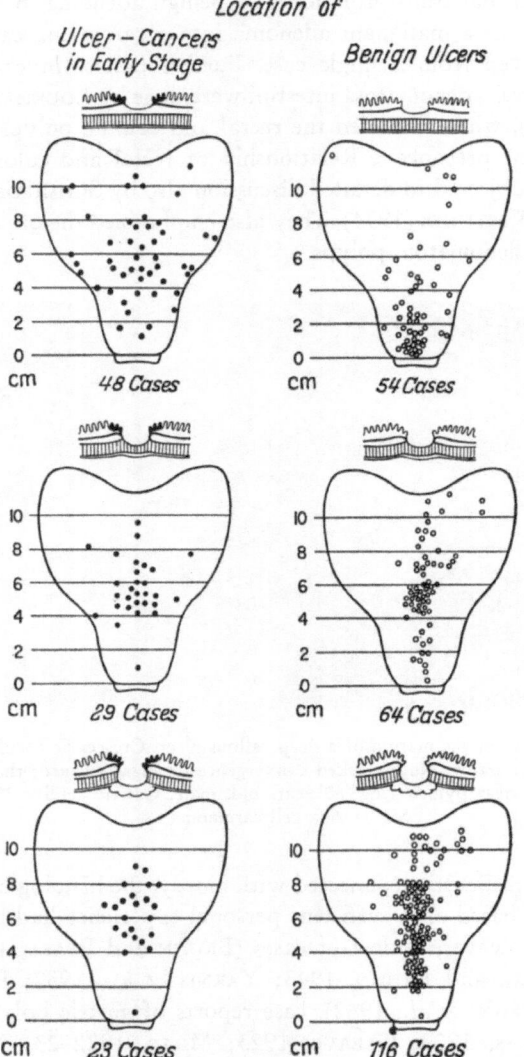

Fig. 12. Comparison of location of ulcer-cancers and benign ulcers. In both diseases, distribution of shallow lesions is more diffuse, whereas that of deep lesions is concentrated to the angular region of the lesser curvature

less frequent accompaniment of metastases in these cases. PAUL and LOGAN (1947) were inclined to separate polypoid carcinomas from the cancerous transformation of the polyps. According to these authors, the former are originally malignant and never arise from benign polyps. STEWART (1929), SPRIGGS (1948), and FLOOD (1961) thought the liability of malignant transformation to be less in the gastric polyposis than in the intestinal polyposis.

However, BERG (1958) claimed the equal possibility of eventual malignant change of adenomas in the large intestine and stomach. Although YARNIS *et al.* (1952) observed in 2 cases malignant degeneration of gastric polyp gastroscopically and roentgenologically, they thought the proof to be lacking. RIGLER and ERICKSEN (1938) also observed in a case the malignant degeneration of

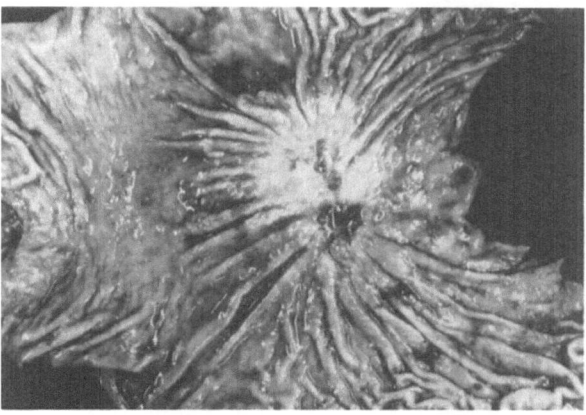

Fig. 13. Superficial spreading carcinoma encircling deep callous ulcer. Cancerous tissue replaces the mucous membrane in obliterating mucosal folds which converge into the ulcer. 66 years old, male. Normacidity. Histology: Undifferentiated adenocarcinoma with signet ring cell formation

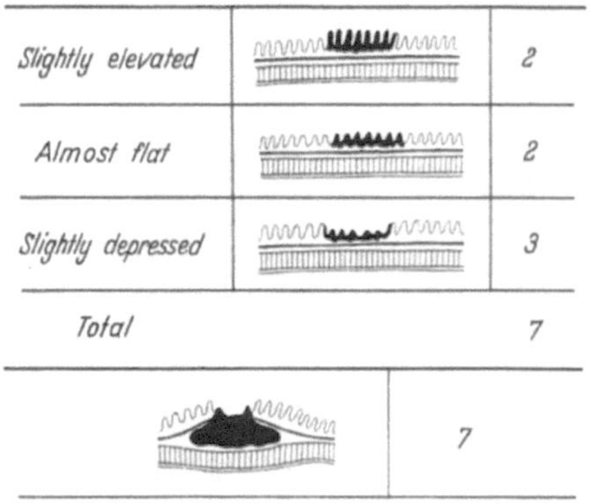

Slightly elevated		2
Almost flat		2
Slightly depressed		3
Total		7
		7

Fig. 14. Classification of *in situ* gastric carcinomas. Appendix: Submucous cancer of stomach

one of multiple polyps in the stomach after 8 months. CAREY and HAY (1950) followed 30 patients with benign polyps from 1 to 9 years and could not confirm in any case malignant degeneration. SPRATT *et al.* (1958) calculated the frequency distributions of adenomatous polyps and cancers in colon and doubted the possibility of transformation of adenomatous polyps into infiltrating, metastasizing carcinomas of the colon. Although they confirmed frequent coexistence of carcinoma in villous adenomas, they excluded these growths from their consideration. In their discussion, some of the above-mentioned

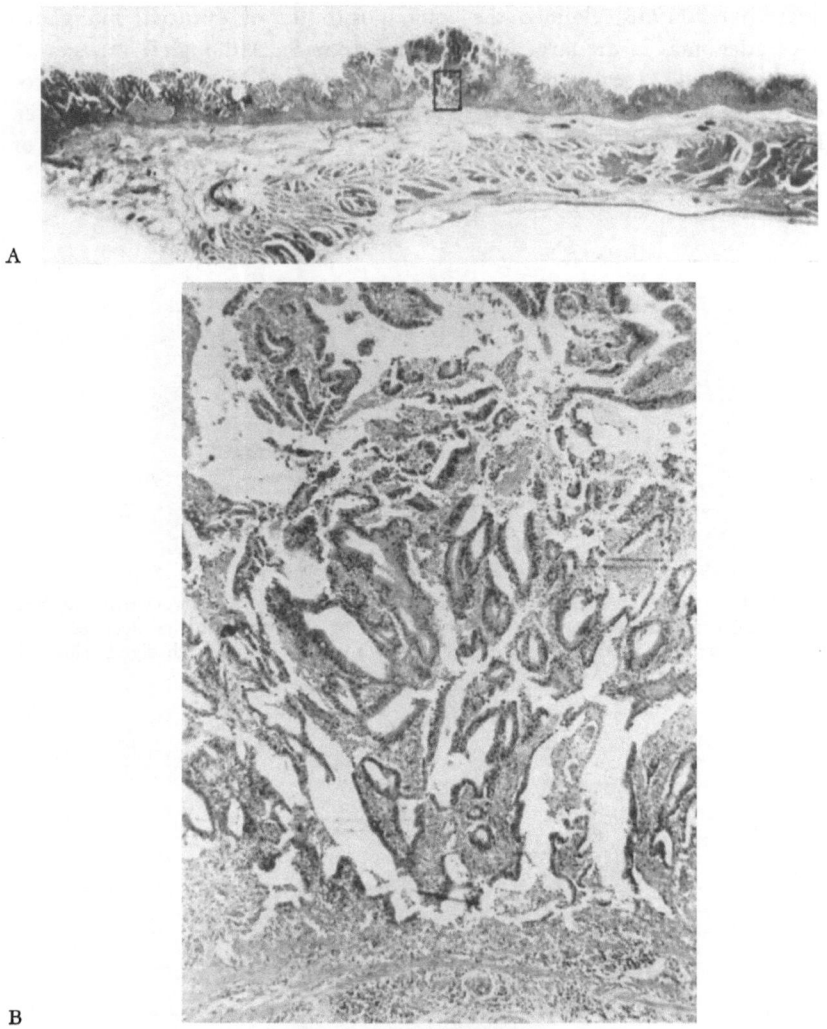

Fig. 15 A and B. Cancerization *in situ* of the gastric mucosa. A. General view. B. Enlargement of the part inside the rectangle in A. Note the deepest part just on the brink of penetrating the muscularis mucosae. 49 years old, female. Gastric anacidity

important references (e.g. LOCKHART-MUMMERY and DUKES, 1928, and WEST-HUES, 1934) escaped quotation.

As mentioned above, in cases of adenomatous polyposis of the large intestine there can be distinguished several stages different in histological feature. There are, on one hand, polyps and/or parts of polyps, which are scarcely distinguishable from normal intestinal mucosa, whereas, on the other hand, those having the properties identifiable with carcinoma. However, so far as a single

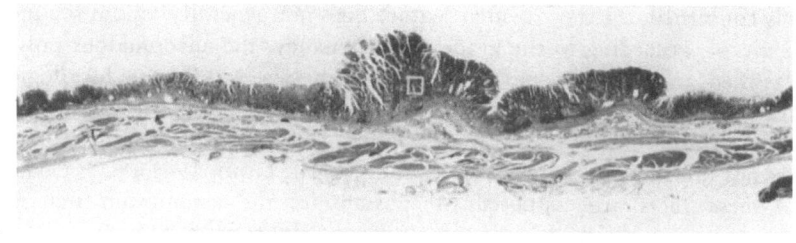

A

B

Fig. 16. Cancerization in situ of the gastric mucosa with slight elevation of muscularis mucosae. 77 years old, female. Gastric anacidity

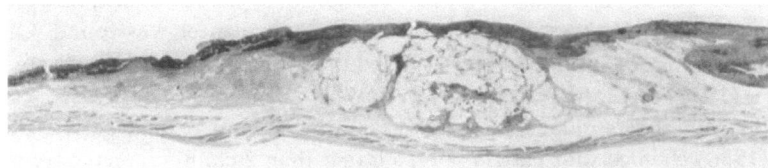

Fig. 17. Gastric carcinoma with mainly submucous location of the focus. 58 years old, male. Gastric anacidity

polyp is concerned, the most benign feature does not generally adjoin the most malignant. If, according to the grade of malignancy, the adenomatous polyps are classified into 3—4 types, the junction between different histological features is usually seen between 2 grades adjoining in the classification. This rule is applicable also to the solitary polyp, in which different histological features not infrequently co-exist (WESTHUES, 1934; DOHI, 1941).

All these facts are supposed to substantiate the assumption that the malignant transformation of the benign adenomas does exist. Moreover, in the intestinal mucosa of the rectal or colonic cancer patients patchy hyperplasias are not infrequently encountered (LOCKHART-MUMMERY and DUKES, 1928; DOHI, 1941). This was interpreted by LOCKHART-MUMMERY and DUKES (1928), and DOHI (1941) as the intermediate between the normal mucosa and the benign adenoma.

However, the opportunity to observe the malignant transformation of the benign polyp into a carcinoma is not frequent. This might be accounted for by the fact, that in spite of the liability to malignant degeneration of certain adenomas, some kind of benign polyps remain benign for a long period of time (CAREY and HAY, 1950; PLACHTA and SPEER, 1957). Therefore, the personal observation of benignancy cannot necessarily rule out the possibility of malignant degeneration in general. In fact LOCKHART-MUMMERY and DUKES (1928) reported a case in which a benign rectal polyp underwent malignant transformation. An analogous case was also seen by one of us (M. K.) and was reported by SUMII (1938). In this case a strawberry-sized pedunculate polyp was found in the sigmoid colon and revealed histologically to be an adenoma. Endoscopic removal was advised, but the patient refused consent. After 19 months the endoscopic examination was repeated. The peduculate polyp was no longer visible and instead an exulcerated infiltrating carcinoma was seen at the same location. In regard to the gastric polyps the opportunity of such verification might have been incomparably scarce, since the gastric biopsy remained long beyond the clinical application. As mentioned above malignant degeneration of benign polyps of the stomach was observed clinically in 2 cases by YARNIS et al. (1952) and in one case by RIGLER and ERICKSEN (1938), although the former authors thought the proof to be lacking. KLEIN and GELLER (1951) reported a case with 3 polyps in the stomach, in which 2 years later carcinoma developed at the site of one of the polyps. SAGAIDAK (1960) presented 152 cases with gastric polyps between 1—2 cm in diameter. Of these 59 were treated by resection. In 8 of the specimens cancer was found. Of the 93 untreated patients, 10 subsequently died of gastric carcinoma. EDWARDS and BROWN (1950) reported a case in which polypoid cancer and an invasive cancer developed in the residual stomach 8 years after removal of a gastric polyp. HAY (1956) claimed that gastric polyps larger than 2 cm in diameter are prone to cancerous transformation, whereas those smaller are not. However, BOWDEN (1962) reported a polypous carcinoma of the stomach smaller than 1 cm in diameter already showing invasive growth. One of the authors (M. K.) also saw a polypous cancer of similar size with invasion.

Histologically there is no essential difference between the gastric and intestinal polyps. The gastric polyps, too, can be classified histologically into several grades in regard to malignancy (HAY, 1953; MONACO et al., 1962). Co-existence of hyperplasia with polyps is not infrequently observed (STEWART, 1929; HAY, 1965; BERG, 1958). Moreover gastric polyps also have a tendency to multiplicity (STEWART, 1929; PEARL and BRUNN, 1943; EDWARDS and BROWN, 1950; HAY, 1956; BERG, 1958; MONACO et al., 1962). In cases of multiple gastric polyps or polyposis, polyps of different histological feature usually co-exist (KONJETZNY, 1940; BERG, 1958). Existence of more than 2 polypous carcinomas in one stomach is not rare (EDWARDS and BROWN, 1950; BERG, 1958). In 3 cases of the present series 2—3 polypous carcinomas were observed in one and the same stomach.

In the present paper 13 cases were classified as polypoid cancers. In these cases coexistence of adenomatous tissue was missed. Histologically all these cases were papillary adenocarcinomas. As will be discussed later, in some of the carcinomas of the "in situ" group, slight elevation of the muscularis mucosae is observed (Fig. 15), so that in later stages they might take the polypoid appearance (NAGAYO et al., 1965). Histological coincidence between both types may support such viewpoint. However, more frequently polypous carcinoma may transform into the polypoid carcinoma, since expulsion of benign cells by more malignant cells is one of the commonest findings encountered in adenomatous polyps (WESTHUES, 1934; DOHI, 1941). Inclusive of these 13 polypoid cancers, all the carcinomas of this group are papillary adenocarcinomas and may be classified into "intestinal cell carcinoma" group according to MULLIGAN and REMBER's (1954) histogenetic classification.

Achlorhydria is observed in the majority of cases with gastric polyps or polyposis (STRAUSS et al., 1928; MILLER et al., 1930; PEARL and BRUNN, 1943; YARNIS et al., 1952; CAREY and HAY, 1948; EDWARDS and BROWN, 1950; HAY, 1953; PLACHTA and SPEER, 1957; MONACO et al., 1962). Atrophic, or atrophic hyperplastic, gastritis (KONJETZNY, 1938; HAY, 1953) and intestinal metaplasia are usually observed in the surrounding mucosa of polypous and polypoid cancers of the stomach (PLACHTA and SPEER, 1957). Development of gastric polyps and polyposis upon atrophic or atrophic hyperplastic gastritis with intestinal metaplasia is generally accepted (KONJETZNY, 1940; MORSON, 1955). All these facts imply that the conditions which facilitate the cancerous transformation of the gastric polyps do not differ in nature from those which facilitate the malignant degeneration of the intestinal polyps. Here, too, the transformation may proceed in the order of; Hyperplasia → benign adenoma → malignant adenoma → carcinoma.

The discussion about the frequency of malignant transformation may be valid when adenomatous polyps of histologically similar potency are considered. That means the result of observation of histologically benign adenomas (such as is done by GAREY and HAY, 1950; or by PLACHTA and SPEER, 1957) might be of little help for determining the prognosis of certain malignant adenomas. In view of the difficulty of the biopsy in the past, histological features of the gastric polyps can never be said to have obtained sufficient considerations up to date. The gastroscope with biopsy curette may answer our earnest desire in this direction.

2. On Ulcer-Cancers

HAUSER (1883) first described a case in which, despite the metastases in the liver and other organs, the primary carcinoma in the stomach had been restricted to the margin of a callous ulcer leaving the large ulcer floor free from cancerous invasion. Since then, demonstration of a gap in the muscularis propria and subsequent formation of the floor with a scar and the restriction of the cancerous focus to the margin of the ulcer without invasion into the ulcer floor were chosen by most pathologists as the criteria for the histological diagnosis of the gastric carcinoma developed upon the callous ulcer (ulcer-cancer). This concept was supported by NEWCOMB (1932—33), who claimed the fusion of the stump of the muscularis mucosae with that of the muscularis propria to be the most reliable finding to conclude the pre-existence of the ulcer.

With the popularization of gastrectomy, the number of cases which satisfy HAUSER's as well as NEWCOMB's criteria gradually increased in gastrectomy cases both operated on as ulcer and as carcinoma (STOERK, 1925; ORATOR, 1925; KONJETZNY, 1938). HOWEVER, STROMEYER (1912) had already pointed out the possibility of taking similar appearance of an originally non-ulcerative carcinoma due to peptic ulceration. Regardless of the severe confutation of STOERK (1925), this opinion was adopted by EWING (1936) and further intensified by MALLORY (1940), who in view of the possible peptic ulceration of carcinoma in situ, considered HAUSER's criteria to be invalid to deduce the ulcerative origin of gastric carcinoma. Recently, general opinion in the United States seems to be more inclined to doubt the close etiologic relationship between callous ulcer and gastric carcinoma (FLOOD, 1961; EISENBERG and WOODWARD, 1963).

However, there are certain questions as to the validity of MALLORY's (1940) objection. Firstly, he anticipated the existence of hyperacidity for the development of peptic ulceration. He admitted he had never observed peptic ulceration in any case with demonstrated anacidity. If, therefore, the peptic ulceration of in situ carcinoma might happen so frequently as to be the most probable source of ulcer-cancers which satisfy HAUSER's criteria, then in proportion to the incidence of ulcer-cancers, hyperacidity must be more frequently observed among cases of in situ carcinoma. This is not the case. For example, 6 of 7 in situ carcinoma cases in our present series were achlorhydric and the other case was hypochlorhydric (Fig. 6 C). Similar to polypous cancers, in situ carcinomas are also thought to develop upon atrophic or atrophic hypertrophic gastritis

(KONJETZNY, 1938; MORSON, 1955). Subsequently, the incidence of gastric anacidity in cases of *in situ* carcinoma should be highly estimated.

Secondly, demonstration of fresh necrosis upon the floor of the ulcer may substantiate the existence of acute exacerbation of peptic ulceration, which is not infrequently observed in ulcer patients, but by no means excludes the possibility of pre-existence of an ulcer to the carcinoma.

Thirdly, in MALLORY's discussion little attention was paid to the coincidence of size between the ulcer-cancers and the callous ulcers. In majority of cases, either lesion has walnut size, when they become subjects of surgical treatment. If most ulcer-cancers be the result of secondary ulceration of *in situ* carcinomas, this kind of carcinoma must be concluded to be especially prone to peptic ulceration when it reaches this size. Moreover, the operation has to be done just at the point, when ulceration has excavated not only the most part of the cancerous tissue but also the muscularis propria, still leaving a thin shell of cancerous tissue. Following STOERK's expression, this might be a *deus ex machina*.

All these facts imply that formation of a cancerous focus such as satisfying HAUSER's criteria as a consequence of secondary ulceration of *in situ* carcinoma might be of exceptionally rare occurrence, if not impossible. On the other hand, if cancerous development really took place in relation to the pre-existent callous ulcer, the ulcer margin should have been the most liable area for the development, as once STOERK (1925), STOUT (1942), and GOLDEN and STOUT (1948) remarked. Distribution of this kind of gastric carcinoma fairly coincides with that of callous ulcers. Both lesions are especially concentrated near the gastric angle of the lesser curvature (NAGAYO et al., 1965; OOTA, 1964). Similar data were obtained also in the present investigation (Fig. 12).

Carcinomatous development upon the margin of shallower ulcers which had no, or only partial, cicatrization of the muscularis propria was first described by STOERK (1925). One of us (KURU, 1953; 1954; 1966a) has also described several cases of chronic ulcer of this kind and described the localized cancerous focus developed near regenerating epithelium in such cases. Needless to mention that in case of cancerous development on such shallow ulcers, not only HAUSER's but also NEWCOMB's criteria become invalid.

KIMOTO (1954) examined in detail 315 consecutive cases of gastric carcinoma operated on in the author's clinic from 1941 to 1953. Special attention was paid by him to the gap of muscularis propria, scar covering the floor of the ulcer, the course and especially the attitude of the stump of the muscularis mucosae, and the accompanying atrophic gastritis in all cases. He discussed the problem of precursors and came to the conclusion that the frequency of the so-called ulcer-cancer is higher than had been assumed by most pathologists (e.g. NEWCOMB, 1932—33; ORATOR, 1925; STOUT, 1943), and might surpass 39 per cent of the examined material (Fig. 18 A). Many pathologists in Japan discussed subsequently the possible incidence of gastric carcinomas related to callous ulcers. The majority of them (NAGAYO and KOMAGOE, 1961; MURAKAMI, 1963; OOTA, 1964; KINO, 1965) are unanimous in assuming the high incidence of ulcer-cancer in the Japanese. Recent observations about early gastric carcinomas strongly support this view (KURU, 1966 a, b; OOTA, 1964; NAGAYO et al., 1963; SANO and KAKIMOTO, 1965). The present investigation of the early cases has also shown the high frequency of carcinoma arising at the margin of

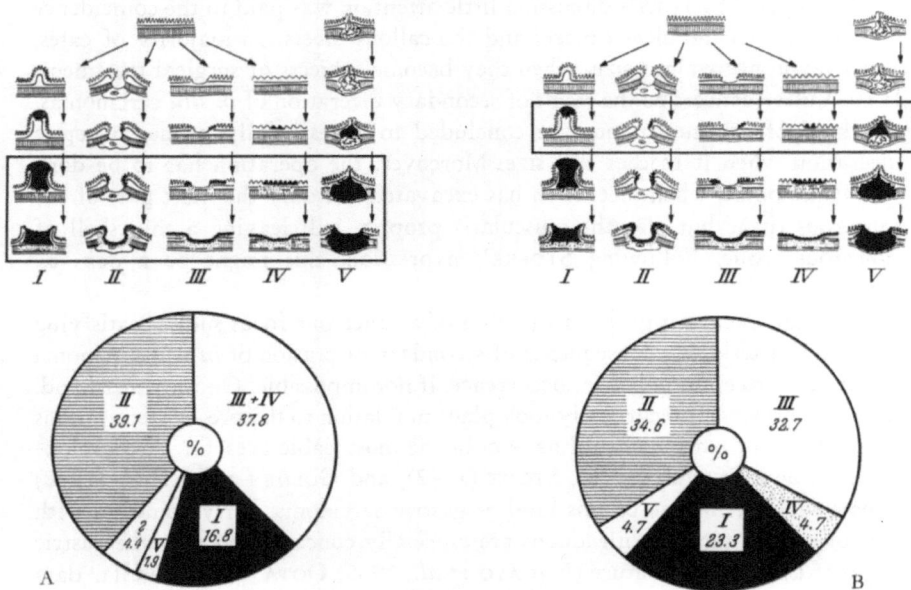

Fig. 18 A and B. Classification of gastric carcinomas into 5 groups according to their origin. Percentage of each group estimated by analysis of 315 advanced cases (A, KIMOTO, 1952) and 150 early cases (B)

the callous ulcer. This view is especially supported by the fact that, the smaller the cancer in this group, the more restricted is the cancerous focus to the margin of the ulcer.

Histologically, papillary carcinomas are rare in this group. Most of the cases over 50 years old belong to the differentiated or undifferentiated adenocarcinoma, whereas the majority of those less than 50 years old are characterized by existence of signet ring cells. Since the former may be identified with a pylorocardiac gland cell type and the latter with a mucinous cell type (MULLIGAN and REMBER, 1954), the above results are in accord with the views of these two authors.

3. On Superficial Spreading Carcinomas

When the diagnosis of gastric carcinoma depended exclusively upon X-ray examination, the majority of small lesions confined to the mucous membrane, making neither a marked prominence nor niche, escaped detection. Attention to such superficial carcinomas of the stomach was called almost simultaneously by GUTMANN *et al.* (1939), KONJETZNY (1940) and STOUT (1942), and the term "superficial spreading" carcinoma was proposed by STOUT (1942, 1943, 1944—45). As the name indicates, this type of carcinomas is characteristic in occupying a wide area despite its less marked invasion into the deeper layers. In STOUT's (1942) first description the accompaniment of ulcers was noted in the majority of cases and the patients had suffered with ulcer symptoms for from one to ten years.

Under a similar title further cases were reported by GOLDEN and STOUT (1948), KONJETZNY (1953), MYHRE (1953), HESS (1956), and NAGAYO *et al.* (1959, 1965). Most of these cases were also accompanied by ulceration.

All the cases in the present series which are classified into this group have open or healed ulcers. However, the depth of the ulcer differs from case to case and it is independent of the size of the superficial lesion. In cases accompanied by deep ulcers with a gap in the muscular coat, convergence of rugae toward the ulcer center is also conspicuous (Fig. 13). The histological features of the ulcer and its surrounding in these cases do not differ from those in the previous group, except for a more marked tendency to superficial spreading. Moreover, the smaller the lesion, the more restricted is the cancerous focus to the ulcer margin, so that the extreme can be hardly distinguished from the typical ulcer-cancer. As STOUT (1942, 1943, 1944—45) has already pointed out, superficial spreading is one of the 3 different modes of carcinomatous expansion. Moreover, since in the present study the absence of cancer cells in the muscularis propria was chosen as the only criterion to distinguish the "early" stage, relatively spread cases were also included, in so far as the spread was limited to the mucous membrane. These circumstances may account for the relatively high percentage of superficial spreading carcinomas in the present series.

It is needless to mention that with inclusion of such more advanced cases, the scrutiny of the nature of the ulcers obviously becomes difficult. Therefore, in spite of the absence of hyperacidity in most of the cases (Fig. 6B), secondary ulceration cannot be completely excluded in cases with more expanded lesions. To be noted, however, is the fact that the majority of cases in this group are not papillary adenocarcinomas, as the cases in the next group are, but are anaplastic carcinomas with signet ring cells.

Here certain considerations should be added about the regenerating epithelium covering the ulcer. Partial or complete healing of an ulcer can result from covering of the ulcer surface with regenerating epithelium (Figs. 9 and 10). Attention should be paid to the infiltration of cancer cells into such regenerating epithelium. If the cancerous focus is sufficiently restricted in such cases (Figs. 9 and 10), we can easily recognize the primary site of cancerization at the margin of the ulcer close to the regenerating epithelium. This appearance was once interpreted by PALMER and HUMPHREYS (1944) as a healing process of a peptic-

ulcerated cancerous focus. However, similar findings have been described by
GUTMANN et al. (1939), GOLDEN and STOUT (1948) and KURU (1953). All these
authors explained these findings as the development of cancer in the mucosa
over the scar of a healed peptic ulcer. The fact that the cancer cells found in
regenerating epithelium were exclusively signet ring cells may support the above
opinion (Fig. 9). In some preparations of this group the ulcer is completely
covered by regenerating epithelium (Fig. 10) as seen in 2 cases of GOLDEN and
STOUT (1948). If superficial spread is sufficiently wide in such cases, healed
ulcers are apt to be overlooked so that these cases might be classified as superficial
spreading carcinomas without ulceration. However, more precise examination
may reveal the site of a primary lesion in the neighbourhood of the regenerated
epithelium with submucous increase of the connective tissue (Figs. 9 and 10).

From the above considerations the majority of superficial spreading carcinomas with ulcers are concluded to be the more advanced stages of ulcer-cancers.

4. Cancerization in situ or Non-polypoid Pre-invasive Carcinoma of the Gastric Mucosa

Mucosal carcinoma of the stomach accompanying neither polyp nor ulcer
was observed only in 7 cases. In these cases the cancerous focus was restricted
to the mucous membrane without any marked change in the course of the
muscularis mucosae. Histologically all cases were classifiable as papillary or
tubular andenocarcinomas and subsequently identifiable with the intestinal
cell carcinoma of MULLIGAN and REMBER (1954). This kind of early gastric
carcinoma had been previously found only fortuitously in autopsy materials
(VERSÉ, 1908; EWING, 1936) or in surgical preparations apart from the main
lesion (GOLDEN and STOUT, 1948; MORSON, 1955). However, GUTMANN et al.
(1939) and MALLORY (1940) called attention to such in situ cancerization and
further analogous cases were reported by MYHRE (1953), MORSON (1955) and
HESS (1956). MORSON (1955) pointed out the cancerous development upon
epithelium with intestinal metaplasia. All five cases in his description were
papillo-tubulary carcinomas, and his case 10 has certain resemblances to the
case shown in Fig. 16. It should be noted that in all of the 7 cases in the present
series atrophic or atrophic hyperplastic gastritis with intestinal metaplasia was
conspicuous in the surrounding area (Fig. 5 C), as seen in MORSON's cases.
Although the size of lesion differed from case to case between 0.7—9.0 cm, in
none of these cases had hyperacidity been demonstrated before the operation.
Moreover, anacidity had been confirmed in 6 of the cases and hypoacidity in
1 case (Fig. 6 C). Therefore, in these cases the probability of peptic ulceration
might be negligibly small, so that transformation of this type into the ulcerative
form with destruction of muscularis propria can scarcely happen. On the
contrary, transformation of these into the polypoid type seems not unlikely, as
NAGAYO et al. (1965) have recently postulated, since as shown in Fig. 16, in two

of these 7 slight elevation of the muscularis mucosae was recognizable corresponding to the papillary elevation of the tumor. As shown in Fig. 15, the smallest carcinoma in this group was 7 mm in diameter. Nevertheless, the deepest part of the lesion was on the brink of penetrating the muscularis mucosae. Multicentric development in this kind of carcinoma was noted by EWING (1936) and HESS (1956).

Here it should be noted, that in Japan pernicious anaemia is only observed rarely. So far as the authors know, there is no report of gastric carcinoma associated with pernicious anaemia. The authors are of the opinion, that the chronic atrophic (or atrophic hyperplastic) gastritis in Japanese is most intimately related to recurrent erosive gastritis (STOERK, 1925). This disease has certain causative factors in common with chronic ulcers. In erosive gastritis, however, due to the intactness of the muscularis mucosae the healing process proceeds incomparably smoothly (MOSKOWICZ, 1924), so that the clinical as well as the histological features differ considerably from those of callous ulcer. To the further elucidation of the relationship between this disease and the chronic atrophic gastritis repeated endoscopical examinations with biopsy of cases of both diseases will contribute much.

5. On Submucous Carcinomas of the Stomach

In the fifth group of gastric carcinomas, the gross appearance differs considerably from the others, in having the main lesion submucously.

Although BEUTLER (1921), EWING (1936) and STOUT (1943) had pointed out the possibility of cancerous development from the heterotopic pancreas in the stomach wall, casuistics with unequivocal histological findings were done only by NICHOLSON (1923), BRANHAM (see GUTMANN et al., 1939) and INOUE (1954). In INOUE's case a structure identifiable with the pancreatic duct was demonstrated inside the adenocarcinoma, which showed mostly submucous growth in the prepyloric region.

In each of 7 cases classified in this group, the major part of the lesion was found in the submucous layer (Fig. 17). However, in none of these 7 could histological evidence be found to substantiate the development from heterotopic pancreas. Histologically papillary (in 1 case), tubular (in 4 cases), undifferentiated (in 1 case) and mucocellular adenocarcinoma (in 1 case, Fig. 17) were encountered.

Conclusions

One hundred and fifty early cancers of the stomach without invasion into the muscularis propria were subjected to detailed histological investigation. The conclusions are:

1. According to their gross appearance they could be classified into 5 completely different categories (Fig. 18).

2. In the first category, the gastric carcinomas had polypous or polypoid appearance. In the majority of this group an adenomatous structure co-existed in or near the carcinoma so that the cancerous transformation of adenoma could be reasonably postulated.

3. The second group was characterized by an accompanying ulcer. In more than the half there was partial or complete defect of the muscularis propria, whereas in the other the defect was confined to the muco-submucous layer. All the cases with a gap in the muscularis propria satisfied HAUSER's and NEWCOMB's criteria and were subsequently identifiable with ulcer-cancers of the classical definition. Regardless of the difference in depth of the ulcer, the smaller the cancer, the more restricted was the cancerous focus to the margin of the ulcer. The conclusion is therefore justified that the carcinoma in this group has developed upon the margin of a pre-existing ulcer.

4. The third group corresponds to the superficial spreading type. However, there was no fundamental difference between this type and the second group except the extent of the superficial lesion, so that the smaller the spread, the more was the appearance indistinguishable from that of the second group. Therefore, most of the so-called superficial spreading carcinomas with ulceration can be identified with the later stages of the second group.

5. The fourth group corresponds to superficial (*in situ*) cancers of the gastric mucosa without polypous or polypoid appearance or ulceration. In all of the 7 cases classified in this group, there was atrophic or atrophic-hypertrophic gastritis with intestinal metaplasia in the surrounding mucosa. Correspondingly in most of the cases, the gastric juice had been proved to be achlorhydric. Therefore, transformation of this type of gastric carcinoma into the ulcer-cancer due to the peptic ulceration seems to be unlikely. However, growth toward the lumen may result in a polypoid appearance.

6. The fifth group differs from the other four, in showing the submucous growth from the beginning. Relation of carcinomas of this group to heterotopic pancreas is postulated.

7. These results imply that the majority of gastric carcinomas in Japanese have a relation to gastric ulcers (Fig. 18 B). They indicate simultaneously that the peptic ulceration of *in situ* carcinoma is not of frequent occurrence.

References

BERG, J. W., Histological aspects of the relation between gastric adenomatous polyps and gastric cancer. *Cancer (Philad.)* 11, 1149—1155 (1958).

BEUTLER, A., Über blastomatöses Wuchern von Pankreaskeimen in der Magenwand. *Virchows Arch. path. Anat.* 232, 341—349 (1921).

BOWDEN, L., Adenocarcinoma in a small gastric polyp. A case report. *Cancer (Philad.)* 15, 468—471 (1962).

BRUNN, H., and PEARL, F., Diffuse gastric polyposis—adenopapillomatosis gastrica. *Surg. Gynec. Obstet.* 43, 559—598 (1926).

CAREY, J. B., and HAY, L. J., Gastric polyps. *Gastroenterology* 10, 102—107 (1948).

CAREY, J. B., and HAY, L. J., Gastric polyps. *Gastroenterology* 14, 280—286 (1950).

DOHI, K., Zur Kenntnis der koexistierenden Polypen in der Schleimhaut der wegen Krebs resezierten oder amputierten Magendarmpräparate, mit besonderer Berücksichtigung des präpolypösen Zustandes. Anhang: Zwei Fälle von Polyposis recti. *Gann* 35, 503—544 (1941).

DOUGLAS, J., Benign tumors of the stomach. *Ann. Surg.* 77, 580—586 (1923).

EDWARDS, R. V., and BROWN, C. H., Benign gastric polyps and their relation to carcinoma of the stomach. *Gastroenterology* 16, 531—538 (1950).

EISENBERG, M., and WOODWARD, E. R., Gastric cancer. A midcentury look. *Arch. Surg.* 87, 810—824 (1963).

EWING, J., The beginnings of gastric cancer. *Amer. J. Surg.* 31, 204—205 (1936).

FLOOD, C. A., Precancerous disease of the gastrointestinal tract. *Amer. J. dig. Dis.* 6, 555—569 (1961).

GLEAVE, H. H., Polyposis of the stomach and duodenum with carcinoma. *J. Path. Bact.* 26, 134—135 (1923).

GOLDEN, R., and STOUT, A. P., Superficial spreading carcinoma of the stomach. *Amer. J. Roentgenol.* 59, 157—167 (1948).

GUTMANN, R. A., BERTRAND, I., and PÉRISTIANY, J., *Le cancer de l'estomac au début.* Paris: Y. Doin & Cie. 1939.

HAUSER, G., *Das chronische Magengeschwür. Sein Vernarbungsprozeß und dessen Beziehungen zur Entwicklung des Magencarcinoms.* Leipzig: J. B. Hirschfeld 1883.

HAY, L. J., Polyps and adenomas of the stomach. *Surgery* 33, 446—467 (1953).

— Surgical management of gastric polyps and adenomas. *Surgery* 39, 114—119 (1956).

HESS, R., Early cancer of the stomach. *Gastroenterology* 86, 365—369 (1956).

INOUE, N., On gastric cancers originating from heterotopic tissues. *Zyuzenkai-Igaku-Zassi* 56, 838—862 (1954) [in Japanese].

KIMOTO, S., Histological studies on precursors of the gastric carcinomas. *Zyuzenkai-Igaku-Zassi* 56, 649—669 (1954) [in Japanese].

KINO, I., A pathological study of scirrhous carcinoma of the stomach with special reference to the relationship of chronic ulcer and ulcer scar as background lesion. *Trans. Soc. Path. jap.* 54, 153 (1965) [in Japanese].

KLEIN, H. C., and GELLER, J. G., Gastric polyp to gastric carcinoma. *Gastroenterology* 17, 442—444 (1951).

KONJETZNY, G. E., *Der Magenkrebs.* Stuttgart: Ferdinand Enke 1938.

— Der oberflächliche Schleimhautkrebs des Magens. *Chirurg* 12, 192—202 (1940).

— The superficial cancer of the gastric mucosa. *Amer. J. dig. Dis.* 20, 91—96 (1953).

KURU, M., On cancers developed upon ulcerative lesions of the stomach. A study of the regeneration of the mucous membrane of the stomach with special reference to its malignant transformation. *Gann* 44, 47—54 (1953).

— Relationship between the gross appearance of gastric cancers and their precursors. *Nihon Rinsho,* Suppl. vol. 182—211 (1954) [in Japanese].

— Pathophysiologie und Früherkennung des Magenkrebses. *Münch. med. Wschr.* 108, 737—747 (1966a).

— *Atlas of early carcinoma of the stomach.* Tokyo: Nakayama-Shoten 1966b.

LOCKHART-MUMMERY, J. P., and DUKES, C. E., The precancerous changes in the rectum and colon. *Surg. Gynec. Obstet.* 46, 591—596 (1928).

MALLORY, T. B., Carcinoma in situ of the stomach and its bearing on the histogenesis of malignant ulcers. *Arch. Path.* 30, 348—362 (1940).

MÉNÉTRIER, P., Des polyadénomes gastriques et de leurs rapports avec le cancer de l'estomac. *Arch. Physiol.,* Sér. IV, 1. tôme, 20, 32—55, 236—261 (1888).

MILLER, T. G., ELIASON, E. L., and WRIGHT, V. W. M., Carcinomatous degeneration of polyp of the stomach. Report of eight personal cases with a review of twenty-four recorded by others. *Arch. intern. Med.* 46, 841—878 (1930).

MILLS, G. P., Multiple polypi of the stomach (Gastritis polyposa): with the report of a case. *Brit. J. Surg.* 10, 226—231 (1922/23).

MONACO, P., ROTH, L., CASTLEMAN, B., and WELCH, E., Adenomatous polyps of the stomach. A clinical and pathological study of 153 cases. *Cancer (Philad.)* 15, 456—467 (1962).

MORSON, B. C., Carcinoma arising from areas of intestinal metaplasia in the gastric mucosa. *Brit. J. Cancer* 9, 378—385 (1955).

MOSKOWICZ, L., Regeneration und Krebsbildung an der Magenschleimhaut. Grundlagen einer biologischen Krebstheorie. *Langenbecks Arch. klin. Chir.* 132, 558—620 (1924).

MULLIGAN, R. M., and REMBER, R. R., Histogenesis and biologic behavior of gastric carcinoma. Study of one hundred thirty-eight cases. *Arch. Path.* 58, 1—25 (1954).

MURAKAMI, T., Ulcer carcinoma. *Proc. 16th General Assembly Jap. Med. Congr.* 3, 110—112 (1963) [in Japanese].

MYHRE, E., Superficial spreading type of carcinoma of the stomach. *Acta chir. scand.* 106, 392—398 (1953).

NAGAYO, T., and KOMAGOE, T., Histological studies of gastric mucosal cancer with special reference to relationship of histological pictures between the mucosal cancer and the cancer-bearing gastric mucosa. *Gann* 52, 109—119 (1961).

— ITO, M., YOKOYAMA, H., and KOMAGOE, T., Early phase of human gastric cancer: Morphological study. *Gann* 56, 101—120 (1965).

— SAWADA, Y., MARUYAMA, K., YOKOYAMA, H., and KOMAGOE, T., Histological studies on superficially-spreading early carcinoma of the stomach. *Trans. Soc. Path. jap.* 48, 29—49 (1959) [in Japanese].

NEWCOMB, W. D., The relationship between peptic ulceration and gastric carcinoma. *Brit. J. Surg.* 20, 279—308 (1932/33).

NICHOLSON, G. W., Studies on tumour formation. *Guy's Hosp. Rep.* 73, 37—64 (1923).

NIEMETZ, D., and WHARTON, K., Benign gastric polyps. *Ann. intern. Med.* 42, 339—344 (1955).

OCHSNER, S. F., and JANETOS, G. P., Benign tumors of the stomach. *J. Amer. med. Ass.* 191, 881—887 (1965).

ORATOR, V., Beiträge zur Magenpathologie II. Zur Pathologie und Genese des Carcinoms und Ulcuscarcinoms des Magens. *Virchows Arch. path. Anat.* 256, 202—229 (1925).

OOTA, K., Histogenesis of gastric carcinoma. *Trans. Soc. Path. jap.* 53, 3—16 (1964) [in Japanese].

PALMER, W. L., and HUMPHREYS, E. M., Gastric carcinoma: Observations on peptic ulceration and healing. *Gastroenterology* 3, 257—274 (1944).

PAUL, W. D., and LOGAN, W. P., Polyps of the stomach with reference to the gastroscopic findings. *Gastroenterology* 8, 592—606 (1947).

PEARL, F. L., and BRUNN, H., Multiple gastric polyposis. A supplementary report of 41 cases, including 3 new personal cases. *Surg. Gynec. Obstet.* 76, 257—281 (1943).

PLACHTA, A., and SPEER, D., Gastric polyps and their relationship to carcinoma of the stomach. *Amer. J. Gastroent.* 28, 160—175 (1957).

RIGLER, L. G., and ERICKSEN, L. G., Benign tumors of the stomach. Observations of their incidence and malignant degeneration. *Radioloy* 26, 6—18 (1938).

RÖSSLE, R., Über einen frühen Oberflächenkrebs der Magenschleimhaut. *Zbl. allg. Path. path. Anat.* 82, 165—170 (1944/45).

SAGAIDAK, V. N., Polyps of stomach: case material of "Herzen". State Oncological Institute. *Vop. Onkol.* 6, 56—61 (1960), Cit. from BOWDEN 1962.

SANO, R., and KAKIMOTO, S., A histopathological study of gastric cancer in early stage. I. The relationship of peptic ulcer and ulcer carcinoma. *Trans. Soc. Path. jap.* 54, 151—152 (1965) [in Japanese].

SCHMIEDEN, V., and WESTHUES, H., Zur Klinik und Pathologie der Dickdarmpolypen und deren klinischen und pathologisch-anatomischen Beziehungen zum Dickdarmkarzinom. *Dtsch. Z. Chir.* 202, 1—124 (1927).

SPRATT, J. S., ACKERMAN, L. V., and MOYER, C. A., Relationship of polyps of the colonic cancer. *Ann. Surg.* 148, 682—698 (1958).

SPRIGGS, E. I., Polyps of the stomach and polypoid gastritis. *Quart. J. Med.* 12, 1—60 (1948).

STEWART, M. J., Carcinoma of the stomach in association with multiple polypoid adenomata. *J. Path. Bact.* 18, 127 (1913—1914).

— The relation of malignant disease to benign tumours of the intestinal tract. *Brit. med. J.* II, 567—569 (1929).

STOERK, O., Zur Frage des Ulkuskarzinoms des Magens. *Wien. klin. Wschr.* 38, 347—352 (1925).

STOUT, A. P., Superficial spreading type of carcinoma of the stomach. *Arch. Surg.* 44, 651—657 (1942).

— Pathology of carcinoma of the stomach. *Arch. Surg.* 46, 807—822 (1943).

— Superficial spreading type of carcinoma of the stomach. *J. nat. Cancer Inst.* 5, 363, (1944/45).

STRAUSS, A. A., MEYER, J., and BLOOM, A., Gastric polyposis. A report of two cases with a review of the literature. *Amer. J. med. Sci.* **176**, 681—690 (1928).

STROMEYER, F., Die Pathogenese des Ulcus ventriculi, zugleich ein Beitrag zur Frage nach den Beziehungen zwischen Ulcus und Carcinom. *Beitr. path. Anat.* **65**, 1—67 (1912).

SUMII, K., Ein Fall von Rektumkrebs, dessen polypöse Herkunft durch sukzessive Untersuchung bestätigt wurde. *Gann* **32**, 459—464 (1938).

VERSÉ, M., Über die Entstehung, den Bau und das Wachstum der Polypen, Adenome und Karzinome des Magen-Darmkanals. *Arb. path. Inst. Leipzig* **5**, 1—167 (1908).

WESTHUES, H., *Die pathologisch-anatomische Grundlage der Chirurgie des Rektumkarzinoms*. Leipzig 1934.

YARNIS, H., MARSHAK, R. H., and FRIEDMAN, A. I., Gastric polyps. *J. Amer. med. Ass.* **148**, 1088—1093 (1952).

Discussion

The following questions were posed by Dr. H. L. STEWART:

1. At what level in the mucosa of the stomach does the neoplastic change take place — surface, midportion, base?

2. In the ulcer-type of cancer, were the arteries fibrosed to any extent in the connective tissue scar below the base of the ulcer?

3. What do you think about the controversy concerning the origin of the ulcer-cancer?

The answers are: —

1. Neoplastic change seems to have taken place at the surface at first.

2. In the case of the deep ulcers with a gap in the muscular coat, endarteritis obliterans is one of the common findings observable in the scar covering the ulcer floor. It was found in 78.3 per cent of the cases.

3. As you remark, controversy prevails in regard to the problem of ulcer-cancer. I know that in the United States Mallory's concept is widely accepted. However, the close relationship between chronic ulcer of the skin (for example lupus) and cutaneous carcinoma is familiar. Recently, cancerous development upon ulcerative colitis has been repeatedly reported. As I have related, it is a fact that a considerable portion of the gastric carcinomas in the Japanese develop at the margin of ulcers. Therefore, it is an important question, whether this is a peculiar circumstance in Japan or not. For the answer to this problem, I eagerly hope, that similar histogenetic examinations will be done in other countries or districts where the incidence of gastric carcinomas is equally high.

The following questions were posed by Dr. E. SAXÉN:

1. How do you distinguish between papillomatous carcinoma and carcinoma arising from adenomatous polyps?

2. What is the percentage of early ulcer-carcinomas in total gastric cancer?

3. Are cancers which perhaps originate in deep ulcers more slowly growing and more differentiated and perhaps more frequent in older persons than those arising from shallow ulcers?

4. Concerning adenomatous polyps and cancers found in them, do you think it is really a cancer? The term "cancer" is originally a clinical term and I think we pathologists are allowed to use it *only* if there is a good correlation between the structural changes seen and the clinical course of the disease. Do

you think that they are real cancers? As you know, some pathologists state that they are always benign.

The answers are: —

1. In the present report, these cases in which carcinoma co-existed with adenoma were classified as polypous carcinomas and those in which adenomatous tissue was no longer recognizable were classified as polypoid cancers. This last may be identifiable with papillomatous carcinoma. We don't believe that these two groups are essentially different in nature, because in cases of polyposis adenomatosa co-existence of both groups is not infrequently observed.

2. As shown in Fig. 18, the percentage of early carcinomas related to deep and moderate ulcers is approximately one-third of the total cases. This fairly coincides with the percentage of so-called ulcer-cancers calculated by analysis of advanced cases.

3. Speed of growth is not easily distinguishable in human stomach carcinomas. However, the average age of the deep ulcer-cancer group is 2 years more than that of the shallow ulcer-cancer group. Moreover, most of the shallow ulcer cases were highly anaplastic cancers with signet ring cells, whereas more differentiated tubular adenocarcinomas was usually encountered in deep ulcer-cancers.

4. Yes, I do think it is a cancer. Not only the cellular atypia, but also the structural irregularity may support this opinion, although invasive growth and metastasis are still absent. I have an example in which a pedunculate adenomatous polyp of the colon transformed into a carcinoma after 19 months, (see the text). It is the earnest desire of us surgeons to detect the cancer at a stage, where neither invasive growth nor metastasis is yet observed.

Etiological Factors in Gastrointestinal Cancer in Man *

JOHN HIGGINSON

International Agency for Research on Cancer, Lyon, France

The wide variation in the incidence of carcinoma of the gastrointestinal tract between countries of relatively similar ethnological background (CLEMMESEN, 1965; HAENSZEL, 1958; SEGI and KURIHARA, 1960) and the change in frequency observed within immigrant populations (HAENSZEL, 1961; HAENSZEL and DAWSON, 1965; TERRIS and HALL, 1963) indicate that environmental factors are significantly involved. However, the failure to demonstrate any

* This study was supported by Public Health Service Grant CA-09615 from the National Cancer Institute.

correlations in geographical distribution between carcinoma of the esophagus, stomach, and large intestine would indicate that different etiological stimuli are involved for each site.

Since substances known or suspected to be carcinogenic to animals have been demonstrated in foodstuffs consumed by humans (CANNON, 1962; HUEPER and CONWAY, 1964, 1965) most etiological studies on gastrointestinal cancer in man have tended logically to concentrate on the role of diet, but except for the relationship between heavy alcohol ingestion and cancer of the esophagus, no specific dietary factors have as yet been implicated. Moreover, few experimental carcinogens produce tumors of the glandular stomach or intestine on oral administration in animals, which makes tests of suspected agents difficult.

In 1959, a retrospective survey was commenced in the greater Kansas City area to investigate the socio-economic and dietary background of patients with carcinoma of the gastrointestinal tract, and the results are presented in this paper. While a strong association with any specific factor could not be demonstrated, the results indicate that certain factors, sometimes considered etiologically important, are unlikely to be of major significance in the Kansas population.

The Kansas population under study was fairly homogeneous, and marked dietary variations were not a feature since the number of immigrants in the Kansas City area was small.

Methodology

Interviews were carried out in hospitals and, following a pilot study, an open-ended interview was used. A total of 93 patients with gastric cancer and 340 patients with cancer of the colon and rectum were available for analysis. Three controls were available for each carcinoma patient in both groups.

Results

Cancer and control patients were matched by age in decades, race and sex (Table I). Unfortunately the number of gastric cancer cases available for study was small. As reported by others, a slightly higher proportion of gastric cancer patients were in the lower socio-economic group. This almost certainly reflects local environmental factors, since incidence patterns in different countries do not consistently correlate with socio-economic levels.

No significant differences were observed between the cases of gastric cancer and controls regarding marital status, religion, occupation, bowel habits, use of tobacco, alcoholic and non-alcoholic beverages, and consumption of individual foodstuffs. However, the dietary patterns of gastric cancer patients indicated a slightly increased use of animal fats, cooked fats, fried foodstuffs, bacon, and decreased use of dairy produce (Tables II, III). The differences,

Table I. *Distribution of cases of gastric, colon, and rectal carcinoma and controls by age, sex, race, height and weight*

	Stomach		Colon and rectum	
	Cancer patients	Controls	Cancer patients	Controls
Total	93	279	340	1,020
Sex (per cent and No.):				
Males	77.4(72)	77.4(216)	57.6(196)	57.6(588)
Females	22.6(21)	22.6(63)	42.4(144)	42.4(432)
Race (per cent and No.):				
White	82.8(77)	82.8(231)	93.8(319)	93.8(957)
Coloured	17.2(16)	17.2(48)	6.2(21)	6.2(63)
Mean age (years):				
Males	65.4	65.8	63.8	63.5
Females	66.1	65.0	63.3	63.3
Mean height (cm):				
Males	172.2	173.5	174.0	174.2
Females	161.5	160.5	163.0	161.5
Mean weight (kg):				
Males	74.8	75.3	76.2	77.1
Females	64.9	62.1	66.8	66.0

however, between patients and controls were not statistically significant. However, when diets were ranked according to content of cooked fat, 57 per cent. of the gastric patients were in the heavy fat group compared with 38 per cent. of the controls. No such differences were seen for patients with cancer of the colon and rectum, and no differences were observed for uncooked fat between the groups.

As previous authors have reported, there was also a tendency for reduced over-all use of fruit and fresh raw vegetables in the gastric cancer group. For cancer of the colon and the rectum, apart from a slight negative correlation between cigarette smoking and cancer, and a more frequent history of constipation and use of laxatives which were of doubtful significance, no obvious differences were observed and the personal dietary habits appeared similar, both in cases and in controls.

Discussion

The present study has only shown mild dietary associations in relation to fat for gastric cancer patients, the number of whom were small, and none for cases of colon and rectum.

As HAENSZEL (1958) has shown, where a retrospective survey has shown some correlation between gastric cancer and an individual dietary pattern, this has only applied to the individual countries examined. For example,

Table II. *Percent distribution of bacon, use of fried foods, and predominant method of cooking meats.*

	Stomach		Colon and rectum	
	Cancer patients	Controls	Cancer patients	Controls
Bacon:				
Never/v. occasionally	9.7	17.9	18.8	19.5
Less than daily	29.0	35.1	33.2	36.9
Daily	60.2	47.0	47.0	43.4
Unknown	1.1	0.0	0.9	0.3
Fried meats:				
Never/v. occasionally	1.1	3.6	6.2	4.7
Less than daily	37.6	43.0	51.8	47.5
Daily	60.3	52.7	41.5	46.8
Unknown	1.1	0.7	0.6	1.0
Fried food at breakfast:				
Never/v. occasionally	14.0	21.5	21.2	24.8
Less than daily	26.9	28.0	32.6	30.9
Daily	58.1	49.1	45.6	43.6
Unknown	1.1	1.7	0.6	0.7
Predom. method of cooking meats:				
Fried	76.3	67.4	62.1	62.6
Boiled and braised	14.0	16.8	15.6	17.4
Broiled and roasted	2.2	3.2	7.9	5.4
Broiled, braised & fried	5.4	10.4	10.9	11.6
Broiled, roasted & fried	1.1	1.1	3.2	2.3
Unknown	1.1	1.1	0.3	0.8

Table III. *Predominant type of fat used in cooking.*

General classification of fat used in cooking	Stomach		Colon and rectum	
	Cancer patients	Controls	Cancer patients	Controls
Present use:				
Predominantly animal	40.9	25.8	25.0	22.1
Predominantly vegetable	25.8	38.4	39.1	44.1
Combination	20.4	26.5	28.8	26.6
Unknown	13.0	9.6	7.1	7.3
Past use:				
Prior predom. animal	39.8	40.9	34.4	42.4
Prior predom. vegetable	1.1	6.8	2.9	5.6
Prior combination	1.1	5.7	2.9	4.1

whereas SEGI *et al.* (1957) found that gastric cancer patients consume more rice than did controls, gastric cancer is significantly high in Iceland and Chile where rice is not widely eaten. Further, no strict correlation has been demonstrated between a high incidence of gastric cancer and any other cereal.

It is possible that the decreased use of fruit and dairy produce reflects the lower socio-economic status of gastric cancer patients. However, HAENSZEL (1958) did not find a consistent pattern between the incidence of gastric cancer and the use of dairy produce and fresh fruit in the United States, Japan and Finland. Further, in Africa the incidence of gastric cancer is very low and the consumption of dairy produce and often fresh fruit and vegetables is less than in the United States (HIGGINSON and OETTLÉ, 1960). The relative absence of urban-rural differences in most countries would also indicate that this factor is not important (WYNDER et al., 1963).

There was, however, a tendency in this present study for more frequent uses by gastric cancer patients of fried foods and animal fats as compared to vegetable fats. STOCKS (1957) also described such an association, but none was found by ACHESON and DOLL (1964). However, such differences in the use of fried foods and animal fats, if only considered in simple quantitative terms, would hardly explain the high incidence of cancer in Japan, Chile, Iceland, and the low incidence in the United States and elsewhere. It is true, however, that the amount of vegetable fats used in the United States has increased over the last 30 years. Attempts to implicate heated fats and cholesterol in experimental alimentary tract carcinogenesis has been almost universally unsuccessful, although heated lard has been shown to have a potentiating effect on the carcinogenic action of 2-acetylaminofluorene (SUGAL et al., 1962).

We have considered the possibility that the addition of antioxidants to the diet might be of value in preventing the formation of carcinogenic oxidative products of cholesterol and similar substances in fats, and thus explain the recent fall in the United States. The degree of increased use of homemade lard, bacon drippings, collected fats, and of reduced use of refrigeration among the gastric cancer patients was insufficient to support such a possibility, nor was the use of supermarkets, as compared to use of home produce, much less — although these would be situations in which autoxidation of fats would be most likely to occur.

Thus while heated or animal fats would appear unlikely as major carcinogenic or cocarcinogenic agents in gastric carcinoma, our findings in association with STOCKS would suggest that they cannot be completely excluded as of etiological significance, since they are widespread dietary items in many communities with a high frequency of gastric carcinomas. Further attention should also be given to consideration of quantitative differences, since the term "heated fats" has little meaning per se, and their nature may differ markedly according to method of preparation (LIJINSKY and SHUBIK, 1965).

In Iceland, DUNGAL (1961) associated gastric cancer with an increased use of smoked fish, due to the presence of polycyclic hydrocarbons, and it is of interest that the countries with the highest incidence (Iceland, Japan and Chile) are all seaboard countries in temperate areas. However, smoked fish is not a consistent item of diet among the Japanese, nor was fish a major feature of the Kansas City diet in gastric cancer patients.

It is still unknown whether the geographical differences in incidence in cancer of the stomach and cancer of the large intestine can be explained by variations in the concentrations of the same carcinogens for each site, or whether different carcinogenic stimuli may be involved in different areas. However, it is feasible to ascribe certain theoretical properties to such stimuli. Exposure to suspected factors should be widespread among both sexes in both urban and rural areas. Variations in incidence by sex, time, and geographical region should bear a consistent relationship to exposure if the same stimuli are involved in all areas. Exposure, however, to carcinogenic stimuli may be so widespread in a community that development of gastrointestinal neoplasia may essentially represent differences in individual susceptibility, rather than in dosage. Here, retrospective surveys of the present type within relatively homogenous populations would be unsatisfactory. It is probable that this is equally true in colon and rectal cancer. The problem is further compounded by lack of convenient methods for measurement of an individual's ingestion of established carcinogens over a long period, or for accurate determination of even present dietary intakes of such carcinogens. Further, in the absence of any definitely suspected agents, concentrated studies on any single stimulus in a prospective study would appear premature.

The possibility of contamination of foodstuffs by carcinogenic chemicals formed in cooking or added to the diet (i. e., food additives or pesticides) has received increasing attention in recent years, but positive proof of a significant role in human carcinogenesis is lacking. Basic data on the ingestion of even known carcinogens are lacking. Further, since the concentration of carcinogenic or cocarcinogenic agents in the same foodstuff might vary according to methods of cooking and preparation, as evidenced by the higher concentration of hydrocarbons in broiled steaks, conclusions based only on the general use of a foodstuff may be misleading. There is no clear correlation between the degree of industrial development, and thus probable exposure to such agents, and temporal and spatial variations in incidence of gastric carcinoma in different countries. In fact, in Chile and Iceland, both with a very high incidence of gastric carcinoma, the degree of industrial development is comparatively low. Certainly, in the United States an increasing use of pesticides and food additives in recent years has not been associated with a similar increase in gastric cancer. Actually, it could be argued that their usage has had a beneficial effect.

In contrast, it is possible to argue that there is some association between colonic and rectal cancer and degree of economic development, a high incidence being predominantly a feature of the better developed countries. A high incidence of colon and rectal carcinoma remains to be reported in a non-industrialized country whose people live on natural diets with large fecal residues. When the proportion of workers employed in each country in the manufacturing trades (1949) was utilized as an index of industrial development, an association with the death rate from rectal and colonic cancer in males (1960—61) was found (HIGGINSON, 1966).

In conclusion, the findings in the Kansas City survey are in accordance with the experience of others in failing to implicate unequivocally any suspected etiological factor in gastric cancer. They do indicate, however, that further more concentrated studies with larger numbers should be undertaken to exclude a relationship between cooked fats and gastric carcinoma in Western countries.

References

ACHESON, E. D., and DOLL, R., Dietary factors in carcinoma of the stomach: A study of 100 cases and 200 controls. *Gut* 5, 128—131 (1964).

CANNON, P., Chemicals in food products. In: *Chemical and biological hazards in food* (AYRES, J. C., KRAFT, A. A., SNYDER, H. E., and WALKER, H. W., eds.) Iowa State University Press. Ames, Iowa. 1962.

CLEMMESEN, J., Gastro-intestinal tract. In: *Statistical studies on the aetiology of malignant neoplasms.* I. Review and results, p. 117. Copenhagen: Munksgaard 1965.

DUNGAL, N., The special problem of stomach cancer in Iceland. *J. Amer. med. Ass.* 178, 789—798 (1961).

HAENSZEL, W., Variation in incidence of and mortality from stomach cancer, with particular reference to the United States. *J. nat. Cancer Inst.* 21, 213—262 (1958).

— Cancer mortality among the foreignborn in the United States. *J. nat. Cancer Inst.* 26, 37—132 (1961).

—, and DAWSON, E. A., An note on mortality from cancer of the colon and rectum in the United States. *Cancer (Philad.)* 18, 265—272 (1965).

HIGGINSON, J., Aetiological factors in gastro-intestinal cancer in man. *J. nat. Cancer inst.* 37, 527—545 (1966).

—, and OETTLÉ, A. G., Cancer incidence in the Bantu and "Cape Colored" races of South Africa. Report of a cancer survey in the Transvaal (1953—1955). *J. nat. Cancer Inst.* 24, 589—671 (1960).

HUEPER, W. C., and CONWAY, W. D., *Chemical carcinogens and cancers*, p. 3, Springfield (Ill.): G. Thomas 1964.

HUEPER, W. C., and CONWAY, W. D., Hydrocarbon residues in cooked and smoked meats. *Nutr. Rev.* 23, 268—270 (1965).

LIJINSKY, W., and SHUBIK, P., Polynuclear hydrocarbon carcinogens in cooked meat and smoked food. *Industr. Med. Surg.* 34, 152—154 (1965).

SEGI, M., FUKUSHIMA, I., FRYISAKU, S., KURIHARA, M., SAITO, S., ASAMO, K., and KAMOI, M., Epidemilogical study on cancer in Japan; a report of Committee for Epidemiological Study on Cancer, sponsored by Ministry of Welfare and Public Health. *Gann* 48, (Suppl) 1—63 (1957).

—, and KURIHARA, M., Cancer in Japan from viewpoint of geographical pathology. *Tohoku J. exp. Med.* 72, 169—193 (1960).

STOCKS, P., Cancer in North Wales and Liverpool Region. In British Empire Cancer Campaign; Thirty-Fifth Annual Report Covering the Year 1957; Suppl. to part II, p. 51 and 95. London 1957.

SUGAL, M., WITTING, L. A., TSUCHIYAMA, H., and KUMMEROW, F. A., The effect of heated fat on the carcinogenic activity of 2-acetylaminofluorene. *Cancer Res.* 22, 510—518 (1962).

TERRIS, M., and HALL, C. E., Decline in mortality from gastric cancer in native-born and foreignborn residents of New York City. *J. nat. Cancer Inst.* 31, 155—162 (1963).

WYNDER, E. L., KMET, J., DUNGAL, N., and SEGI, M., An epidemiological investigation of gastric cancer. *Cancer (Philad.)* 16, 1461—1496 (1963).

The Epidemiology of Cancer of the Stomach in Japan with Special Reference to the Role of Diet

Takeshi Hirayama

Epidemiology Division, National Cancer Center Research Institute, Tokyo, Japan

1. Size of the Problem

Mortality. Cancer ranks second in the list of major causes of death in Japan. It is the leading cause of death between age 35 to 54, the most productive age in one's life. In 1965, 58,786 men and 47,585 women died of cancer, the mortality rate per 100,000 population being 121.7 and 95.2 respectively. The most common site of cancer in Japan is cancer of the stomach, in both males and females. The death rate in 1965 was 59.2 for males and 35.5 for females. The percentage of stomach cancer to total sites of cancer is 48.6 for males and 37.3 for females.

Morbidity. In 1960, a Cancer Morbidity Survey was conducted by the Ministry of Health and Welfare in 4 prefectures (The Second National Cancer Survey). The total number of cancer patients who visited all the medical institutions in the district during the previous year was studied. According to this study, the number of stomach cancer cases per 100,000 population was calculated as 86.6 for males and 47.7 for females, the relative frequency being 52.8 and 25.7 per cent respectively.

Autopsy Figures. Out of 16,363 male autopsied cancer cases and 13,523 female autopsied cancer cases in the period 1958 to 1963 in Japan cancer of stomach was found in 25.1 per cent of males and 16.2 per cent of females.

Mass-Screening Data. Between 1961 and 65, 15,148 adults were examined by mass-stomach-X-rays by the Japan Cancer Society in various parts of Japan. Out of these, 65 or 430 per 100,000 were found to have cancer of the stomach.

Summary: The high frequency of cancer of the stomach thus shown by mortality, morbidity, autopsy and mass-screening figures makes this type of cancer of particular importance in Japan.

2. Selected Epidemiologic Phenomena

Age. The rates for stomach cancer were noted to go up with the advance of age, as shown by mortality, morbidity and mass-X-ray-screening statistics (Fig. 1).

Sex. The male preponderance was observed in each of these statistics. The male preponderance, however, was far smaller than that for cancer of the esophagus in all age groups.

International Comparison: The frequency of stomach cancer in Japan was noted to be one of the highest in the world by comparing age specific death rates (Segi and Kurihara, 1966).

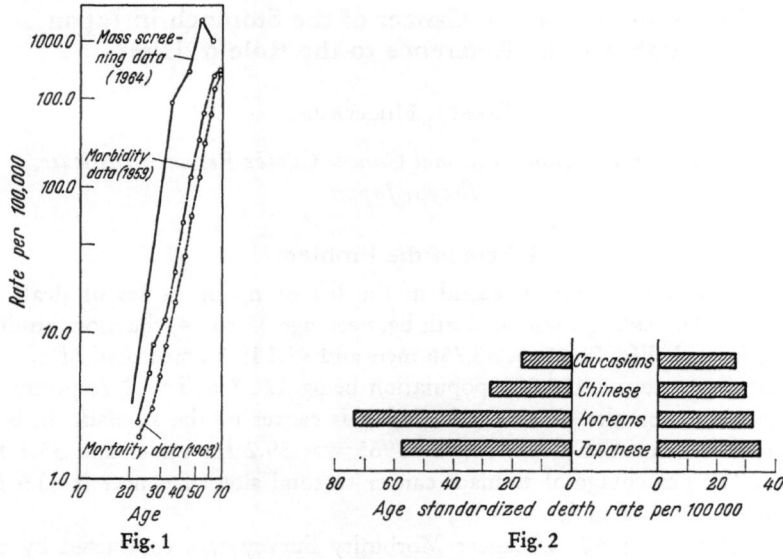

Fig. 1

Fig. 2

Fig. 1. Age distribution of cancer of the stomach

Fig. 2. Age standardized death rate for stomach cancer according to different ethnic groups in Japan 1955—1963

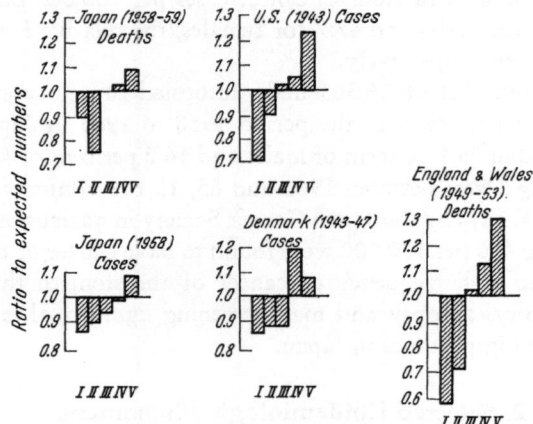

Fig. 3. Stomach cancer incidence according to five socio-economic classes

Race. Among various ethnic groups in Japan, the age standardized death rate for stomach cancer was noted to be much higher among Japanese and Koreans, as compared to Caucasians and Chinese (Fig. 2).

Socio-Economic Variation: Both mortality and morbidity rates were found to become higher with the decrease in socio-economic status, resembling the tendency in U.S., England & Wales and Denmark (Fig. 3). (HIRAYAMA and

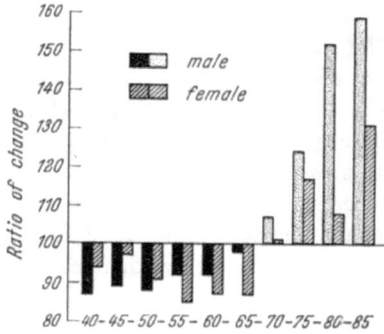

Fig. 4. Ratio of change in death rate for stomach cancer in Japan from 1955 to 1964

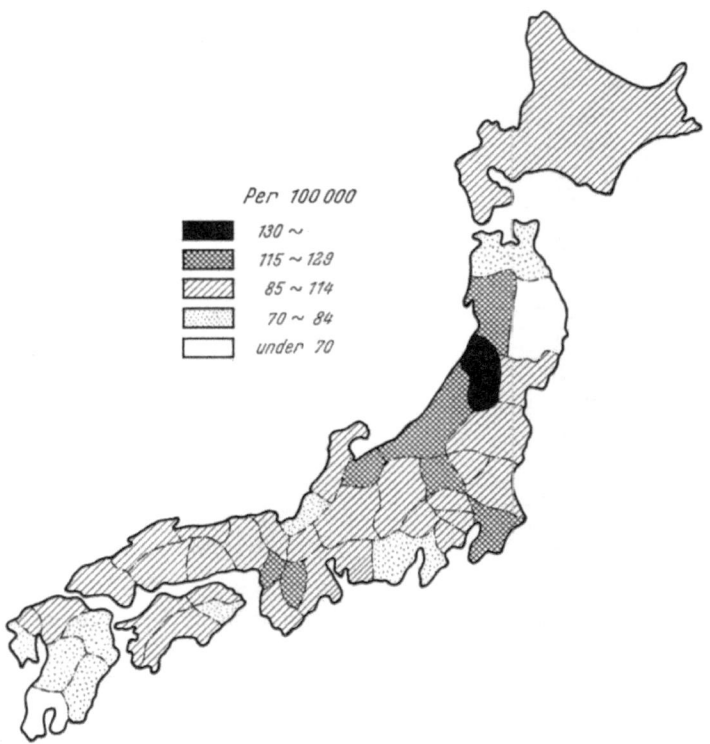

Fig. 5. Age standardized death rate of cancer of the stomach (1955)

YUSA, 1963; Registrar-General, 1958; CLEMMESEN and NIELSEN, 1951; DORN and CUTLER, 1959; HIRAYAMA, 1963.)

Annual Trend. Just as among Japanese in the U. S., the age specific death rates of stomach cancer in Japan also started to decrease since 1955, except in the age group over 70 (Fig. 4).

ʹ *Regional Variation.* The observation of age standardized death rate of stomach cancer by villages, towns and cities clearly indicated a significant geographical aggregation showing a high endemicity in the northern district facing Japan Sea (Tohoku and Hokuriku) (Fig. 5), (HIRAYAMA, 1963).

Summary. All of these epidemiologic phenomena suggest a significant effect of environmental factors which probably operate more strongly in males, stronger in Japanese, stronger in lower socio-economic strata and stronger in the northern part of Japan. The decreasing trend in recent years also indicates the strong effect of post-war environmental change.

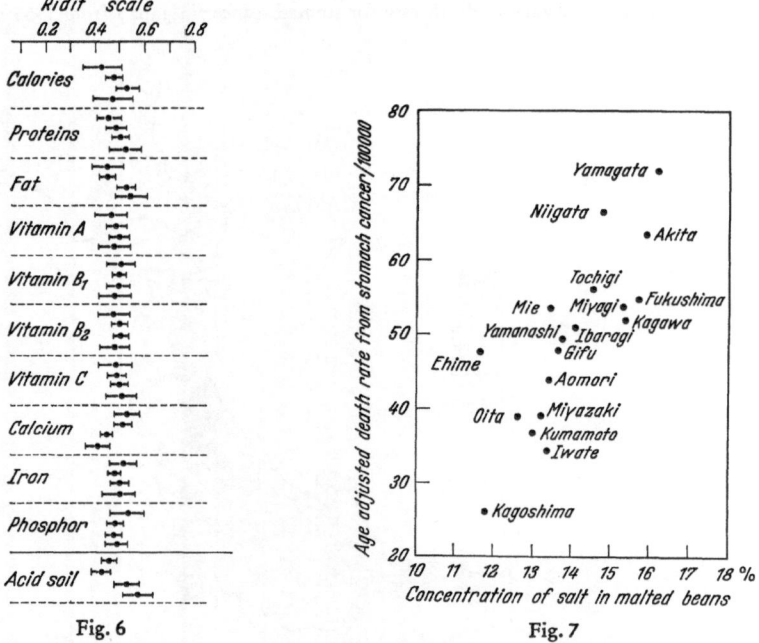

Fig. 6   Fig. 7

Fig. 6. Age standardized death rate from stomach cancer according to the amount of intake of nutritional elements. 690 counties in Japan

Fig. 7. Age-adjusted death rate from stomach cancer according to the concentration of salt in malted beans (rural prefectures only)

3. Correlation Studies

The age standardized death rate of stomach cancer, in 690 counties where the National Nutritional Survey was conducted, was found by HIRAYAMA (1963) to be significantly higher in counties where the average amount of calcium intake is quite low (Fig. 6). A positive correlation was also observed between the concentation of salt in the soy-bean paste consumed and the age standardized death rate for stomach cancer in each prefecture (Fig. 7). The quality of the soil in the endemic area was found in general more acidic than in the less endemic area (Fig. 6).

4. Controlled Case Studies

In our series of controlled case studies a close association was clearly shown between the pattern of diet and the incidence of cancer of the stomach.

Study in Kanagawa Prefecture. In 1960 and 61, 454 cases of stomach cancer and the same number of controls exactly matched, by age, by sex and by

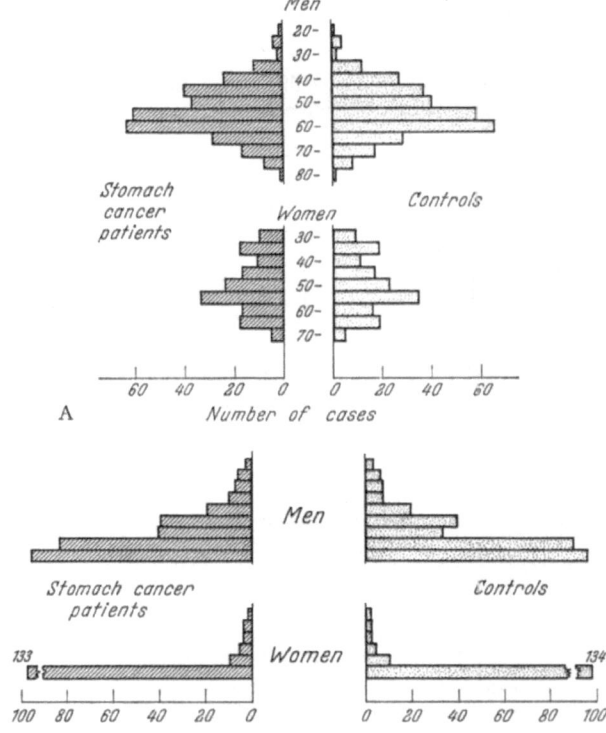

Fig. 8 A and B. Sex and occupation composition of study group (454 cases) and control group (454 cases)

occupation (Fig. 8 a, 8 b), were compared as to the habits of eating and smoking in Kanagawa Prefecture (HIRAYAMA, 1963). Stomach cancer patients were found to drink significantly less milk than control patients (Fig. 9), while the use of salty food was significantly higher in stomach cancer patients than in controls (Fig. 10). There was no difference at all in the extent of cigarette smoking in these two groups (Fig. 11). The result of further analysis revealed that the effect of the intake of milk and that of salty food were mutually independent (Figs. 12, 13).

Study in Six Selected Prefectures. In 1963, the diet pattern (of three years before) was compared between 1,524 stomach cancer patients and 3,792 control patients, matched by sex, by age and by occupation, in 6 selected prefectures

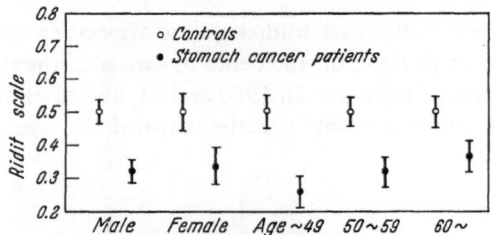

Fig. 9. Comparison of the extent of drinking milk among stomach cancer patients and the controls (Ridit analysis)

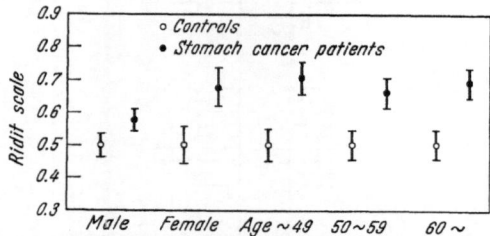

Fig. 10. Comparison of the extent of taking salty food between stomach cancer patients and the controls (Ridit analysis)

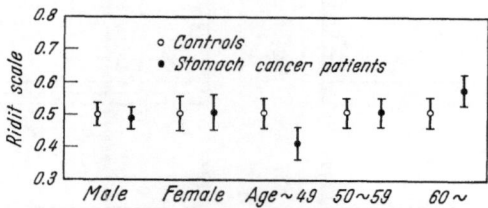

Fig. 11. Comparison of the extent of smoking cigarettes between stomach cancer patients and the controls (Ridit analysis)

in Japan (The Third National Cancer Survey) (Fig. 14). Stomach cancer patients were found to follow the conventional diet pattern more frequently than did the controls (Fig. 15).

Comparison with Multiple Matched Controls. In order to standardize various host and environmental conditions, controls were reselected so as to match to the study group not only as to sex, age and occupation, but also as to place of residence, personal medical histories and family medical histories. Then, a detailed comparison of habits of eating, smoking and drinking was done

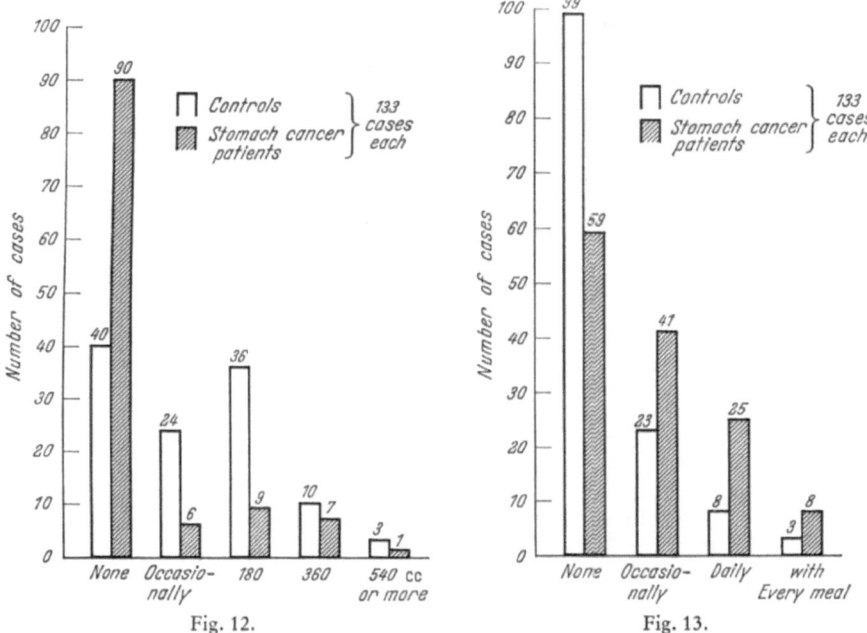

Fig. 12.   Fig. 13.

Fig. 12. Comparison of the use of milk between stomach cancer patients and controls matched
as to sex, age, occupation and the use of highly salted food

Fig. 13. Comparison of the use of highly salted food between stomach cancer patients and
controls matched as to sex, age, occupation and the use of milk

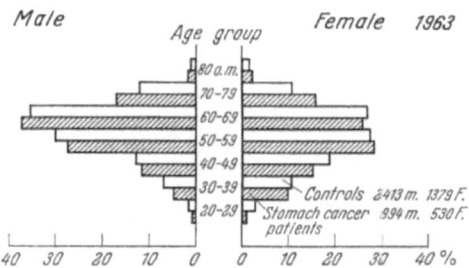

Fig. 14. Age composition of stomach cancer patient group and control group

between 652 stomach cancer patients and the same number of multiple matched
controls (Fig. 16).

It was revealed that the stomach cancer patients consume highly salted
pickles (tsukemono) in significantly higher frequency than the controls while
the frequency of milk intake is significantly lower in stomach cancer group
compared to the controls. No significant difference was observed with regard to
the frequency of intake of other items such as rice, soybean paste soup, fish

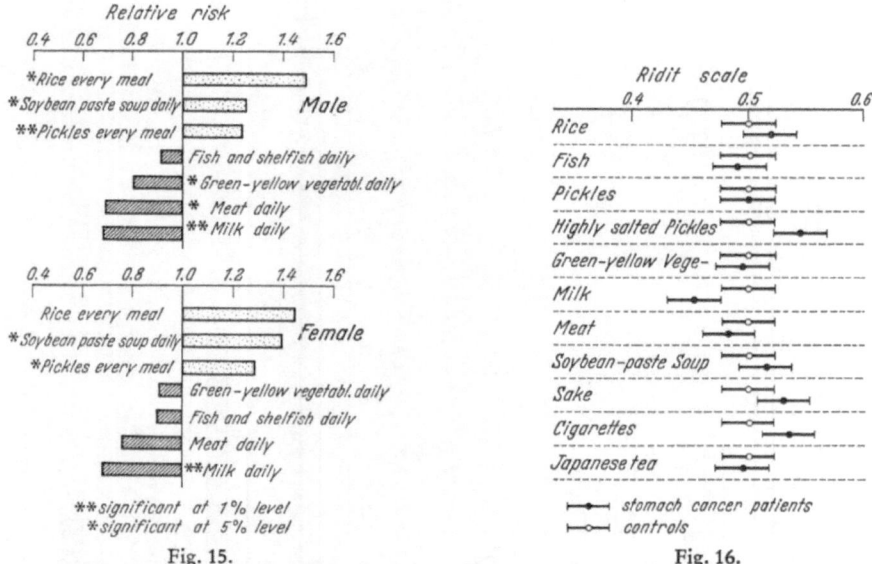

Fig. 15.   Fig. 16.

Fig. 15. The relative risk of stomach cancer according to the frequency of intake of various foods

Fig. 16. Frequency of intake of various foods, comparison between 652 stomach cancer patients and 652 controls matched as to sex, age, occupation, place of residence, past medical history and family history. Japan 1963

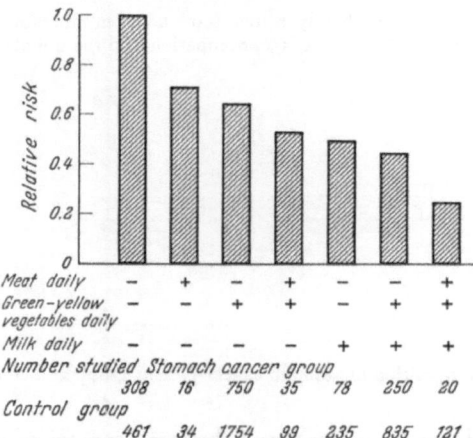

Fig. 17. The relative risk of stomach cancer according to the different combination of foods

and hot green tea. No striking association was observed with the habit of smoking and drinking. From this result it is apparent that the excess intake of highly salted pickles and the lesser intake of milk associate most closely with the occurrence of stomach cancer.

Test of Independence. As the habit of drinking milk is considered as an index of the modernized diet and the habit of frequent intake of pickles is considered as representing the older type of diet, the test of independence in the effect of each factor was felt necessary. The result of this cross-tabulation clearly showed that the percentage of persons with a daily intake of milk was significantly lower among the patient groups than among controls, irrespective of the habit of taking pickles. On the other hand the percentage of persons taking pickles with every meal was found significantly higher among the patient groups than among controls, regardless of the habit of drinking milk.

The Minimum Risk. The relative risk was calculated using Cornfield's method according to the various combination of intake of milk, meat and green-yellow vegetables (Fig. 17). The risk of stomach cancer among people who take all of these foods daily was found to be the lowest, being only one-fourth of the risk among people who take none of these foods daily. In this observations, it was apparent that milk was the single strongest dietary factor in lowering the risk of stomach cancer. However, it was also clear that the beneficial effect did not come solely from the daily intake of milk. The daily intake of meat and/or green-yellow vegetables appeared to lower the risk of stomach cancer, at least to some extent, even in the absence of daily intake of milk.

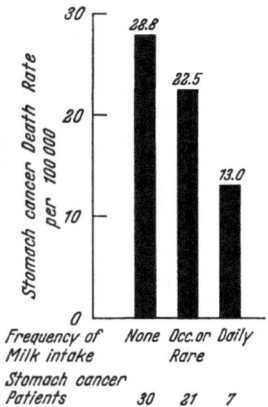

Fig. 18. Milk drinking and stomach cancer, prospective population study, Jan. to June, 1966

5. Population Prospective Studies

Since the fall of 1965 a prospective population study covering 265,118 adults age 40—69 (over 91 per cent of all the inhabitants of that age in each district) has been in progress in 29 Health Center Districts in 6 prefectures in Japan. Although it is premature to report the result of this study, preliminary analysis of stomach cancer deaths in the first six months in this population already shows that the frequency is significantly higher among non-drinkers of milk (Fig. 18). It is expected that the role of diet in the epidemiology of stomach cancer will be confirmed through this co-operative study.

Discussion

It is of special interest that the closest association with stomach cancer was observed between (1) the lesser frequency of milk intake and (2) the excess intake of salty pickles. These two dietary factors were noted to be closely associated with stomach cancer, especially when study groups were compared to multiple-matched controls. The cross-tabulation of milk intake and intake of pickles showed that these factors were mutually independent in their association with stomach cancer.

A similar tendency was shown in the case-control study among Japanese in Hawaii and also in the mass-screening survey for stomach cancer conducted by Japan Cancer Society in 1961—65 (Fig. 19) (HIRAYAMA, 1963).

The effect of the excess intake of salty pickles could be interpreted as causing chronic irritation and damage on the mucus membrane of the stomach as was shown in animal experiments (SATO *et al.*, 1959; MINOWA *et al.*, 1960).

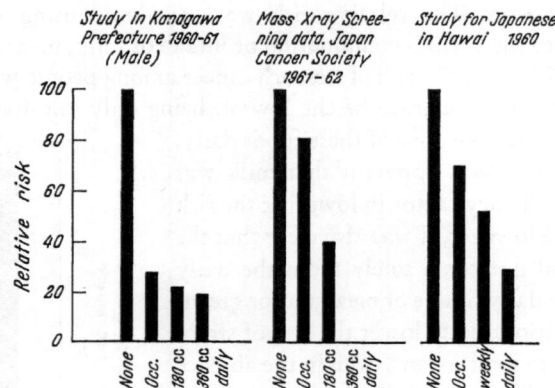

Fig. 19. Relative risk of stomach cancer by the frequency of milk intake

With regard to the reason of apparent protective effect of milk, its nutritional quality, in addition to its physico-chemical characteristic, should be considered to be responsible for its outstanding beneficial effect on stomach cancer in view of the observation of a risk gradient according to the various combination of milk, meat and green-yellow vegetables (STOCKS and MARY, 1933; SUGIURA, 1951; HOCH-LIGETI, 1946; HIRAYAMA, 1963).

The dietary pattern of the Japanese people is now in the process of dramatic change. The per capita milk consumption increased as much as ten times from 1949 to 1963. The basic change in the methods of preserving food, together with the growing popularity of westernized food, is now creating a new pattern of Japanese diet. It is speculated that such change in diet will result in a decline of the incidence of stomach cancer in Japan. Although it is still one of the most important diseases in the nation, the age-adjusted death rate of stomach cancer has been on a downward trend since 1959 for both males and females. The rate of decrease appeared to be correlated with the increase of milk consumption in each district in Japan (Fig. 20), in line with similar results from comparison between countries in the world as well as between states in the U. S. (Fig. 21) (HIRAYAMA, 1963).

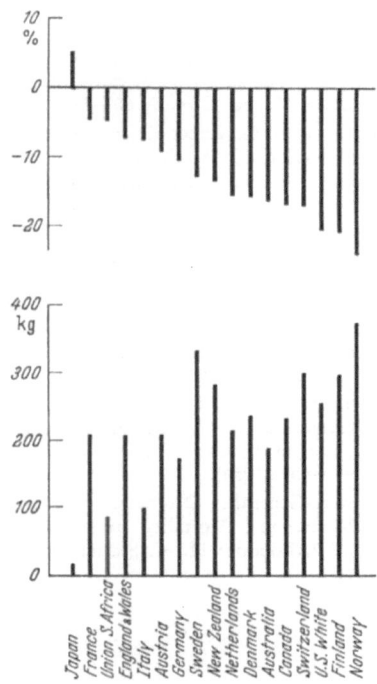

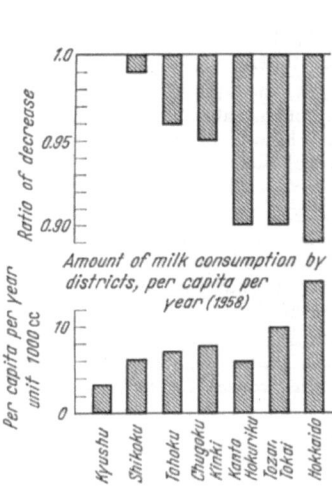

Fig. 20. The mortality rate for stomach cancer by districts, comparison between 1958 and 1963

Fig. 21. Ratio of change in age-adjusted death rate from stomach cancer in various countries, 1952—53 and 1958—59

Summary

The excess intake of highly salted food was found to be an important factor related to the high incidence of stomach cancer in Japan, while daily drinking of milk was noted to have a beneficial effect on the incidence of this leading type of cancer in Japan. The improvement of diet pattern, especially the increase of milk consumption, therefore, should be encouraged as a possible preventive measure for cancer of the stomach in Japan, in parallel with the early case finding programs currently in progress.

References

Bross, I. D. J., *Biometrics*. The Biometric Soc. vol. 14, No 1, p. 18—88, March 1958.

Clemmesen, J., and Nielsen, A., The social distribution of cancer in Copenhagen, 1943—1947 *Brit. J. Cancer*, 5, 159—171 (1951).

Dorn, H. F., and Cutler, S. J., Morbidity from cancer in the United States. Public

Health Monograph, No 56. Washington, D. C.: U. S. Government Printing Office. 1959.

Haenszel, W., Variation in incidence of and mortality from stomach cancer with particular reference to the United States. *J. nat. Cancer Inst.* 21, 213 (1958).

Hirayama, T., A study of epidemiology of stomach cancer, with special reference to the effect of diet factor. *Bull Inst. Publ. Health* 12, 85—96 (1963).

HIRAYAMA, T., and YUSA, Y., The occupational-social class risks of cancer in Japan. *Jap. J. Cancer Clin.* 9, 66—74 (1963).

HOCH-LIGETI, C., Effect of fresh milk on the production of hepatic tumors in rats by dimethylaminoazobenzene. *Cancer Res.* 6, 563 (1946).

MINOWA, S., TAKAHASHI, H., KANO, T., MATSUYAMA, K., ARAKI, Y., and YAGI, T., Studies of the relation between cancer and calcium. Histological study on injury by salt in stomach mucosa and efficacy of calcium against it. *Kita Kanto Igaku* 10, (3), 713—718 (1960).

QUISENBERRY, W. B., TILDEN, I. L., and ROSENGARD, J. L., Racial incidence of cancer in Hawaii. *Hawaii med. J.* 13, 449—451 (1954).

Registrar-General's Decennial Supplement. Occupational Mortality part II, vol. 1 and 2. London: H. M. Stationery Office 1958.

SATO, T., FUKUYAMA, T., SUZUKI, T., TAKAYANAGI, J., MURAKAMI, T., SHIOTSUKI, N., TANAKA, R., and TSUJI, R., Studies of the causation of gastric cancer. *Bull. Inst. Publ. Health,* 8, 187 (1959).

SEGI, M., and KURIHARA, M., Cancer mortality for selected sites in 24 countries, No 4 1962—63. Dept. of Publ. Health, Tohoku Univ., School of Med., Sendai, Japan 1966.

STOCKS, P., and MARY, N. K., Co-operative study of the habits, home life dietary and family histories of 450 cancer patients and an equal number of control patients. *Ann. Eugen. (Lond.)* 5 (3/4), 237 (1933).

SUGIURA, K., On the relation of diets to the development, prevention and treatment of cancer, with special reference to cancer of the stomach and liver. *J. Nutr.* 44, 345—360 (1951).

WYNDER, E. L., KMET, J., DUNGAL, N., and SEGI, M., An epidemiological investigation of gastric cancer. *Cancer (Philad.)* 16, 11 (1963).

Discussion

Dr. SAXÉN asked:

The per capita consumption of milk and milk products is one of the highest in the world in Finland and so also is the incidence of stomach cancer. How could this be explained from the beneficial effects of milk which you have been proposing?

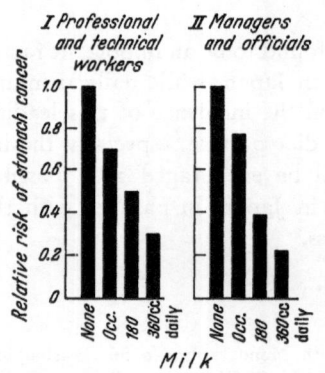

Fig. 22. Relative risk of stomach cancer according to the frequency of milk intake

Dr. HIRAYAMA replied:

I am well aware of the facts you just mentioned. As I showed in my presentation (Fig. 21), the magnitude of decline in the age adjusted death rate from stomach cancer is world highest in Norway and Finland.

I consider this particular phenomenon must be the reflection of the world highest consumption of milk in these countries. I should like to emphasize that any protective factor, such as milk consumption in this case, does not govern the absolute level of the incidence but gives strong influence on the magnitude of its change.

Dr. Saxén then asked the following question:

Could it be that in Japan the use of milk in the diet is correlated with a higher standard of living, which would be responsible for the decrease in stomach cancer and not the consumption of milk per se?

Dr. Hirayama replied:

The lower risk of stomach cancer among daily drinkers of milk could not be considered as just the reflection of the fact that they belong primarily to the higher socio-economic strata as a clear-cut dose-effect relationship was observed between the extent of milk intake and the relative risk of stomach cancer in each of such higher socio-economic groups as is shown in Fig. 22.

The Different Incidence of Gastric Cancer all over the World and Possible Reasons for this Difference

E. A. Saxén and M. Hakama

Finnish Cancer Register, Helsinki, Finland

It is well known that the incidence of gastric cancer varies in different countries; that there are differences within them and that in most countries the incidence of stomach cancer is decreasing. It has also been well established that many of these differences and changes are real, not being due to variations in standards of diagnosis and treatment.

Before going further, we should like to stress two points. Firstly, no far-reaching conclusions are justified, since figures compiled from all over the world can only be interpreted properly by those who have collected them, who know their reliability and the possible sources of errors. Secondly, there is no reason to suppose that the cause of gastric cancer is the same all over the world. Also, multiple etiologic factors in the development of gastric cancer must be taken into consideration. Experimental cancer research has clearly shown how great a number and variety of causative agents exists. They may act simultaneously or consecutively and vary at different stages of the neoplastic disease.

As already pointed out by Segi, one of the most interesting facts about stomach cancer is the decrease in incidence observed in most countries. This decrease in the risk of stomach cancer is not an artefact, at least not in all countries, induced by changes in standards of diagnosis, but a real one (Haenszel, 1958). If the number of physicians per population can be regarded as a measure of standard of diagnosis, we can see in Fig. 1 that there is no marked association between the standard of diagnosis and stomach cancer.

We have calculated some figures also from Finland, illustrating this decrease in stomach cancer incidence.

Age specific incidence rates and percentage of decrease in the incidence by age groups (females) are shown in Fig. 2.

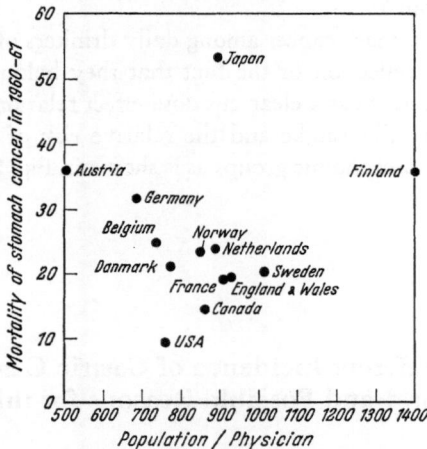

Fig. 1. Correlation between age adjusted mortality rates of stomach cancer in 1960—61 and the number of inhabitants per physician in 1960—62 in different countries

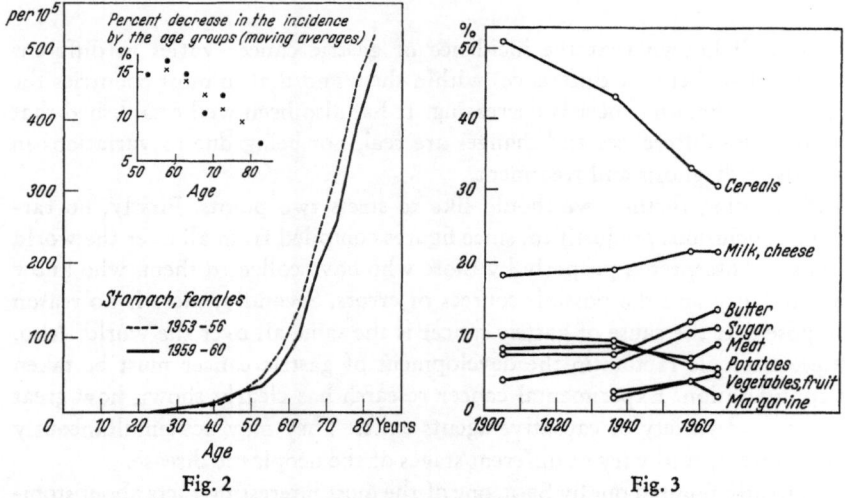

Fig. 2
Fig. 3

Fig. 2. Age specific incidence rates of stomach cancer in 1953—56 and 1959—1960; per cent decrease in incidence by the age groups (moving averages). Finnish females

Fig. 3. The percentage of major foodstuffs in the total energy intake in Finland

Thus also the figures from Finland show that the older the age group, the lesser the decrease. This is consistent with the hypothesis that the factor or factors, to which the older age groups were exposed decades ago, no longer affect the people, or at least not to the same degree. The decrease has usually been connected with nutritional improvement.

As seen in Fig. 3, changes in food habits in Finland have been very great (PEKKARINEN et al., 1964).

The causes of gastric cancer may well be different in different countries. Therefore, it is perhaps useless to try to find one single hypothesis which would fit all the facts for geographical variations and variations in time. However, if the causative factor is one and the same, then the factor should have a different prevalence in countries of different stomach cancer incidence, that is to

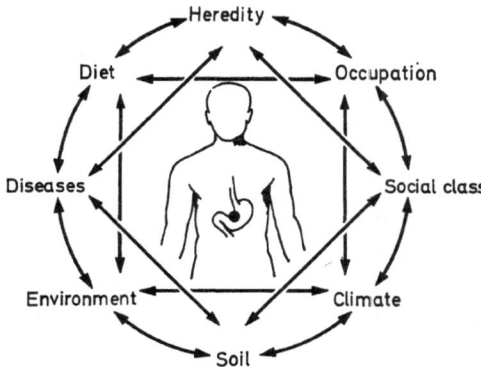

Fig. 4. Schematized presentation of interrelationships of etiological factors affecting stomach cancer incidence

say the geographical distribution of the factor should be consistent with the geographical distribution of stomach cancer. A substantial change in the occurrence of the factors should result in a change in the incidence of stomach cancer. The possibility of multiple factors should be borne in mind in this connection and the real difficulty relates to possible weaker factors, none of which by themselves have a marked effect on the stomach cancer incidence, but which together could very greatly affect the incidence rates. The greatly schematized Fig. 4 shows some groups of factors and how interrelated they often are. It also illustrates how difficult it is at this level to distinguish between the different factors or so-called causes of cancer.

The following list shows some of the factors allegedly associated with high stomach cancer incidence, as reported in world literature (CLEMMESEN, 1965). They are not few and it is not our intention to deal with all of these suggestions.

Soil: acidic soil
meadow soil
peat soil
lowlying clay areas
igneous rocks near the surface
deep ground water
mineral balance high zinc/copper ratio

Climate: northern countries
heavy rainfall
low temperature

Environment: rural areas
grain dust
iron dust

6*

		Dietary factors:	irregular meal times
	inorganic dust with		excess zinc, copper
	free silica		deficiency in iron,
Occupation:	farmers		molybdenum
	workers in quarries		deficiency in vitamins A, B₁,
	low social class		B₁₂, C.

Dietary factors: irregular meal times
excess zinc, copper
deficiency in iron, molybdenum
deficiency in vitamins A, B_1, B_{12}, C.
tobacco
alcohol
liquid paraffin (purgative)

Occupation: farmers
workers in quarries
low social class

Diseases: stomach ulcer
chronic gastritis
adenomatoid polyps
intestinal metaplasia
hyposecretion
pernicious anemia
Plummer Vinson
dental caries

Diet: high intake of starchy foods rice, cereals, potatoes
highly brined food, homecured bacon, salami sausage
smoked food, salted food, fried food
hot food
low protein diet
low consumption of fruit and fresh vegetables

Heredity: blood group A
race (Mongolian, Japanese, Finnish etc.)

The most natural explanation for differences in stomach cancer incidence is that it reflects differences in the environment, most probably food habits. In the proceedings of the last UICC Symposium on Geographical Pathology of Gastro-intestinal Cancer (1961) held in Copenhagen less than ten years ago in 1958, we read on this subject: "The study of environmental factors in gastro-intestinal cancer is the most promising line of investigation in solving the problem of etiology. It has often been suggested that diet may affect the incidence of gastric carcinoma. The symposium found that such a relationship has not been established and recommended further investigation."

Relatively few studies have been performed on the nutritional background of patients with stomach cancer. In a recent joint study (WYNDER *et al.*, 1963) undertaken concurrently in New York, Iceland, Japan und Yugoslavia by WYNDER, KMET, DUNGAL and SEGI, no constant differences were revealed either of excess or deficiency in regard to dietary factors between the study group and the control group in any of the countries. The authors conclude, therefore, that it may be more pertinent to compare dietary factors in populations with different rates of gastric cancer, rather than to compare patients and controls within a given population.

In this connection, we shall report some calculations of only one very simple variable, namely that of cereal consumption (HAKAMA *et al.*, 1967). It has been observed that one common characteristic for areas of high gastric cancer incidence is low intake of fresh vegetables and fruits and a high consumption of rice, cereals and potatoes, that is, of starchy foods.

Our calculations may thus be concentrated under two hypotheses:

The consumption of cereals in populations with high stomach cancer incidence should be higher than in populations with low stomach cancer incidence.

If the incidence of stomach cancer is decreasing more rapidly in one population, there should be in the same population a decrease in cereal consumption
at a greater rate than in another population where the decrease is slower.

An unknown time lag between the cause and effect must of course be supposed in each of the hypotheses.

Fig. 5 shows the correlation between mortality of stomach cancer in 1960
—1961 and consumption of cereals per capita in 1934—38[1]. The time lag has
thus been supposed to be 20—30 years. There seems to be a relatively high
correlation between these variables.

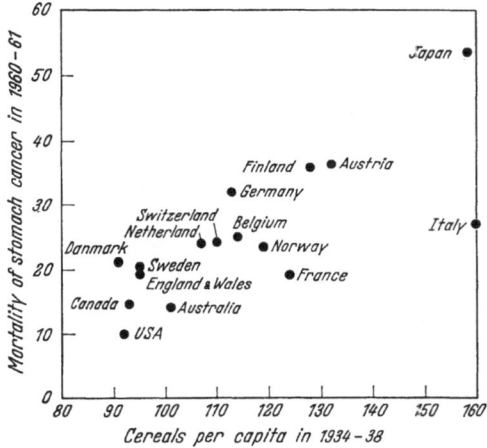

Fig. 5. Correlation between age-adjusted mortality rates of stomach cancer in 1960—61 and
the cereal (flour) consumption per capita in 1934—38 in different countries

In figure 6 we have calculated the correlation between the per cent change
in death rates for stomach cancer from 1952—53 to 1960—61 and the per cent
change in cereal consumption per capita from 1934—38 to 1960—61.

Also this figure gives the impression of a relatively high correlation between
the variables studied. No tests have been performed for statistical inference,
because of the suggestive nature of the hypotheses. The nature of this relationship remains completely obscure. However, as the correlation of this specific
dietary habit and stomach cancer mortality was so striking, we thought the
reporting of these calculations may be justified. Of course, the high consumption of cereals correlates with many other things, e. g. with some other factors
connected with low standard of living.

In conclusion, we should like to say that we are confident that the striking
differences in the incidence of gastric cancer, which exist throughout the world,
as also the rapid decrease in stomach cancer incidence, can provide vital clues
to the understanding of the etiology of the disease. The causative factors could

[1] We have used Professor Segi's data (1964) for mortality and U. N. Statistical Yearbook
(1964) for data of cereal consumption.

be characterized, possibly eliminated from the environment and the disease perhaps prevented.

So far, these remarkable international variations in stomach cancer incidence have been the concern primarily of geographical pathologists, whose main interest has often been in the description and verification of the patterns.

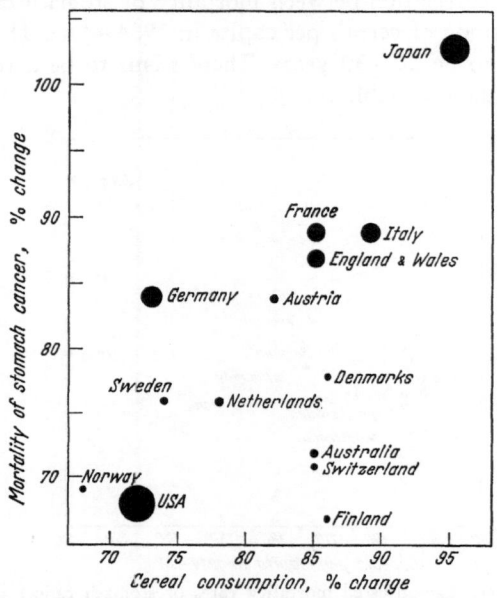

Fig. 6. Correlation between per cent change in age adjusted death rates for stomach cancer from 1952—53 to 1960—61 and percent change in cereal (flour) consumption per capita from 1934—38 to 1960—61

Now it is time for analytic studies designed to test the various hypotheses by which the patterns can be explained. Such studies are still lacking. They are certainly not easy to perform. However, we have great faith in the modern biomathematical methods and hope that problems like these can be solved.

References

CLEMMESEN, J., Statistical studies in malignant neoplasms. Köbenhavn: Munksgaard 1965.

Geographical pathology of gastro-intestinal cancer. Acta U.I.C.C. 17, 3 (1961).

HAENSZEL, W., Variation in incidence and mortality from stomach cancer, with particular reference to the United States. J. nat. Cancer Inst. 21, 213—262 (1958).

HAKAMA, M., and SAXÉN, E. A., Cereal consumption and gastric cancer. Int. J. Cancer 2, 265—268 (1967).

PEKKARINEN, M., SEPPÄNEN, R., and ROINE, P., Näringsforskning Nr. 4, 139—149 (1964).

SEGI, M., and KURIHARA, M., Cancer mortality for selected sites in 24 countries, No 3, 1960/61. Dept. Public Health, Tohoku Univ., School of Med., Sendai, Japan 1964.

WYNDER, E. L., KMET, I., DUNGAL, N., and SEGI, M., An epidemiological investigation of gastric cancer. Cancer (Philad.) 16, 1461—1496 (1963).

The following question was posed by Dr. J. HIGGINSON:

What is the importance of cereal consumption and how can you explain the high consumption of cereals in Africa and the low incidence of stomach cancer?

The following response was given:

I really do not know whether the high use of cereals simply reflects a low standard of living and the possible deficiencies connected with it, or whether perhaps cereals contain some carcinogenic factors, for example aflatoxins or some other agents connected with poor storage perhaps. As to the low incidence of stomach cancer in Africa, I can only repeat that figures from different countries can only be properly interpreted by those who have collected them and know their reliability. I should also like to repeat that there is, in my mind, no reason to expect the so-called cause of gastric cancer to be the same all over the world.

Stomach Cancer among the Japanese

WILLIAM HAENSZEL and MITSUO SEGI

*National Cancer Institute, National Institutes of Health, Bethesda, Maryland, 20014, U.S.A. and
Tohoku University School of Medicine, Sendai, Japan*

Stomach Cancer Among the Japanese

Epidemiological observations have provided to date most of the information bearing on the etiology of stomach cancer. The lack of a suitable animal in whom carcinomas of the glandular stomach could be readily induced by oral administration of known carcinogens has impeded development of a well-rounded experimental program.

A role for host factors in this disease has been suggested by two types of observations: (a) an excess risk for persons of blood group A (AIRD et al., 1953; BILLINGTON, 1956; BUCKWALTER et al., 1957; SPEISER, 1956; WHITE and EISENBERG, 1959); (b) clustering of stomach cancer cases within families, the collective evidence from several studies suggesting that stomach cancer risks among relatives of probands are 2—3 times those for relatives of index controls (STATE et al., 1947; VIDEBAEK and MOSBECH, 1954; MACKLIN, 1955; WOOLF, 1956). Familial aggregation studies have been criticized on a variety of technical grounds and some uncertainty exists about the true magnitude of the excess risks (GRAHAM and LILIENFELD, 1958). It has been further pointed out that familial aggregation is a necessary, but not sufficient, condition for the presence of a genetic component, since this phenomenon could also arise from differences among families in exposures to environmental agents. Observations which point to environmental factors include the large differences in stomach cancer risks between countries and the very rapid decline in incidence and mortality during the past quarter century in several countries, notably the United States (HAENZEL, 1958).

The Japanese offer unusual opportunities to investigate the relative contributions of host characteristics and environmental exposures as determinants of stomach cancer risk. International comparisons of mortality leave no doubt that Japan must be included with other high risk countries such as Chile, Finland and Iceland (SEGI and KURIHARA, 1964). For over 50 years Japanese have migrated in substantial numbers to Hawaii and the continental United States, thus providing information on the course of stomach cancer in a high-risk population migrating to a country where much lower risks prevail. STEINER and others have emphasized the importance of migrant populations as a study resource (STEINER, 1954).

From necropsy findings in Los Angeles County General Hospital STEINER was impressed by the high relative frequency of stomach cancer among Japanese compared to the cancer site distribution for other ethnic groups. His necropsy data yielded no direct measure of the position of U.S. Japanese relative to the risks prevailing in Japan and among U.S. whites. Suggestive data on this point were reported by SMITH, who found the stomach cancer mortality of U.S. Japanese as of 1949—52 to be about 80 percent of that expected on the basis of rates in Japan, with adjustment for age and sex distribution of the migrant population; similarly, the U.S. Japanese had mortality over 3 times that for the host population of U.S. whites (SMITH, 1956). One might conclude, therefore, that while stomach cancer mortality had been displaced downward among Japanese migrants their experience still conformed more closely to that of the home population than to the host population. The data for Japanese migrants agreed with observations on several other groups migrating from Europe to the United States. This particular pattern of displacement is quite specific for stomach cancer and not duplicated in the results for other cancer sites.

More recent data from California (BUELL and DUNN, 1965) and for the total United States for 1959—62 (HAENSZEL and KURIHARA, in preparation) have confirmed and elaborated the earlier observations on stomach cancer mortality. Furthermore, it has been possible to distinguish between migrants (Issei) and their U.S. -born descendants (Nisei). This feature could not be introduced in the earlier material, since only a small fraction of the Nisei at that time had reached the ages of high stomach cancer risk. Fig. 1 relates the risks among Issei and Nisei to the home and host populations as of 1959—62. The drift in Issei risks away from those prevailing in Japan continued during the intervening 10-year period. As of 1959—62 the overall Issei risk was 67 percent of that prevailing in Japan; the Nisei figure was lower still, 42 percent. While the overlap in age distributions of Issei and Nisei is not great, the configuration of the age-specific rates would suggest that the Issei-Nisei differential for stomach cancer will persist in future years.

To emphasize the different behavior of stomach and other sites within the digestive tract, Fig. 2 presents the corresponding data for cancer of the large

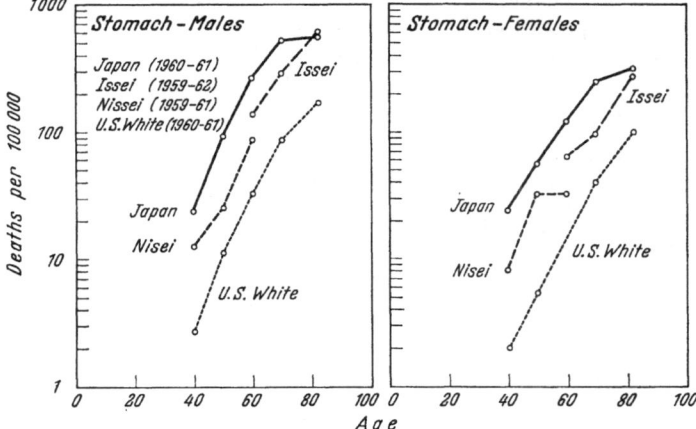

Fig. 1. Age-specific death rates from cancer of the stomach

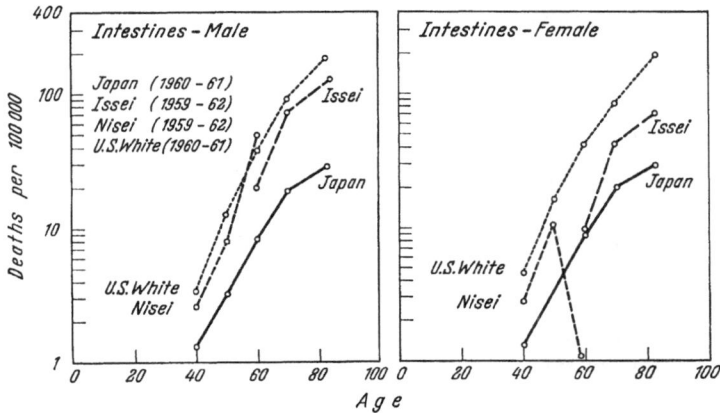

Fig. 2. Age-specific death rates from cancer of the large intestine

intestine. There is an obvious upward displacement in risk to the U.S. white level for the latter site, particularly among males, accompanied by minimal differences between Issei and Nisei. The transition in risk for colon appears to occur within the lifetime of the migrants. The experience of Japanese migrants for intestines is consistent with observations on migrants from Poland, where low risks have also prevailed for colon (STASZEWSKI and HAENSZEL, 1965).

The observations on stomach cancer mortality among U.S. Japanese appear generally consistent with incidence data from the Hawaii cancer register

QUISENBERRY *et al.*, 1966) and do not immediately rule out hypotheses invoking environmental and/or host factors. The effects noted are not trivial and should be amenable to exploitation. The basic strategy is to see whether changes in stomach cancer risks among the Japanese migrants can be associated with changes in customs, occupation and other environmental exposures due to migration, with the expectation that observations on migrants and home and host populations will permit inferences not possible from data collected within a single population. For example, one may look at the difference in risk between Japan and U.S. Japanese and ask whether it is numerically compatible with the gradients in exposures to factors thought to be associated with stomach cancer in these populations. To this end the following pieces of information are needed: (a) stomach cancer risks in Japan and among the U.S. Japanese; (b) the relative risks for stomach cancer for a variety of population characteristics and exposures in Japan and among U.S. Japanese; (c) measures of displacement in exposure to suspect items. Information on (a) comes from existing mortality and incidence data; (b) can be estimated from case-control studies underway in two prefectures of Japan and in Hawaii and California; (c) can be derived from interviews of persons 35 years and over in representative samples of households in Hiroshima and Miyagi prefectures, Hawaii and California. The household surveys in addition to providing data for inter-area comparisons represent another source of controls for data obtained from stomach cancer patients.

Data Collection

In conduct of the case-control interviews and household surveys care was taken to co-ordinate and maintain comparability in procedures used in Japan and the United States. For the household surveys in Japan a representative sample of households already prepared for Hiroshima and Miyagi prefectures was used. The U.S. Bureau of the Census drew samples of Japanese households in Hawaii and California from the 1960 population census returns. The selection rule for hospital controls is simple and leaves little ambiguity in designation of control patients. The general rule in all areas is to interview two controls for each diagnosed case, one being the next older, and the other the next younger person, of the same sex in the same hospital service on the day the case was interviewed. (In Hawaii and California Japanese comprise only a small proportion of hospital admissions and the rule was modified to permit use of other hospital services as a source of controls.) Persons with diagnoses of gastric ulcers, other diseases of the stomach, and other cancers of the digestive system were excluded from the control series.

A major portion of the interviews for stomach cancer patients and controls was devoted to a diet history. All reviews of stomach cancer epidemiology conclude that the evidence points to some connection with diet, although there is no consensus on the foods or methods of preparation involved. The present study was viewed as a screen to secure leads on existing associations rather than to test specific hypotheses, which suggested that coverage of a wide range of food items be attempted. Dietary histories are notoriously difficult to elicit, but the presence of profound contrasts between Japanese and Western food habits encouraged us to proced. The interview was structured to secure information on phasing-out of Japanese-style foods and phasing-in of Western foods so that the populations might be classified and ordered by degree of transition in diet.

We adopted "frequency of use" — the number of meals the item was used per day, week, month — as the basic measuring device. To attempt recording of amounts used appeared impractical except in special situations, such as noting rice consumption in bowls.

The questionnaires used in Hawaii and California were bilingual and the interviewers conversed in English and Japanese. The bilingual schedule represented more than an administrative convenience for data collection. Shades of meaning are difficult to convey in translation and the bilingual schedule has contributed to inter-area comparability of data.

The diagnostic record for each stomach cancer patient covered the standard range of information to permit classification by certainty of diagnosis. In Miyagi prefecture and Hawaii a supplementary pathology protocol for surgical and necropsy specimens from stomach cancer patients, was developed by a group of collaborating pathologists (Professor K. AKAZAKI, formerly of Tohoku University School of Medicine; Dr. G. STEMMERMANN, Kuakini Hospital, Honolulu; Dr. K. HERROLD, National Cancer Institute). The pathology protocol is an integral part of the study in these two areas and represents one of the few instances in which patient interview data and pathology findings can by systematically collated and examined.

Results — Miyagi Prefecture

Interviewing of patients and hospital controls continues in Hawaii and California, but the volume of data accumulated there does not warrant analysis at this time. Field work began first in Miyagi prefecture and an initial set of tabulations for stomach cancer patients, hospital controls and households has been completed for this prefecture. A brief summary of these results follows to illustrate the nature of the findings and problems in interpretation and to reinforce the contention that studies on diet and stomach cancer cannot be successfully carried out within a single geographical area.

Relative risks have been computed in a conventional manner (MANTEL and HAENSZEL, 1959; CORNFIELD and HAENSZEL, 1960) to describe the association of stomach cancer with "high" or "low" consumption of individual food items. The procedure is described in more concrete terms for rice: the diagnosed cases, hospital controls and household respondents were classified into two groups —

eat rice at 3 or more meals daily, 2 or fewer meals daily. Comparison of the distributions for cases and controls can provide an estimate of the stomach cancer risk among persons eating rice 3 or more times daily relative to a unit risk for those using rice less frequently. The objective is to estimate the difference in risk that would be revealed by a prospective study, where one first classifies a population by frequency of rice consumption and then observes the subsequent appearance of stomach cancer among individuals in each cohort.

Table I summarizes the relative risks for individual foods yielded by comparison of cases with hospital controls. On initial screening the major concern is with identification of large effects and the results have been grouped into three categories: higher risks for "above-average" users; smaller and less substantial differences between "above-" and "below-average" users (1.30 > relative risk > 0.75); lower risks for "above-average" users. The table deals only with estimated magnitude of effects and does not consider tests of statistical significance. For rice and miso higher risks among "above-average" users were suggested. Above-average consumption of items associated with lower risks includes pork, beef and some fruits.

In principle, reliance on more than one set of controls confers advantages. The use of hospital controls may enhance comparability of replies. The same person normally interviews the case and matching controls, sometimes without knowledge of their identity, and the clinical setting facilitates patient rapport and encourages more accurate recall. Selection factors influencing hospital admission will also tend to balance out in case-control comparisons, particularly when many diagnoses are included in the control series, a practice followed in the present study. The use of general population controls will protect against failure to identify items because they are associated with a wide spectrum of diseases and hospital admissions. The latter is more than a theoretical possibility. For example, it has been observed in retrospect that case-control investigations of cigarette smoking and lung cancer estimated smaller excess risks for cigarette smokers than those reported by later prospective studies. The reason appears to be the association of cigarette smoking with other diseases, including coronary artery disease and certain respiratory disorders, represented in the control series.

It should be noted that comparisons of cases with more than one set of controls will yield different estimates of relative risk. In a well-behaved universe one may hope for concordance in relative risk estimates derived from the several control series. When this occurs, interpretation of the results becomes more straightforward, since explanations based on the unrepresentative nature of a single control series may be discarded. However, in Miyagi prefecture the hospital and general population controls did not yield consistent estimates for all foods and Table II indicates the scope of these inconsistencies. The much lower relative risks for pickled foods (radish, hakusai, cucumber) from the general population contrasts, for example, might mean nothing more than that many ill people tend to reduce consumption of such foods. However, more detailed study of the results will be required before a general synthesis and reconciliation can be attempted.

It is well-known that the probability of hospital admission will vary by age, sex and place of residence. Sendai residents are overrepresented in admission to Sendai hospitals and residents of outlying rural areas of Miyagi prefecture under-represented. If urban-rural differences in patterns of food use are present, failure to control for residence would affect relative risk esti-

Table I. *Relative risk* of stomach cancer for "above-average" users (risk for "below-average" users = 1.00) for selected food items; estimated from diagnosed cases and hospital controls, Miyagi prefecture*

High risks	No important difference (0.75 < R.R < 1.30)	Low risks
Rice (3+/day vs. ≤ 2/day) 1.84	raw fish, shrimp, fish products, eggs, laver, soybeans, bean curd, fermented soybeans, hakusai, daikon, eggplant, mushrooms, yams, pickled hakusai, tomatoes, chicken, ham and bacon	Pork (10+/mo. vs. ≤ 9/mo.) 0.71
Miso (13+/wk. vs. ≤ 12/wk.) 1.80		Beef (5+/mo. vs. ≤ 4/mo.) 0.61
		Smoked fish (3/mo. vs. ≤ 2/mo.) 0.67
		Bread (4/wk. vs. ≤ 3/wk.) 0.74
		Lettuce (5/mo. vs. ≤ 4/mo.) 0.70
		Pineapple (1/mo. vs. ≤ 0/mo.) 0.63
		Plum (3/mo. vs. ≤ 2/mo.) 0.63
		Grape (10/mo. vs. ≤ 9/mo.) 0.75
		Peach (10/mo. vs. ≤ 9/mo.) 0.71
		Pear (10/mo. vs. ≤ 9/mo.) 0.75

* Adjusted for sex, age, urban-rural residence.

mates from the case-hospital control comparisons. We attempted to minimize these extraneous factors by controlling for sex, age, and place of residence in the computation of relative risks presented in Tables I and II.

There is the further possibility that some differences in relative risk estimates might be reduced by control for social class and other variables. Studies in white populations have consistently revealed an inverse gradient in stomach cancer with social class (DORN and CUTLER, 1959) and a similar social-class gradient may hold within Japanese populations as well. The data presented in Table III do not support the expectation that adjustment for social class would substantially modify the relative risk estimates. The substitution of social class for residence or simultaneous adjustment for residence and social class had surprisingly little effect on most of the relative risk estimates, whether based on hospital or general population controls. The behavior of the relative risks for rice is a possible exception worth noting; replacing residence by social class, reduced the relative risk from 2.5 to 1.9 (population controls), but with adjustment for sex, age, residence and social class the relative risk returned to 2.5.

The meaning of these data is presently obscure and their interpretation must await additional analyses. The use of certain food items can be correlated positively or negatively, so that attention should be directed to estimating relative risks for individual foods with control for the presence or absence of other foods in the diet. This is difficult to carry out on data collected within a single locality because of the common dietary background shared by all

Table II. *Foods (partial list) for which hospital controls and general population controls yielded divergent relative risk estimates, Miyagi prefecture*

	Relative risk*	
	Hospital Controls	Population
Rice	1.84	2.48
Soba	0.75	1.54
Raw fish	0.98	1.55
Pickled radish	0.92	0.29
Pickled hakusai	0.93	0.30
Pickled cucumber	1.00	0.58
Persimmon	1.03	0.47
Strawberry	0.82	1.78
Tomato	0.86	1.88
Chicken	1.15	2.05
Ham, bacon	0.89	1.56
Beef	0.61	0.99

* Adjusted for sex, age, urban-rural residence.

Table III. *Changes in relative risk estimates for selected food item introduced by adjustment for social class Miyagi prefecture*

	Hospital controls, adjusted for			Population controls, adjusted for		
	Sex, age, residence	Sex, age, social class	Sex, age, social class, residence	Sex, age, residence	Sex, age, social class	Sex, age, social class, residence
Rice	1.84	1.81	1.70	2.5	1.94	2.5
Miso	1.80	1.80	1.67	1.50	1.27	1.54
Soba	0.75	0.75	0.81	1.54	1.72	1.51
Raw fish	0.98	0.96	0.94	1.55	1.48	1.49
Hakusai	0.88	0.94	0.90	1.13	0.99	1.15
Ham, bacon	0.89	0.90	0.93	1.56	1.69	1.47

inhabitants. This is the problem that confronted WYNDER and collaborators (1963) in the investigations of diet and stomach cancer in Japan, Iceland and other countries. Investigations of dietary hypotheses can best be carried out when greater heterogeneity in food practices prevails within the study population and the changes in diet among Japanese in Hawaii and California may provide the key to permit successful attack on this problem.

Summary

The downward displacement in stomach cancer mortality among Japanese migrants to the United States and their descendants provides an opportunity to see whether the changes in risk can be associated with changes in customs, occupation or other environmental exposures traceable to migration. Case-control studies in two prefectures of Japan and in Hawaii and California undertaken with this objective in mind are described. Some preliminary results from interviewing in Miyagi prefecture on the association of selected items of diet with stomach cancer are presented and discussed.

References

AIRD, I., BENTALL, H. H., and ROBERTS, J. A. F., A relationship between cancer of stomach and the ABO blood groups. *Brit. med J.* 1953 I, 799—801.

BILLINGTON, B. P., Gastric cancer-relationships between ABO bloodgroups, site and epidemiology. *Lancet* 1956 II, 859—862.

BUCKWALTER, J. A., WOHLWEND, C. B., COLTER, D. C., TIDRICK, R. T., and KNOWLER, L. A., The association of the ABO blood groups to gastric carcinoma. *Surg. Gynec. Obstet.* 104, 176—179 (1957).

BUELL, P., and DUNN jr., J. E., Cancer mortality among Japanese Issei and Nisei of California. *Cancer (Philad.)* 18, 656—664 (1965).

CORNFIELD, J., and HAENSZEL, W. M., Some aspects of retrospective studies. *J. chron. Dis.* 2, 523—534 (1960).

DORN, H. F., and CUTLER, S. J., Morbidity from cancer in the United States; Part I and part II combined. *Public Health Monograph* 56, Washington, D. C.: U. S. Government Printing Office, 1959.

GRAHAM, S., and LILIENFELD, A. M., Genetic studies of gastric cancer in humans: An appraisal. *Cancer (Philad.)* 11, 945—958 (1958).

HAENSZEL, W. M., Variation in incidence of and mortality from stomach cancer, with particular reference to the United States. *J. nat. Cancer Inst.* 21, 213—262 (1958).

MACKLIN, M. T., Role of heredity in gastric and intestinal cancer. *Gastroenterology* 29, 507—511; disc. 512—514 (1955).

MANTEL, N., and HAENSZEL, W. M., Statistical aspects of the analysis of data from retrospective studies of disease. *J. nat. Cancer Inst.* 22, 719—748 (1959).

QUISENBERRY, W. B., BRUYERE, P. T., and ROGERS, M. G., Ethnic differences in cancer in Hawaii. *Milit. Med.* 131, 222—223 (1966).

SEGI, M., and KURIHARA, M., Cancer mortality for selected sites in 24 countries, No. 3, (1960/61). Sendai, Japan, Tohoku University School of Medicine 1964.

SMITH, R. L., Recorded and expected mortality among Japanese of the United States and Hawaii, with special reference to cancer. *J. nat. Cancer Inst.* 17, 459—473 (1956).

SPEISER, P., Bestehen mathematisch gesicherte Beziehungen zwischen der A-B-0 Gruppen, des Rhesusfaktors Rh$_0$ (D) und des Geschlechtes zu Carcinoma ventriculi, Ulcus ventriculi und Ulcus duodeni? *Krebsarzt* 11, 344—348 (1956).

STASZEWSKI, J., and HAENSZEL, W. M., Cancer mortality among the Polishborn in the United States. *J. nat. Cancer Inst.* 35, 291—297 (1965).

STATE, D., VARCO, R. L., and WANGENSTEEN, O. H., Attempt to identify likely precursors of gastric cancer. *J. nat. Cancer Inst.* 7, 379—384 (1947).

STEINER, P. E., *Cancer: Race and geography.* Baltimore: Williams & Wilkins Co. 1954.

VIDEBAEK, A., and MOSBECH, J., Aetiology of gastric carcinoma elucidated by study of 302 pedigrees. *Acta med. scand.* 149, 137—159 (1954).

WHITE, C., and EISENBERG, H., ABO blood groups and cancers of the stomach. *Yale J. Biol. Med.* 32, 58—61 (1959).

WOOLF, C. M., Further study on familial aspects of carcinoma of stomach *Amer. J. human. Genet.* 8, 102—109 (1956).

WYNDER, E. L., KMET, J., DUNGAL, N., and SEGI, M., An epidemiological investigation of gastric cancer. *Cancer (Philad.)* 16, 1461—1496 (1963).

A Statistical Study of Mortality from Cancer of the Stomach in Selected Countries

Mitsuo Segi

Department of Public Health, Tohoku University,
School of Medicine, Sendai, Japan

On the basis of the data kindly supplied by the central statistical bureaus of 24 countries, we have computed the age-adjusted death rates for cancer of selected sites every 2 years since 1950 (Segi, 1960, 1962, 1964, 1966). The standard population used for the computation is the total population (including males and females) of the 46 countries around 1950. The latest rates calculated by us are for 1962—63.

By using the data for cancer mortality which were published by the W.H.O. (1963, 1964, 1965), we were able to calculate death rates for cancer of 13 more countries or areas other than the 24 countries for 1960—61 (Table I). We are going to make some observations on the death rates of these countries.

Age-adjusted Death Rates for Cancer of the Stomach in 37 Countries in 1960—61

The death rate for stomach cancer among males is highest in Chile (71.00), and Japan (69.50) is on the same level with her. The rate is third highest in Hungary (46.40) followed by Australia (45.55), Finland (45.17), Czechoslovakia, Germany, F.R., Poland, Italy and Venezuela. The lowest rate is in Egypt (2.43). Next come Ceylon (5.21), Mexico (8.72), U.S. White (11.46), Greece (15.17), Australia (18.38), New Zealand (19.01) and Canada (19.45). The rate of each of these countries which belong to the lowest bracket is less than one third of the rates for Chile or Japan.

The rate among females, as among males, is highest in Chile (45.79) and the second highest is in Japan (36.80). There is a marked difference between the rates of these two countries and that of Austria (26.49), the third highest. Austria, Hungary (26.11) and Finland (26.07) are on the almost same level. Next come Czechoslovakia (23.97) and Germany, F.R. (23.22). The order of rates of the countries among both males and females is quite similar.

The lowest rate is seen among females in Egypt (1.49), as among males, and U.S. White (5.81), Ceylon (8.16), Mexico (8.58) and U.S. Nonwhite (8.89) also belong to the lowest bracket. The rates of these countries are less than one fourth of Chile or Japan.

Age-adjusted Death Rates for Cancer of the Stomach in Iceland

Since Dungal's reports (1955 a, b; 1963) it has become a well-known fact that Iceland has a high incidence of stomach cancer. Recently the data (Pop ...

Table I. *Age adjusted death rates for cancer of the stomach in 37 countries in 1960—61*

Male		Female	
Country	Rate	Country	Rate
1. Chile	71.00	1. Chile	45.79
2. Japan	69.50	2. Japan	36.80
3. Hungary	46.40	3. Austria	26.49
4. Austria	45.55	4. Hungary	26.11
5. Finland	45.17	5. Finland	26.07
6. Czechoslovakia	43.59	6. Czechoslovakia	23.97
7. Germany, F. R.	39.95	7. Germany, F. R.	23.22
8. Poland	39.79	8. Venezuela	21.96
9. Italy	34.56	9. Poland	19.39
10. Venezuela	33.00	10. Italy	18.49
11. West Berlin	32.72	11. Colombia	18.35
12. Belgium	31.44	12. Belgium	18.14
13. Portugal	31.30	13. Spain	18.09
14. Netherlands	31.10	14. Switzerland	17.60
15. Switzerland	30.41	15. West Berlin	17.54
16. Spain	30.37	16. Norway	17.45
17. Norway	29.11	17. Portugal	17.37
18. South Africa	28.62	18. Ireland	16.74
19. Northern Ireland	27.88	19. Netherlands	16.45
20. Scotland	26.83	20. Northern Ireland	16.35
21. Sweden	26.12	21. Denmark	16.26
22. Denmark	25.96	22. Scotland	16.09
23. England and Wales	25.44	23. South Africa	15.84
24. France	25.44	24. Israel	14.97
25. Ireland	23.79	25. Sweden	14.30
26. Israel	22.29	26. England and Wales	13.26
27. Taiwan	21.86	27. France	12.74
28. Yugoslavia	21.72	28. Yugoslavia	12.70
29. Colombia	21.20	29. Taiwan	11.93
30. U.S. Nonwhite	20.14	30. Australia	9.65
31. Canada	19.45	31. Canada	9.61
32. New Zealand	19.01	32. Greece	9.47
33. Australia	18.38	33. New Zealand	9.22
34. Greece	15.17	34. U.S. Nonwhite	8.89
35. U.S. White	11.46	35. Mexico	8.58
36. Mexico	8.72	36. Ceylon	8.16
37. Ceylon	5.21	37. U.S. White	5.81
38. Egypt	2.43	38. Egypt	1.49

1964) published from this country enabled us to calculate age-adjusted death rates for cancer in 1951—1960 for this country. The rates for a 10 year period in this country rank third among both males and females of the 37 countries in 1960—61. The rate among males (64.98) is a little lower than that among males in Japan (69.50) and the rate among females (28.44) also follows Japan (36.80). The rates in Iceland, as compared with Norway, are 80 per cent higher for males and 30 per cent for females.

Trend in the Age-adjusted Death Rates for Cancer of the Stomach

The trend in the biennial age-adjusted death rates for 24 countries in 1950—51 through 1962—63 is to be discussed here (Table II). Data for 1952—53 being not furnished us, the trend for Chile is not shown for this period.

Trend in the rates among males shows a decreasing tendency in almost all countries. The rate in Japan began to descend with a peak in the year 1958—59. Among the countries having high rates, Finland shows a most remarkable decrease. The decrease of the rates in Switzerland, Denmark, Australia and Norway is also remarkable. The fall of mortality in U. S. White, the lowest-rated country of the 24, is most dramatic. The rate of U. S. White fall from 17.26 in 1950—51 to 9.78 in 1962—63, which is about a 40 per cent decrease. However, the rates in England and Wales, Italy and Germany, F. R. are decreasing slowly.

Among females, the trend in the rates in almost all countries has been showing a more marked decrease than for males. The rates in Japan began to decrease slightly since 1956—57. Of the countries having high rates, Finland shows a most marked decrease, which enables us to surmise that the rates in Finland will be lower in the near future than those of Germany, F. R. The fall of mortality in Switzerland, Denmark, Sweden, Canada, Norway and New Zealand is also marked. The rate of U. S. White, a country having the lowest rate as males, falls 9.31 in 1950—51 to 5.10 in 1962—63, showing a 40 per cent decrease as males.

Trend in the Death Rates for Cancer of the Stomach Classified by Age Group

In many countries the death rates for stomach cancer by age group are declining remarkably in the younger age groups. On the contrary, the rates in the older age groups are either slightly decreasing or still increasing. This has been already pointed out by CLEMMESEN (1965), HAENSZEL (1961) and STOCKS (1958), and cohort analysis has proved this also. The fact that age-adjusted death rates have been rapidly decreasing in almost all countries (Fig. 1) forecasts that the rates in the older age groups in some countries may decline at some future time. The period from 1950—51 through 1962—63 which we have been studying may be just a passage in the long history of the death rates for stomach cancer. However, it seems possible to suppose, from this tendency of the short time, a change of the rates in the near future.

Let us illustrate the trend in age-specific death rates of three countries (Table III).

The rates for Japanese males are decreasing in the age groups of 60—64 years and above 65 years, but they are still increasing in the age groups of 70—74 years and above 75 years. Among females, the rates in the age groups

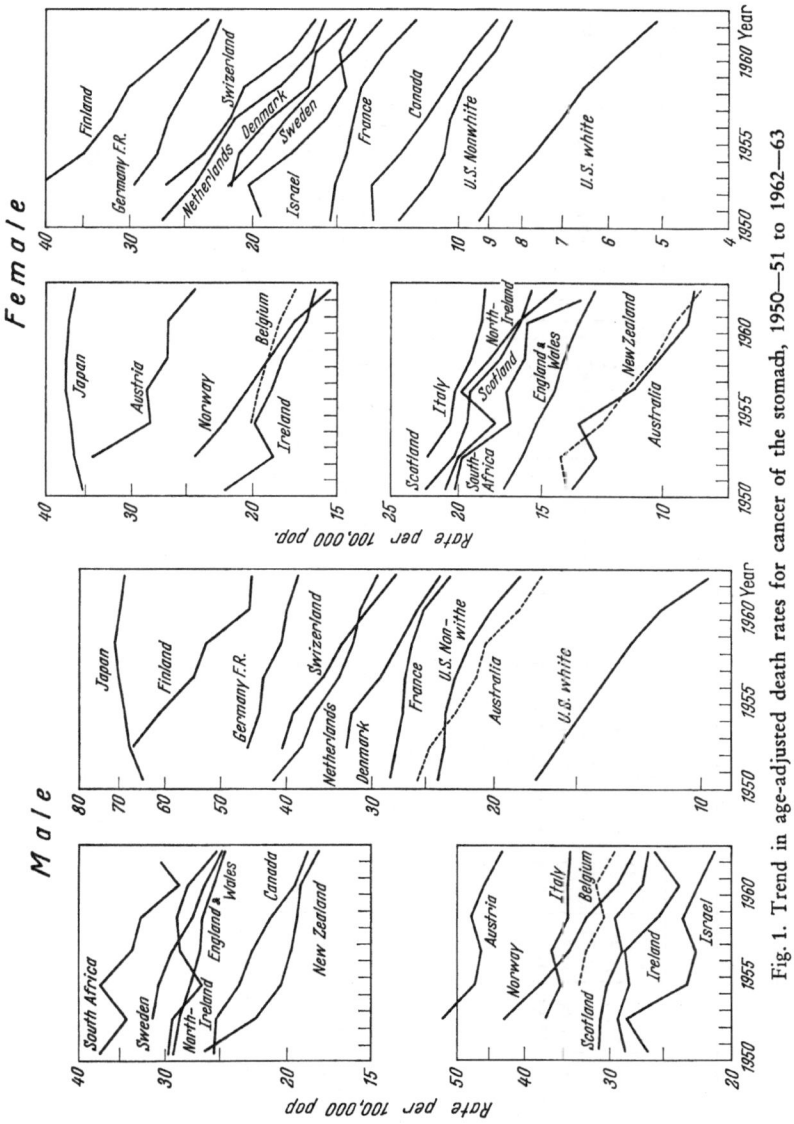

Fig. 1. Trend in age-adjusted death rates for cancer of the stomach, 1950—51 to 1962—63

of 65—69 years and younger are decreasing, as males, but they are still increasing in the age group of 70—74 years.

The male rates in the age group of 70—74 years in England and Wales are decreasing, and a peak is seen in the rates of the age groups of 80—84 years and above 85 years during our study years. Female rate in this country is decreasing remarkably in the age group of 80—84 years, but no decrease is seen in the age group above 85 years.

5*

Table II. Age-adjusted death rates for cancer of the stomach in 1962—63. The figures in ( ) show rank order

Country	Male							Female							Sex ratio of age-adjusted death rate in 1962—63
	1950—51	1952—53	1954—55	1956—57	1958—59	1960—61	1962—63	1950—51	1952—53	1954—55	1956—57	1958—59	1960—61	1962—63	
South Africa	37.47	34.07	37.14	33.51	32.44	28.62	*30.33 (8)	20.27	19.71	16.83	16.96	15.91	15.84	*13.14 (17)	*231
Canada	25.50	25.37	23.49	22.48	21.05	19.45	18.69 (21)	13.36	13.39	12.13	11.20	10.45	9.61	8.76 (23)	213
Chile	73.59	—	69.71	71.20	70.84	71.00	64.63 (2)	52.10	—	47.63	47.03	43.54	45.79	41.04 (1)	157
United States, White	17.26	16.06	14.87	13.68	12.69	11.46	9.78 (25)	9.31	8.58	7.72	7.07	6.50	5.81	5.10 (25)	192
United States, Nonwhite	24.06	23.64	23.49	22.75	21.69	20.14	18.12 (22)	12.23	11.23	10.52	10.32	9.83	8.89	8.26 (24)	219
Israel	26.19	28.25	23.10	22.44	23.48	22.29	21.05 (20)	19.45	20.27	17.52	15.64	14.64	14.97	14.17 (16)	149
Japan	64.38	67.05	68.30	69.88	70.63	69.50	67.96 (1)	35.17	36.09	36.59	37.24	37.10	36.80	35.99 (2)	189
Germany, Fed. Repub.	—	45.57	43.82	43.38	40.63	39.95	38.41 (5)	—	29.53	27.20	26.31	24.72	23.22	22.08 (5)	174
Austria	—	52.77	47.22	46.10	47.77	45.55	43.04 (4)	—	34.10	28.01	28.39	26.56	26.49	24.22 (3)	178
Belgium	—	—	33.22	32.46	30.57	31.44	29.46 (10)	—	—	20.03	19.57	18.90	18.14	17.25 (8)	171
Denmark	—	32.68	32.13	29.21	27.54	25.96	23.93 (18)	—	21.52	20.88	18.82	16.64	16.26	14.41 (15)	166
Finland	—	66.75	61.11	54.58	52.62	45.17	44.80 (3)	—	40.28	34.65	31.94	29.86	26.07	22.96 (4)	195
France	28.26	27.68	27.03	26.98	26.38	25.44	23.03 (19)	15.33	15.08	14.53	14.15	13.86	12.74	11.57 (20)	199
Ireland	28.30	29.06	28.04	28.77	25.53	23.79	25.68 (14)	21.93	18.68	19.82	18.81	18.01	16.74	16.22 (9)	158
Italy	—	37.34	35.14	36.25	34.52	34.56	34.22 (6)	—	22.10	20.69	20.31	19.05	18.49	18.24 (6)	188
Norway	—	42.94	37.97	34.40	32.41	29.11	27.67 (12)	—	24.25	22.04	20.48	18.74	17.45	15.30 (13)	181
Netherlands	41.82	37.99	36.34	33.87	32.02	31.10	29.50 (9)	26.95	24.22	22.82	21.30	18.06	16.45	15.64 (11)	189
Portugal	—	—	—	28.29	30.20	31.30	32.60 (7)	—	—	—	17.18	17.67	17.37	17.99 (7)	181
England and Wales	29.20	28.65	27.54	26.76	26.50	25.44	24.69 (17)	17.09	16.02	15.22	14.34	13.94	13.26	12.57 (19)	196
Scotland	31.11	31.04	30.27	28.87	29.25	26.83	26.20 (13)	22.24	20.39	19.39	19.15	17.24	16.09	15.47 (12)	169
Northern Ireland	29.63	29.23	26.52	28.57	28.67	27.88	25.30 (15)	20.98	20.02	17.51	19.76	17.91	16.35	14.45 (14)	175
Sweden	—	31.42	30.83	29.36	27.32	26.12	24.83 (16)	—	21.60	19.46	17.89	16.08	14.30	12.98 (18)	191
Switzerland	—	40.45	39.03	35.62	33.44	30.41	27.81 (11)	—	26.77	23.18	21.44	20.65	17.60	16.05 (10)	173
Australia	25.76	24.78	22.74	21.17	20.65	18.38	17.06 (24)	13.91	14.02	12.24	11.27	10.13	9.65	8.93 (22)	191
New Zealand	26.86	22.26	20.31	19.74	19.24	19.01	17.90 (23)	13.65	12.41	13.20	11.10	10.03	9.22	9.00 (21)	199

* 1962 only.

Table III. *Death rates for cancer of the stomach classified by age groups in Japan, England and Wales and U. S. White in 1950—51 and 1962—63*

	Male		Female	
	1950—51	1962—63	1950—51	1962—63
Japan:				
All ages	47.25	57.32	28.88	35.10
—20	0.08	0.11	0.09	0.12
20—24	0.70	1.43	0.96	1.49
25—29	2.35	3.28	3.26	4.48
30—34	7.12	7.49	8.55	9.98
35—39	15.96	15.89	16.11	17.33
40—44	35.19	31.83	28.50	28.80
45—49	72.77	62.95	45.12	42.73
50—54	126.95	113.76	67.75	65.63
55—59	218.83	194.34	107.20	94.03
60—64	325.31	308.11	156.40	136.90
65—69	444.98	450.02	220.57	198.88
70—74	483.08	567.11	247.25	275.14
75—79	399.15	609.28	236.25	323.06
80—84	} 250.83	529.64	} 162.28	294.40
85 and over		343.20		217.61
England and Wales:				
All ages	38.30	34.00	28.49	24.50
—20	0.03	0.03	0.05	—
20—24	0.42	0.10	0.30	0.24
25—29	1.04	0.40	0.94	0.74
30—34	1.97	1.55	1.83	1.19
35—39	5.60	3.87	3.87	2.38
40—44	13.23	8.24	6.61	4.43
45—49	27.28	17.30	12.70	8.12
50—54	46.35	34.63	19.65	15.15
55—59	77.74	67.67	32.43	24.63
60—64	122.11	104.15	59.64	42.97
65—69	180.49	151.74	101.59	68.19
70—74	248.44	216.58	150.91	103.57
75—79	301.88	271.43	216.54	160.45
80—84	300.30	301.86	272.51	222.00
85 and over	251.97	269.99	262.09	261.32
U. S. White:				
All ages	19.99	12.00	11.69	7.45
—20	0.03	0.01	0.01	0.01
20—24	0.10	0.10	0.10	0.07
25—29	0.39	0.18	0.35	0.20
30—34	0.94	0.78	1.05	0.43
35—39	2.59	1.60	1.77	1.26
40—44	5.32	3.20	3.45	2.29
45—49	11.47	6.06	6.05	3.91
50—54	21.52	11.82	10.93	5.93
55—59	40.64	20.44	19.52	10.03
60—64	67.30	34.00	31.77	15.09
65—69	106.53	57.97	49.96	26.63
70—74	151.77	85.33	80.15	41.30
75—79	204.47	122.13	119.42	60.38
80—84	245.84	161.53	158.54	93.63
85 and over	264.82	185.41	180.47	129.41

In the U. S. White the fall in mortality is very marked in every age group. The rates decrease to half in the age groups 50—64 years, and even in the age group of 85 years and over the rates decrease by 30 per cent. Decrease of female rates is more marked than in males. In the age group of 60—64 years the rates decrease to less than half, and in the age groups of 65—79 years they decrease to almost half, although a tendency of declining in the age group of above age of 85 is almost same as males, by 30 per cent.

Sex Ratio of the Age-adjusted Death Rates for Cancer of the Stomach

When one observes the age-adjusted death rates for stomach cancer in 37 countries in 1960—61, it is worthy of attention that the sex ratio for Ceylon only is below 100, showing 64. This means that the female rate is higher than the rate among males in Ceylon. No marked difference is seen between male and female rates in Mexico (102) and Colombia (116) either. In both Ireland (142) and Israel (149) the difference between the rates among males and females is larger, as compared with the countries mentioned above. In Venezuela and other countries the rates among males are 150 per cent more than those among females. France (200), Canada (202), Poland (205), New Zealand (206) and U. S. Nonwhite (227) are given as the countries whose male rates are twice as high as those among females. The rates among females for stomach cancer in many countries are decreasing more markedly than those among males. Consequently the sex ratio is gradually becoming larger in many contries.

Percentage Distribution of Death from Cancer of the Stomach to All Cancer Deaths

Among males, percentage distribution of stomach cancer deaths to all cancer deaths in 1962—63 is 49.4 per cent in Japan and 42.8 per cent in Chile. In addition to these two countries, Israel, Ireland, Italy, Norway, Portugal and Sweden show the highest ratio of stomach cancer of all cancer deaths. In some other countries the ratio of lung cancer occupies the first position. The ratio of stomach cancer in U. S. White, however, ranks fourth highest in the list.

Among females, percentage distribution of deaths from stomach cancer is highest in Japan (37.7 per cent) followed by Chile (29.8 per cent). Deaths from stomach cancer still head the list in each of Germany, F. R., Austria, Finland, Italy, Norway and Portugal. Except for U. S. Nonwhite, however, there are a lot of countries where the first position of deaths from cancer is breast cancer followed by cancer of the stomach. It may be noticed that deaths from stomach cancer in U. S. White is in the fifth place, a little lower than the deaths from ovarian cancer.

Geographical Correlation between Ulcer of the Stomach and Stomach Cancer

We computed age-adjusted death rates for ulcer of the stomach for 24 countries (Table IV), observing the correlation between age-adjusted death rates for stomach cancer and the rates for ulcer of the stomach in 1962—63, one will note

Table IV. *Age-adjusted death rates for ulcer of the stomach in 24 countries in 1962—63*

Male		Female	
Country	Death rate	Country	Death rate
1. Japan	16.00	1. Japan	5.85
2. Portugal	9.65	2. Portugal	2.52
3. South Africa	6.98	3. Ireland	2.39
4. Chile	6.89	4. Chile	2.39
5. Finland	6.27	5. South Africa	2.15
6. Germany, F. R.	5.43	6. Austria	2.06
7. Austria	5.17	7. Denmark	2.00
8. Ireland	4.90	8. England and Wales	1.99
9. Italy	4.74	9. Sweden	1.99
10. U. S. Nonwhite	4.49	10. Scotland	1.97
11. England and Wales	4.41	11. Finland	1.70
12. Sweden	4.40	12. Australia	1.67
13. Scotland	4.40	13. Switzerland	1.64
14. Denmark	4.28	14. Northern Ireland	1.59
15. Belgium	4.22	15. New Zealand	1.55
16. Northern Ireland	4.16	16. U. S. Nonwhite	1.49
17. U. S. White	3.91	17. U. S. White	1.42
18. Australia	3.57	18. Canada	1.31
19. Canada	3.57	19. Germany, F. R.	1.26
20. New Zealand	3.53	20. Norway	1.20
21. Switzerland	3.46	21. Netherlands	1.16
22. France	3.20	22. Israel	1.13
23. Netherlands	3.11	23. Belgium	1.11
24. Israel	2.38	24. Italy	0.97
25. Norway	2.29	25. France	0.74

that the rates among males for both of these are extremely high in Japan, and Chile and Finland belong to the same group as Japan. Portugal having high rates for stomach ulcer belongs to the middle bracket in cancer of the stomach.

Among females, Japan and Chile also have high rates for both stomach cancer and ulcer. In view of the results so far achieved, we find that Japan stands in a similar position to Chile in relation to stomach cancer and ulcer.

References

CLEMMESEN, J., Statistical studies in the aetiology of malignant neoplasms, I. Copenhagen 1965.

DUNGAL, N., *Ann. Coll. Surg. Engl.* 16, 211 (1955 a).
— *Schweiz. Z. allg. Path.* 18, 550 (1955 b).

DUNGAL, N., *Schweiz. Z. allg. Path.* **16**, 634 (1963).

HAENSZEL, W., End results and mortality trends in cancer. *N.C.I. Monograph* No 6 (1961).

SEGI, M., Cancer mortality for selected sites in 24 countries No 1. Department of Public Health, Tohoku University School of Medicine, Sendai 1960.

— *Ibid.,* No 2, Sendai 1962.

— *Ibid.,* No 3, Sendai 1964.

— *Ibid.,* No 4, Sendai 1966.

Statistical Bureau of Iceland, Population and vital statistics in Iceland, 1951—1960. Reykjavik 1964.

STOCKS, P., *Cancer,* vol 3, chapt. 4, London: Butterworth & Co. 1958.

World Health Organization, Annual epidemiological and vital statistics 1960. Geneva 1963.

World Health Organization, *Ibid.,* 1961. Geneva 1964.

World Health Organization, World health statistics annual 1962, 1. Geneva 1965.

Cancer of the Stomach in the U.S.S.R.

ALEXANDR CHAKLIN

*Department of Epidemiology, Institute for Experimental
and Clinical Oncology of Academy of Medical Science, U.S.S.R.*

In most parts of U.S.S.R. cancer of the stomach occupies first or second place in the structure of malignant tumour morbidity and mortality. The obligatory information about every new case of malignant tumour all over the country and sufficient information about all deaths from cancer give cancer researchers in the country a great opportunity to study the epidemiology of cancer of the stomach. The 260 oncological dispensaries and 2,300 oncological cabinets are now keeping cancer registries summarizing data about all cases of cancer. In outpatient departments is a center for dispensarization for all patients with pre-tumour processes. The frequency of gastritis, ulcer and polyposis is studied and the patients are followed up, to see how often gastric cancer could develop on the soil of different gastric diseases.

A study of geographic differences of gastric cancer was organized from 1952 in several parts of the country with differences in the nutrition, the types of foods produced and consumed, the amount of fruit and vegetables eaten, the ways in which the food is prepared, the rhythm and manner of feeding, the drinking of alcohol and other important factors. Now we have a national study center for gastric cancer epidemiology in the Cancer Institute in Vilnius.

The Problem Commission for Cancer Epidemiology of the Academy of Medical Sciences of the U.S.S.R. in Moscow developed a special program for the study of stomach cancer epidemiology. This program included both retrospective and prospective studies. The main attention is given to a study of the history of diseases, family position, working and living conditions, habits and customs and other aspects. The analysis of the results of this study is not yet completed.

From published material in the country we see that morbidity from cancer of the stomach is very much different in different parts of the country. The morbidity rate for stomach cancer per 100,000 population is 60.0 in Leningrad, 68.5 in Gorki, 68.0 in Frunze. It is comparatively higher in men than in women; for example in Krainita it was 52.1 for men and 46.6 for women in 1960. Mortality from stomach cancer in the age group after 60 is 10—15 times higher than in the age group of 30—39. The age standardized rates per 100,000 in men is 0.62 in age under 30, 12.5 in age 30—39, 35.5 in age 40—49, 161.0 in age 50—59, 289.6 in age 60 and older, in women it is 0.58 in age under 30, 10.2 in age 30—39, 35.5 in age 40—49, 88.0 in age 50—59, 149,3 in age 60 and older.

In the Republic of Armenia it was demonstrated that cancer of the stomach is relatively rare (15.0 for 100,000 for both sexes, 17.3 for men and 12.7 for women in 1959). A high amount of magnesium was found in the soil and in the water, in lake Sevan 45.2 mg of magnesium was found in 1 liter of the water (K. L. BASICIAN). It was demonstrated that some occupational factors play an indirect role in the development of stomach cancer. We think, however, that the main factors affecting stomach cancer are the complex of dietary peculiarities of the population and also the composition of the soil and others.

A Comparative Study of Histochemical Patterns in Non-Neoplastic and Neoplastic Gastric Epithelium[1]

A Study of Hawaii Japanese

G. N. STEMMERMANN[2]

*Kuakini Hospital, and Department of Pathology,
University of Hawaii School of Medicine, Honolulu, Hawaii, U. S. A.*

Gastric disease in the Japanese people of Hawaii has distinct characteristics which distinguish it from that encountered in other racial groups in these islands. Benign gastric ulcer is very common and gastric cancer is their most common malignant neoplasm. They very rarely suffer from pernicious anemia, a known precursor of gastric carcinoma. This disease pattern more closely resembles that of native Japanese than that of Caucasians in the United States and Northern Europe. This histochemical investigation is part of a parallel study of the clinical, epidemiological and pathological characteristics of gastric cancer in native and migrant Japanese[3]. It was undertaken to determine whether the

[1] A revised version of this paper, with colored plates, will appear in *J. nat. Cancer Inst.*

[2] I am deeply indebted to Dr. KATHERINE HERROLD, Dr. S. SPICER, and Dr. G. GLENNER for their advice and assistance in planning this study and the preparation of this paper.

[3] This project was supported in part by NCI Research Contract PH43-63-558, to the University of Hawaii, Honolulu, Hawaii.

cells of stomach cancers occurring in these people might show any distinctive characteristics and whether these characteristics might indicate the non-neoplastic gastric cell from which they are derived.

Material Studied

The non-neoplastic mucosa and tumor tissue from 80 patients with gastric cancer were stained for mucosubstances. Enzymes were assessed in 26 of these cases. The enzymes and mucosubstances in the mucosa and the ulcer margins were studied in twelve stomachs removed from adults with benign gastric ulcer. Gastric mucosal enzymes and mucosubstances were studied in twelve stomachs removed at necropsy from fetuses and newborn infants.

Methods Empolyed

Mucosubstances. Paraffin sections were prepared from tissue samples removed from the following sites: four portions from each carcinoma and four sections from the margins of benign ulcers. Mucosal strips were taken from the entire length of the lesser and greater curvatures of both benign and malignant stomach specimens. These sections were stained by the methods of SPICER and co-workers (1966): Periodic Acid Schiff (PAS), Alcian Blue (AB) at pH 2.5 and pH 1, High Iron Diamine-AB, with and without Periodic Acid, Aldehyde Fuchsin-AB, Periodic acid-phenylhydrazine-Schiff (PHS), Periodic Acid Diamine (PAD), AB pH 2.5-PAS, AB pH 2.5-PAS after Sialidase digestion. Control sections of mouse stomach and salivary glands were used to gauge the effectiveness and uniformity of the techniques employed.

Enzymes. Samples from the same areas were frozen and cut on a cryostat. They were stained to demonstrate the following enzymes: Aminopeptidase [L-leucyl-4methoxy β Naphthylamide method (NACHLAS et al., 1960)] Lactic Dehydrogenase [Tetrazolium-Nitro BT method (PEARSE, 1960)], Acid and Alkaline Phosphatase [Naphthyl AS-BI Phosphate method (BURSTONE, 1962)].

The intensity of the staining reactions of both inter- and extracellular mucosubstances and of intracellular enzymes was roughly graded as follows: 0 = no staining, 1 = faint staining, 2 = definite, but submaximal staining, 3 = intense staining. A rough approximation of the number of tumor cells showing any reaction was coded as follows: 0 = none, 1 = 1—33 per cent, 2 = 34—66 per cent, 3 = 67—100 per cent.

Results: The staining reactions noted in the various sites are as follows:

Non-neoplastic Epithelium

Mucosubstances: The stains for mucosubstances produced consistent patterns among the various non-neoplastic gastric cells. These are summarized in Table I. Some reactions merit description in greater detail, either because they have not previously been recorded or because they differ in some respects from the results reported by other workers.

The surface epithelial cells of the infant differed from those of the adult in that they contained acid mucosubstances rather than neutral mucosubstances. The characteristic adult reaction appeared in the surface epithelium of the antrum before that of the gastric body. The infant surface epithelium resembled the epithelium of the adult neck cells and regenerating epithelium at ulcer margins. The mucosubstances at these three sites were resistant to sialidase, although the mucus neck cells in mouse control sections were sialidase sensitive.

The antral glandular cells resembled surface cells, but differed from them in certain respects: a) They lose the infantile acid mucosubstance reaction after surface cells. b) They are not quite so intensely PAS positive as adult surface cells. Comparable reactions are noted with PAD.

The chief cells of the adult corpus glands stained faintly with PAS, red with aldehyde fuchsin and black with PAD, indicating the presence of a sulfomucin at this site. These reactions were not found in some specimens, but when one of the reactions was positive, all were positive. This variability of staining from case to case may reflect variability in the amount of stored mucosubstance, which would, in turn, depend upon the state of secretion or the ability of the cells to store this material.

Two mucosubstances were identified in intestinalized epithelium. One was PAS positive, stained dark brown with high iron diamine-AB, dark red with aldehyde fuchsin-AB, and was PAS positive in the AB-PAS sequence. This mucosubstance was most abundant in the superficial portions of the cells. It occurred in small aggregates and surrounded the goblets. The mucosubstance of the goblets was PAS positive, stained blue with AB at pH 2.5, blue with aldehyde fuchsin-AB, red with PHS, and blue with high iron diamine-AB and blue with AB-PAS. The two types of mucin merged at the goblet margins. This pattern was not found in all intestinalized epithelial cell groups, some lacking the first of these mucosubstances. This was the only non-uniform reaction found in non-neoplastic cells. It would seem likely that the first of these muco-substances is a sulfomucin and that of the goblet a sialomucin. The deep red PHS stain of the goblet mucus of intestinalized epithelium was the best marker to separate these cells from other gastric cells. The use of PHS consistently showed intestinal cells in the pylorus of the fetal and neonatal stomach. These occurred in very small groups and sometimes only one intestinal cell was found in a gland. The presence of these isolated cells was not suspected in routine histologic preparations.

Enzymes. The characteristic localization of maximal activity of different enzymes in different gastric epithelial cells is well documented and was con-firmed by this study. There was intense acid phosphatase activity in chief cells and LDH activity in parietal cells, whereas LAP and alkaline phosphatase activity was restricted to intestinalized areas. The localization of acid and alkaline phosphatase activity within individual cells was not the same for each enzyme. The former was found deep in the cytoplasm and in intestinalized cells was often paranuclear in position. The alkaline phosphatase activity was almost entirely a surface phenomenon. The enzyme activity of the cells of the antral glands served as an additional means of differentiating these cells from surface cells, which were otherwise similar to them. These antral cells were found to show more acid phosphatase and LDH activity than surface cells.

Carcinoma Cells

The staining reactions of cancer cells was even more inconsistent than might be expected after reference to Table I. For example, although most tumors contained acid mucosubstances which were stained blue by AB at pH 2.5, there were four tumors which contained no such material. The cells of individual tumors also showed this inconsistency. All of the cells of the 27 tumors showed this reaction, but in 23 instances the reaction was noted in less than a third of the

Table I. *Histochemistry — Gastric epithelium*

	New-born sur-face	Adult sur-face	Neck	Chief	Pa-rietal	An-tral gland	Ulcer mar-gins	Meta-plasia	Carcinoma
Alk P'tase	0	0	0	0	0	0	0	red	0-red
Acid P'tase	red	red	red	dark red	0	red	red	red	red, dark red
LAP	0	0	0	0	0	0	0	blue	0, blue
LDH	0	0	0	light blue	dark blue	light blue	0	light blue	0, dark blue
PAS	red	red	red	pink	0	red	red	red	red
AB at pH 2.5	blue	0	blue	0	0	0	blue	blue	blue
AB at pH 1	0	0	0	0	0	0	0	light blue	0, light blue and blue
AB pH 2.5—PAS	red, purple	red	red	pink	0	red	red	red, blue	red, blue
PHS	pink	pink	pink	0	0	pink	0	red	0, pink, and red
Ald. Fuchs, AB	blue	0	blue	red	0	0	blue	red, blue	red, blue
PAD	brown	brown	brown	black	0	brown	brown	brown	0, brown, black
Hi Fe Diam, AB	blue	0	blue	0	0	0	blue	blue, black	blue, black
Hi Fe Diam, AB, HIO	brown	brown	brown	0	0	brown	brown	brown	brown

cells and in the remaining cases the number of cells stained represented from 33 to 66 per cent of the cancer cell population. Among the stains for muco-substances, only the PAS reaction and the High Iron Diamine-PAS reaction showed consistent staining of at least some neoplastic cells in all tumors. The constituent cells of some tumors showed a variety of staining reactions, among which surface, chief, neck and intestinal patterns could be identified. These different cell types tended to be segregated into groups of cells containing similar mucosubstances. Comparable inconsistency was noted with the enzyme preparations. All tumors contained at least some cells showing acid phosphatase activity. In eleven of 26 cancers, there was no aminopeptidase activity; in seven this activity was maximal in all cells and the remaining cancers were inter-mediate between these extremes. In seven cancers there was no alkaline phosphatase activity, and in seven this activity was maximal in all cells, and the remainder were intermediate. Eight tumors showed no LDH activity in any cells and only one showed maximal activity in all cells.

An attempt was made to determine whether carcinoma cell types (e. g. signet ring, well-differentiated adenocarcinoma, undifferentiated adenocarcinoma) could be correlated with any pattern of enzyme activity or mucoprotein pro-duction. This could not be done inasmuch as groups of morphologically similar tumor cells, even in the same cancer might display different staining patterns.

Stains for mucosubstances showed consistent staining of the chromatin of cancer cell nuclei during the metaphase of mitosis, but at no other time. In spite of the wide variety of reactions seen among cytoplasmic mucins, the staining of these mitoses was the same for all mitotic figures. They stained red with AB-PAS, brownish-black with PAD, brown with High Iron Diamine-AB, red with PHS and red with PAS.

Discussion

The histochemical characteristics of the various gastric epithelial cells are well documented (CORREIRA et al., 1963; HESS et al., 1958; LEV, 1965; NACH-LAS et al., 1958; PLANTEYDT and WILLIGHAGEN, 1960; SALENIUS, 1962), al-though more attention has been devoted to enzymes than to mucosubstances. SALENIUS (1962) has shown that mucous neck cells, chief cells, parietal cells, surface cells, pyloric gland cells and intestinal cells can be identified in the stomach by the 13th week of fetal life. The presence of acid mucosubstance in the surface epithelium of a newborn stands in sharp contrast to that of the neutral mucus of the adult surface epithelium. This acid mucosubstance gra-dually disappears, first from the pylorus and later from the corpus, suggesting that functional development continues for some time after birth. The staining reactions of the surface cells and pyloric gland cells of the newborn so closely resemble those of the adult neck cells and regenerating cells at ulcer margins, that this appearance may well mark sites of cell replication. This impression is consistent with the evidence that regeneration of rat gastric mucosa appears to be from cells of the mucous neck type and that these, in turn, serve as a source of parietal and chief cells (TOWNSEND, 1961).

The presence of a material resembling sulfomucin in human chief cells is consistent with the observation of SPICER and his associates (1967) that sulfated mucosubstance occurs in the canine chief cells. The presence of cancer cells with these characteristics suggests that functional development in this direction may also occur in neoplastic cell lines.

This study also confirms the observation of SALENIUS that intestinal cells are normally present in the pylorus during fetal and neonatal life. This raises the question as to whether intestinal epithelium in the adult stomach is metaplastic and/or whether it is formed from cells already at the site. Some of these intestinal cells are probably derived from the reparative epithelium, such as that at ulcer margins, and have differentiated along one of the several lines which lead to a cell type normally found in the stomach. Nor does this occur infrequently. Intestinal type cells are found in the pylorus of all of our patients with benign gastric ulcer and may also be found in the mucosa which has recovered ulcer craters. The intestinalization of the pyloric mucosa which accompanies carcinoma does not differ, in either extent or degree, from that found with ulcer, and in either condition intestinal cells may line the entire mucosa. These studies support the opinion of PLANTEYDT (1961) and PLANTEYDT and WILLIGHAGEN (1965) that both intestinalization and carcinoma arise from undifferentiated cells of the gastric mucosa, possibly the result of the same stimuli. Two enzymes — aminopeptidase and alkaline phosphatase — are not found in the non-intestinal gastric epithelium but are consistently found in intestinal cells. They are inconsistently found in carcinoma cells which have the staining characteristics of chief cells, mucous neck cells, intestinal cells and antral gland cells. Groups of cells within the same cancer may resemble different non-neoplastic gastric epithelial cells. The presence of cancer cells with the enzyme and mucosubstances of gastric cells does not rule out the possibility that these tumors are derived from an intestinal epithelium, but this finding imposes the requirement that they develop as a result of reverse metaplastic change from intestinal epithelium. A simpler explanation of the inconsistent staining patterns found in these stomach cancers by both PLANTEYDT and our studies would be based on the existence of an undifferentiated stem cell, capable of transmitting a variety of functional capabilities to descendants. The occurrence of groups of cells of the same tumor with differing enzymes and mucosubstances could then be explained by diverging cell lines. Carcinoma composed of cells with the histologic and histochemical characteristics of intestinal epithelium have been found to arise in stomachs of rodents which show no evidence of metaplasia in non-neoplastic areas. This indicates that metaplasia is not an obligatory precursor of gastric carcinoma, even when the tumor has intestinal properties (PLANTEYDT et al., 1962).

This study of stomach cancer in Hawaii Japanese showed it to be histochemically similar to the tumors described by PLANTEYDT among Northern Europeans, in spite of the dissimilarity of the gastric disease patterns found in these two populations.

The distribution of the various mucosubstances in normal metaplastic and cancerous epithelium is summarized in Table II. This is an adaptation from the classification of mucosubstances proposed by SPICER et al. (1966).

Table II. *Examples of epithelium with histochemically distinguishable mucosubstances*

I. Neutral mucosubstance — neutral glycoproteins, immunologic glycoproteins, fucomucins, mannose-rich mucosubstance: *Gastric surface epithelium, carcinoma cells.*

II. Acid mucosubstance

   A. Sulfomucins

      1. Periodate unreactive or weakly reactive — *Gastric chief cells, carcinoma cells.*

      2. Periodate reactive — *intestinalized epithelium, carcinoma cells.*

   B. Nonsulfated mucosubstances

      1. Sialomucins

         a) Quickly digested by sialidase

         b) Slowly digested by sialidase

            1. Periodate reactive

            2. Periodate unreactive

         c) Sialidase resistance altered by saponification

         d) Other acid mucosubstances * — resistant to sialidase

            1. Periodate reactive — *mucus neck cells, newborn surface epithelium, regenerating epithelium at ulcer edges, carcinoma cells, intestinalized epithelium.*

            2. Periodate nonreactive

* Spicer classifies such acid mucosubstances as sialidase resistant sialomucins. Some may not be sialic acid, proof depending upon correlated biochemical assays.

One other finding merits further attention — the presence of mucosubstances in the chromosomes of cancer cells during mitotic metaphase. This change was not observed in the mitotic figures of non-neoplastic small intestinal mucosa. The absence of this reaction in non-neoplastic intestinal epithelial mitoses and the uniformity of the staining reaction, in contrast to the lack of uniformity in the staining of cancer mucosubstances, suggests that this change is not the result of coating of the chromosomes with cytoplasmic mucosubstance after the breakdown of the nuclear membrane. YOUNG and BRODY (1966) have shown that mitotic figures in the human testis and in a number of tumors studied are periodic acid-Schiff (PAS)-positive. In the testis, the PAS reaction of chromosomal figures is abolished by diastase. In tumors the mitotic figures are diastase-fast, but nonetheless give positive staining with Best's carmine, and the Bauer-Feulgen reaction. These authors believe that a role of DNA in these reactions could be excluded. The mitotic figures of tumors still gave a positive PAS stain after extraction of all the Feulgen-positive material (DNA) from resting nuclei. In their reactions, the mitotic figures of tumors showed some of the histochemical properties of the amylopectin type of glycogen found in type IV (Cori) glycogen disease. Companion studies with material from such a case have been carried out, with striking similarity in behavior of the abnormal glycogen and the substance reacting in the mitoses of the tumors.

Summary

1. The distribution of mucosubstances and enzymes in the gastric carcinoma cells of Hawaiin Japanese was studied and compared with the distribution of these substances in the normal gastric epithelial cells of adults and of children; and in the regenerating epithelial cells of the margins of benign gastric ulcers.

2. The mucosubstances of the surface epithelial cells of the infant differed from those of the adult in that they stained as acid mucosubstances rather than neutral mucosubstances. This characteristic was lost by the body epithelium after that of the antrum.

3. The pylorus of the fetus and the newborn infant contained isolated cells with the histologic and histochemical characteristics of intestinal cells. Intestinal epithelium was found in the pylorus of all patients with gastric cancer and gastric ulcer.

4. The chief cells were found to have a distinctive staining pattern with some stains for mucosubstance, which suggested that they contained a sulfomucin. Some cancer cells also showed these reactions.

5. The enzymes and mucosubstances noted in the gastric carcinomas varied from patient to patient and even from cell to cell in the same tumor. They did not consistently resemble any one non-neoplastic gastric or intestinal epithelial cell; nor could the histochemical characteristics of a tumor be correlated with the degree of its morphologic differentiation.

6. These studies suggest that cell regeneration after injury may proceed from a stem cell along several lines, permitting the development of mature gastric and intestinal cell types and of carcinoma. They also support the view that intestinal metaplasia is not an obligatory precursor of gastric cancer.

7. This study also demonstrated that chromosomes of gastric carcinoma mitotic figures are PAS, PAD and PHS positive. These reactions are not found in non-dividing cancer nuclei or in non-neoplastic nuclei at any time. Studies to determine the precise chemical reason for this intriguing reaction, and to assess its frequency in this, and other tumors, are obviously indicated.

References

BURSTONE, M. S., Enzyme histochemistry and its application in the study of neoplasms, p. 276. New York: Academic Press 1962.

CORREIRA, J. P., FILIPE, M. I., and SANTOS, J. C., Histochemistry of the gastric mucosa. *Gut* 4, 68—76 (1963).

HESS, R., SCARPELLI, D. G., and PEARSE, A. G. E., The cytochemical localization of oxydative enzymes. *J. biophys. biochem. Cytol.* 4, 753—760 (1958).

LEV, R., The mucin histochemistry of normal and neoplastic gastric mucosa. *Lab. Invest.* 14, 2080—2100 (1965).

NACHLAS, M. M., MONIS, B., ROSENBLATT, D., and SELIGMAN, A. M., Report on improvement in the histochemical localization of leucine aminopeptidase with a new substrate. *J. biophys. biochem. Cytol.* 7, 261—264 (1960).

—, WALKER, D. G., and SELIGMAN, A. M., A histochemical method for the demonstration of diphosphopyridine nucleotide diaphorase. *J. biophys. biochem. Cytol.* 4, 29—36 (1958).

PEARSE, A. G. E., *Histochemistry* 2nd ed., p. 911. Little, Brown & Co. 1960.

PLANTEYDT, H. T., Een histochemisch onderzoek. (Doctoral Thesis) *"Maag en maagcarcinom"*, University of Leiden 1961.

—, LEEMHUIS, M. P., and WILLIGHAGEN, R. G. J., Enzyme histochemistry of gastric tumors in animals. *J. Path. Bact.* 83, 31—38 (1962).

PLANTEYDT, H. T., and WILLIGHAGEN, R. G. J., Enzyme histochemistry of the human stomach, with special reference to intestinal metaplasia. *J. Path. Bact.* 80, 317—323 (1960).

— — Enzyme histochemistry of gastric carcinoma. *J. Path. Bact.* 90, 393—398 (1965).

SALENIUS, P., The ontogenesis of the human gastric epithelial cells. *Acta anat. (Basel)* 50, Suppl. 46, 1—75 (1962).

SPICER, S. S., HORN, R. G., and LIPPI, T. J., *Histochemistry of connective tissue mucopolysaccharides.* Monograph, Internat. Academy of Pathology. Baltimore: Williams & Wilkins Co. (in press) 1966.

—, SUN, D. C. H., and HOLLANDER, F., Carbohydrate histochemistry of gastric epithelial secretions in dog. *Ann. N. Y. Acad. Sci.* in press (1967).

TOWNSEND, S. F., Regeneration of gastric mucosa in rats. *Amer. J. Anat.* 109, 133—147 (1961).

YOUNG, I., and BRODY, H., Glycogen and glycogen-like substances in chromosomes. *Amer. J. Path.* 48, Abstr. p. 14a—15a (1966).

Experimental Cancer of the Glandular Stomach. A Review

HAROLD L. STEWART

National Cancer Institute, Bethesda, Maryland, U. S. A.

Genuine progress has been made in the experimental induction of adenocarcinoma of the glandular stomach during the 6 years that have elapsed since the interim meeting of the International Union Against Cancer in Tokyo in 1960. At that meeting I gave a preliminary report of the induction of this neoplasm in rats by the administration of a fluorenamine compound, N,N'-2,7-fluorenylenebisacetamide (2,7-FAA) in the diet. Since then, other chemical agents of different classes have also been found that induce this neoplasm when administered orally, intragastrically, intraperitoneally or intravenously. This report reviews the various regimens that have been employed to induce adenocarcinoma and related lesions of the glandular stomach and the possible mechanisms involved. A number of studies have also revealed information on the precancerous changes that occur in the glandular stomach of animals treated with gastric carcinogens and these are reviewed.

Polycyclic Hydrocarbons

Of the various carcinogenic polycyclic aromatic hydrocarbons (LORENZ et al., 1940) tested for the induction of cancer of the glandular stomach in laboratory animals at the National Cancer Institute (STEWART, 1953), the intramural injection of a uniform dose of 3-methylcholanthrene (3-MCA) in an aqueous methocel suspension was most frequently used. Each cubic centimeter of this suspension contained 30 mg of 3-MCA so that the injection of 0.01 cc of the suspension delivered 0.3 mg of 3-MCA into the submucosa of the wall of the glandular stomach of mice. Of 472 mice from six inbred strains that received this dose of 3-MCA into the antrum and that were allowed to live out their life span, 221 developed a precancerous lesion, 23 adenocarcinoma, 7 adenoacanthoma, 46 mixed adenocarcinoma and sarcoma, 5 mixed adeno-acanthoma and sarcoma, and 39 sarcoma (STEWART and BENNETT, 1953). No primary neoplastic lesion was found in the glandular stomach of the other 131 mice autopsied. The C3H and C3Hb strains of mice were the most susceptible to the induction of carcinoma and sarcoma, and next in order were the strain A and strain BALB/C mice. The C57BL strain mice were somewhat less susceptible to the induction of carcinoma but considerably less susceptible to the induction of sarcoma when compared with the C3H or the C3Hb strain mice. There appeared to be no sex difference. Of 68 DBA mice only 3 developed a malignant tumor of the glandular stomach, 1 a mixed adenocarcinoma and sarcoma, and 2 sarcoma. These findings indicate a genetic factor operating in the suscep-tibility to the induction of experimental gastric cancer in mice by this method and relative low susceptibility for this site by comparison with other tissues as for example the subcutaneous tissues and lung.

SAXÉN and STEWART (1952) examined histologically 156 sarcomas of the stomach of mice that had been induced by the injection of one or another carcinogenic polycyclic aromatic hydrocarbon into the wall of the viscus. They classified them as leiomyosarcoma 51 per cent, fibrosarcoma 19.3 per cent, rhabdomyosarcoma 8.9 per cent, malignant Schwannoma 3.4 per cent and sarcoma, not otherwise specified, 17.4 per cent. The carcinogen, vehicle and strain of mouse seemed not to influence the histologic type of the tumor. When however larger doses of carcinogen were employed there was a corresponding increase in the occurrence of areas of adenocarcinoma in the sarcomas.

Changes in Mucosal Cells at Site of Injection of 3-MCA

A number of observers have set forth their views on the development of cancer of the stomach in man from heterotopic intestinal epithelium (MORSON, 1955; JÄRVI, 1961). Many believe that the large majority of gastric carcinomas in man originate from such areas of heterotopic intestinal epithelium in the stomach. JÄRVI (1961) based his belief on the presence in the carcinomas of cells with a brush border, like those in the intestine, goblet cells and mucus that stains like intestinal epithelial mucus with mucicarmine and not as gastric mucus stains with Best's carmine stain. WATTENBERG (1959) found amino-peptidase, an intestinal but not a gastric enzyme, present in 50 per cent of gastric carcinomas that he examined.

JÄRVI (1961) studied the histopathogenesis of experimental carcinoma of the glandular stomach of the mouse following the intramural injection of 3-MCA. He based his study on material, consisting of specimens from our work here, which I sent to him and he supplemented these with specimens of mouse stomachs in which he had induced adenocarcinomas by the same technique. He found no evidence of intestinal epithelium in these mouse stomachs which were undergoing cancerization with infiltration of neoplastic gastric epithelium into the connective tissue and muscular coats of the viscus. He found three types of cells in the invading epithelium: tall cells of the surface epithelial type of the glandular mucosa, shorter cells of the neck cell type and cells like the cells of the pyloric glands. The pyloric gland cells formed buds which opened into microcavities bordered by the surface cells and neck cells. Goblet cells were also observed in the surface epithelium of the glandular stomach but these cells did not participate in the process of cancerization. In the invading epithelium JÄRVI (1961) noted and illustrated balloon-like secretory vacuoles perched on the surface of the tall cells. Where the vacuole was attached to the cell wall a pseudobrush border could be seen but this structure had no relation whatever to the true brush border cells of the intestine. JÄRVI (1961) also described "tuft cells" which occurred as isolated cells particularly at the points where the epithelium invaded the deeper layers of the stomach. He also identified this cell in apparently normal mucosa in treated and untreated mice. The "tuft cell" had a characteristic appearance with a tuft-like bunch of tall, divergent, bristles on the apical surface and these bristles continued into the body of the cell to terminate at the level of the nucleus. The "tuft cell" was clearly distinguishable from the intestinal cell with a brush border. JÄRVI (1961) observed "tuft cells" in the gall-bladder, in the ducts and acini of the pancreas and in the duodenal mucosa of mice in which a 3-MCA coated thread had been sewn into the wall of the stomach. Similar cells have been observed in the rabbit, dog, cat, rat and golden hamster. They have been interpreted as resorptive cell types of various sites in the digestive tract because of a system of channels that connect with supra-nuclear vacuoles and open on the surface of the cell between the bristles.

PLANTEYDT et al. (1962) considered the types of cells induced by 20-methyl-cholanthrene in the mucosa of the glandular stomach of mice as described by JÄRVI and KEYRILÄINEN (1955), JÄRVI and LAURÉN (1951) and SUGIMACHI (1959) and in their histochemical studies PLANTEYDT et al. (1962) found certain resemblances between abnormal cells in the gastric mucosa and intestinal epithelium and certain differences as well. They found alkaline phosphatase and 5-nucleotidase present in intestinal epithelium and also in the apical border of some gastric cancer cells. On the other hand aminopeptidase activity was not found in the gastric cancer cells, whereas in intestinal epithelium a high activity of this enzyme was demonstrated. These 3 enzymes are absent from the epithelial cells of the normal gastric mucosa. PLANTEYDT and associates (1962) think that in the gastric tumors in mice induced by 20-methylcholanthrene there is a differentiation to several types of cells, some of which are comparable with different types of epithelium normally occurring in the gastrointestinal tract. They did not find highly differentiated cells such as chief cells and parietal cells in the invading portions of the tumors. Their observation that in gastric tumors of mice a high activity of some enzymes is found that are completely absent in the normal mucosa but present in the intestinal epithelium, suggests a differentiation of the gastric tumor cells in the direction of intestinal epithelium.

Mucosal Changes in Glandular Stomach of Mice Ingesting Carcinogenic Polycyclic Aromatic Hydrocarbons

STEWART and LORENZ (1949) reported that a few of their experimental mice that ingested the carcinogenic hydrocarbons 3-MCA or dibenz [a, h] anthracene showed areas of gastritis and occasionally extensions of portions of this altered glandular mucosa into the submucosa. None of the mucosal extensions penetrated completely through the wall of the stomach and therefore did not meet their criterion for genuine carcinoma. Even more severe glandular mucosal changes were observed in C57 black mice that ingested 3-MCA with or without Tween 80 in high fat diets in the experiments of WONG, DANUTE, and WISSLER (1959). Their mice showed both atrophic and proliferative changes in the mucosa of the glandular stomach and they described the changes in detail. The atrophic changes involved the entire extent of the glandular mucus membrane and consisted of a decrease in the thickness of the mucosa, loss of parietal cells, replacement of normal gastric glands by mucus-secreting glands of the intestinal type and a slight to moderate increase in the fibrous tissue in the mucosa, muscularis mucosae and submucosa. The proliferative changes increased the thickness of the mucosa up to 4 times. The glands here were also of the intestinal type and were hypertrophic, hyperplastic, tortuous, cystic and irregular in pattern. The nuclei were hyperchromatic, crowded, depolarized and often in mitosis. The atrophic changes in the mucosa of the glandular stomach were limited to the early part of their experiment and the proliferative changes to the later part, thus corresponding to an initial suppressive effect followed by a late enhancing effect on cell growth. The mucosa of the glandular stomach went through an initial phase of atrophic changes, together with a conversion of the highly specialized gastric glands to the simple intestinal type of glands and then progressed to a final phase of proliferative changes. The proliferative changes appeared earlier and more frequently and were more severe in the mice that had ingested both the 3-MCA and Tween 80 than in those that ingested only 3-MCA. In one animal with severe proliferative changes in the mucosa there was extension of glands below the muscularis mucosae but none of the animals developed genuine cancer.

Intramural Injection of 3-MCA in Rats

In rats, the injection of 0.02 cc of the aqueous methocel suspension containing 0.6 mg of 3-MCA into the wall of the glandular stomach produced adenomatous diverticula and cancers. The adenomatous diverticulum is a type of precancerous lesion not observed in other species including man (STEWART and HARE, 1950; HARE et al., 1952). The wall of the adenomatous diverticulum consisted of fibrous and muscular elements of the stomach. The external surface was nodular and covered by glistening peritoneum, except where adhesions attached to it. The mucosal surface was composed of atypical glandular structures, cysts, polypoid nodules and areas of inflammation, producing a histologic picture resembling somewhat the lesion of inflammatory diverticulitis of man but having neoplastic features in addition. Some areas of adenomatous diverticula contained patches of glands and squamous cell metaplasia both of which were distinctly neoplastic in appearance. The stroma of some such areas contained deposits of metaplastic bone. A few adenomatous diverticula were composed of even more aggressive hyperplastic glands and thus suggested a transition to genuine carcinoma.

When two areas of the glandular stomach of the same rat were tested for neoplastic response to the intramural injection of 3-MCA, the antral site (1st site) was found to be considerably more susceptible to the induction of carcinoma and of the adenomatous diverticulum than was the acid-secreting fundic site (2nd site), whereas the fundic site was more susceptible to sarcoma. In man, spontaneous gastric carcinoma occurs more frequently in the antrum than in the fundus; hence, man and the rat are strangely similar in this respect. Of 265 rats tested in this experiment, an adenomatous diverticulum occurred at the first or at the second or at both injection sites 273 times in 220 rats. There were 28 malignant tumors in 26 animals as follows: 4 adenocarcinoma, 4 adenoacanthoma, 3 mixed carcinoma and sarcoma, 16 sarcoma and 1 unclassified malignant tumor. The carcinomas extended through the wall of the stomach onto the peritoneum and into the pancreas and implants and metastases were found in diaphragm, lymph node, liver, and lung.

In an earlier experiment of this type HOWES and DE OLIVEIRA (1948) sutured a thread impregnated with 3-MCA into the wall of the stomach. It is not possible to determine how many tumors they obtained but they did give a clear description of the tissue reactions that occurred around the thread. GRANT and IVY (1955) mentioned 6 carcinomas as occurring in their 117 rats following the implantation of hydrocarbon carcinogens in the gastric submucosa. Later WONG and GRANT (1966) implanted crystals of dimethylbenz[a]anthracene (DMBA) adherent to a small strip of Gelfoam submucosally in the glandular stomach of rats to study the gastric tissue response to this localized injury. They observed the sequence of events between 1 day and 17 weeks which they regarded as the precancerous period. They reported an initial lack of fibroblastic response, the sustained presence of fibrinoid necrosis and necrotizing vasculitis with subsequent mucosal ulceration prior to atypical epithelial regeneration. This confirmed previous observations made in mice by STEWART (1953).

BENKO and associates (1957) injected 0.1 mg of benzo[a]pyrene in oil into the wall of each of 150 albino rats. A number of the rats developed the adenomatous diverticulum and sarcoma but none developed genuine adenocarcinoma. These results are probably explicable on the use of a smaller dose of a less potent carcinogen than HARE and his associates (1952) used (0.6 mg of 3-MCA into two sites in the glandular stomach).

SKORYNA and RITCHIE (1960) reported the highest yield yet of gastric carcinomas in this type of experiment in rats. In the series of rats kept longest after the initial procedure, they reported 21 per cent with carcinoma. They attributed the higher yield of tumors in their experiments to the placement of the 3-MCA impregnated threads into the submucosa of the glandular stomach on three separate occasions over a span of 6 months, and the fixations of these threads *in situ* by sutures. They believe this technic kept the carcinogen in contact with the mucosa for a long time. However, their high yield of carcinomas is in part due to their failure to adhere to strict criteria for diagnosis. HARE and his associates (1952) accepted as genuine carcinomas only those lesions that invaded all coats of the stomach and infiltrated onto the peritoneum or into contiguous viscera or metastasized. Any lesion falling short of these criteria was classified by HARE and associates (1952) as diverticulum. It is difficult to try to determine the objective criteria SKORYNA and RITCHIE (1960) used. They stated: "The differentiation between diverticula and adenocarcinomas was not always easy nor was any simple means of differentiation found." One gathers from reading their report that they relied heavily on the histologic appearance of the lesion and on the presence of invasion, but they did not define the structures invaded. They said the carcinomas did not infiltrate far beyond their macroscopic limits. We know that in animal pathology limited invasion may be a manifestation of a perfectly benign lesion, as for example the adenomatous hyperplastic lesion of the glandular stomach of Strain I mice. Their reliance on the histologic appearance of the lesion for a diagnosis of cancer in their rats is not entirely justified for we know that in man and lower animals many lesions that are perfectly benign may exhibit cellular atypicality and an anaplastic appearance of varying degree when examined under the microscope. One would like to believe that their technic is an improvement on the other technics for the induction of adenocarcinoma of the glandular stomach but until the results of such experiments are judged by criteria similar to those that were used to evaluate the results of other experiments one must withhold judgment.

Fluorenamine Compounds

Chemical compounds of different classes including some of the fluorenamine group, were fed to different species and strains of laboratory animals at the National Cancer Institute without inducing cancer of the glandular stomach until we (MORRIS et al., 1961; STEWART et al., 1961) obtained positive results with N,N'-2,7-fluorenylenebisacetamide (2,7-FAA). These results with 2,7-FAA have been confirmed by NAGAYO (1965). In their first experiment in which N-2-fluorenylacetamide (2-FAA) on oral administration to rats was demonstrated to be a carcinogen for many tissues, WILSON, DE EDS, and COX (1941) reported finding an adenoma of the glandular stomach in one rat. Later, RICHARDSON (1956) reported the induction of adenocarcinoma of the glandular stomach with metastasis in 2 of a large group of Sprague-Dawley rats that ate a basal semisynthetic diet containing 0.1 per cent of 2-FAA and had their stomachs also lavaged with 1 to 2 cc. of an alcoholic solution of 2-FAA. Other lesions of the glandular stomach reportedly found in 47 of 89 rats necropsied from RICHARDSON's experimental group of 137 rats, were adenomatous diverticulum and atypical proliferation in 23, persistent ulcer in 11, and gastritis in 22. This report by RICHARDSON (1956) appeared as an abstract and was presented orally at the 47th meeting of the American Association for Cancer Research, but we have seen no later publication with illustrations and so cannot objectively assess the lesions he reported. More recently MILLER and associates (1964) have shown that the administration of the N-hydroxymetabolite of 2-FAA, N-hydroxy-2-fluorenylacetamide induced an anaplastic adenocarcinoma of the glandular stomach in a mouse.

In our first experiment with the feeding of 2,7-FAA to rats we found four carcinomas of the glandular stomach, three at the pylorus and one at the fundus (STEWART et al., 1961) and a number of precancerous lesions also. These 4 rats with gastric adenocarcinoma were among a group of 72 male and female AxC and Buffalo strain rats that ingested the 2,7-FAA and from 47 of these the stomach was examined both grossly and histologically. Apart from the stomach, and as might be expected, a variety of tumors arose in different organs and tissues and atrophic changes appeared in the sex organs and in many endocrine and exocrine glands. All of the gastric carcinomas formed a neoplastic mass on the peritoneum of the stomach and variously infiltrated the fibro-fatty tissue of the mesentery and the pancreas. This was our first experience with the induction of carcinoma and precancerous lesions of the glandular stomach by the oral administration of a chemical carcinogen in the diet. Precancerous lesions in the form of plaques, umbilicate lesions and hyperplastic foci of the mucous membrane of the fundic, antral and pyloric mucosa of the glandular stomach were observed in approximately one-half of the 47 animals. Moreover, in all 47, some degree of atrophic gastritis was observed and was frequently associated with cellular atypism, intestinal metaplasia and inflammatory changes. The atrophy was more pronounced in the fundic than in the antral mucosa, on the lesser than on the greater curvature, and in the zymogen than in the acid cells. With pronounced depletion of both zymogen and acid cells, the mucous cells, many of which contained hyperchromatic nuclei, extended part way down the gastric glands or lined the glands from surface to base. A few large acidophilic cells with numerous granules were seen. These resembled Paneth cells that are described in lesions of atophic gastritis in man. The deep portion of the gastric glands of many of the rats became lined with hyperchromatic cells. The lamina propria underwent atrophy in some and in others showed edema, inflammatory cells, and an increase in hyalin in the stroma between the glands.

The two types of precancerous lesion, the plaque-like and the umbilicate, occurred in 17 of the 47 rats. The plaque-like lesion was found in 8 rats and in 2 of these, umbilicate lesions were also present. Five of the plaque-like lesions were located on the lesser curvature of the glandular stomach near the limiting ridge, one on the superior, and the other on the inferior surface of the antrum. The plaque-like lesion was superficial and was confined to the mucous membrane in 6 rats while in the other 2, it infiltrated a thickened collagenous muscularis mucosae in one, and the submucosa and muscularis propria in the other. This in our opinion justified the designation of precancerous for the plaque-like lesion. One or more umbilicate lesions were found in 11 rats, in the fundus in two and in the antrum in the others. Some of the umbilicate lesions were confined to the mucous membrane, while the atypical glands of others had extended into the submucosa, muscularis propria, and subserosa, thus indicating its neoplastic nature. At all levels the stroma about the glands of the umbilicate lesions was increased, often infiltrated with inflammatory cells, and sometimes hyalinized. At the pyloric ring five rats showed pronounced cellular hyperplasia and atypism of the gastric and duodenal glands of the surface mucosa and of the Brunner's glands as well. These atypical glands infiltrated the deep coats at the pylorus but did not extend onto the serosa. The three genuine carcinomas that were located at the pylorus could, therefore, have originated from the surface mucosa of the stomach or duodenum, or the Brunner's glands, or from any two or from all three of these sources.

To test whether, in order to induce gastric carcinomas by the 2,7-FAA, it is necessary to administer the compound by the oral route, or whether it is effective by some other route, an experiment was designed in which the compound was injected through the abdominal wall into the peritoneal cavity of 19 Buffalo strain rats (MORRIS et al., 1962). Three of these rats developed carcinoma of the glandular stomach (two at the pylorus and one at the fundus), 7 developed precancerous lesions and the majority of them had atrophic gastritis. Thus the 2,7-FAA was about equally effective as a carcinogen for the mucosa of the glandular stomach administered orally in the food or injected into the peritoneal cavity. These, to our knowledge, were the first gastric adenocarcinomas to be induced by the administration of a chemical compound by a route (intraperitoneal injection) by which there was no initial contact between the chemical and the gastric mucosa.

We carried out another experiment which showed the effects of two different carcinogens in the same rat, the oral administration of 2,7-FAA and the intra-mural injection of 3-MCA at the fundic and antral sites of the glandular stomach (STEWART et al., 1965). As described, 2,7-FAA administered orally to rats induces gastric carcinoma and precarcinomatous lesions but not sarcoma, whereas the 3-MCA injected intramurally into the glandular stomach of rats induces carcinoma, sarcoma, carcinosarcoma, and precarcinomatous and pre-sarcomatous lesions. The combination of 2,7-FAA feeding and 3-MCA injection induced an increased number of gastric sarcomas over that which would be expected from the injection of 3-MCA alone and more carcinomas than the sum of those that would be expected from the administration of either 2,7-FAA or 3-MCA alone, but the additional carcinomas were frequently mixed with sar-coma. With injections of 3-MCA alone into the fundic and antral sites of the glandular stomach most of the sarcomas arose at the fundic site, whereas with the combined treatment most of the sarcomas were located at the antral site. Hence the combined treatment reversed the susceptibility of these two sites to sarcoma. Moreover, the number of the cancers induced by the combined treat-ment exceeded the sum of the cancers that would be expected to be induced by either method alone and they appeared earlier. Hence this is an example of the synergistic effects of two carcinogens on the glandular stomach.

A closely related fluorenamine compound N,N'-2,7-fluorenylenebis-2,2,2-trifluoroacetamide (2,7-FAA-F_6) was synthesized and administered orally to Buffalo strain rats because from assumptions from previous experiments we though this compound might prove to be a very active carcinogen (MORRIS et al., 1963). Although in this assumption we were mistaken, it is nevertheless interesting to review the reasons for the assumption. They were based upon the results of experiments in which the substitution of the halogen, fluorine, for the hydrogens of the acetyl side chain of N-2 fluorenylacetamide (2-FAA), yielded the compound, N-(2-fluorenyl)-2,2,2-trifluoroacetamide (2-FAA-F_3), which proved to be a more potent carcinogen for the liver, mammary gland, and some other sites than 2-FAA itself (MORRIS et al., 1960). Moreover, in a later experiment, the addition to 2-FAA of a second acetylamide group, as in 2,7-FAA also resulted in an increased carcinogenic activity of that compound over 2-FAA, as indicated by the development of many more intestinal tumors and tumors at such unusual sites as the glandular stomach, salivary glands, and cranial nerves (MORRIS et al., 1957, 1961; SNELL et al., 1961 a and b; STEWART et al., 1961). We reasoned, therefore, that if the halogen element fluorine was substituted for the hydrogens of the acetyl groups of both side chains of 2,7-FAA, the resulting compound, 2,7-FAA-F_6, might be an even more potent carcinogen than the 2,7-FAA, an expectation that was not borne out. In the experiment in which the 2,7-FAA-F$_6$ was fed to 20 rats, 7 of them developed lesions of the glandular stomach that were like those that we diagnosed as precarcinomatous in the experiment in which 2,7-FAA was fed but no genuine carcinomas arose. However, one rat did develop a sarcoma of the glandular stomach. In one of our previous unpublished experiments in which N-benzoyl-2-aminofluorene was fed to rats, one animal developed a neurilemmoma of the wall of the stomach.

Mechanism of Gastric Carcinogenesis by 2,7-FAA

When we first considered the mechanism for the induction of gastric adenocarcinoma by the feeding of 2,7-FAA, we wondered whether the lesions of atrophic gastritis and neoplasia resulted from direct contact between the mucous membrane of the glandular stomach and the 2,7-FAA that was swallowed or from the effects of the 2,7-FAA or its metabolites after they were absorbed from the alimentary tract and returned to the stomach by way of the circulating blood or a combination of both. It is well known that certain carcinogenic chemical compounds may be absorbed from the intestine and enter the circulation and be carried to the liver and other organs and later returned to the alimentary tract. During this circulation, these compounds may be modified to become either more potent or less potent carcinogens. While an immediate direct effect of the 2,7-FAA on the mucosa in its passage through the stomach cannot be denied, one must bear in mind the failure of the gastric glandular mucosa to undergo a cancerous change when powerful carcinogenic polycyclic aromatic hydrocarbons are administered in the drinking water, under which circumstances the exposure of the mucosa was virtually continuous for many months. One of the hydrocarbons, benzo(a)pyrene, was shown to penetrate full thickness of the glandular mucosa (SETÄLÄ and ERMALA, 1951) and yet not induce gastric adenocarcinoma. These failures with oral administration are in contrast to the ease with which adenocarcinoma can be induced when the polycyclic hydrocarbons are injected intramurally at the base of the gastric mucosa of mice and rats. Moreover, the polycyclic hydrocarbons are themselves proximal carcinogens whereas the fluorenamine compounds require metabolic activation. With the orally administered 2,7-FAA, therefore, it is not unreasonable to be sceptical of the theory of a direct contact mechanism and to consider the importance of the transport to the stomach of 2,7-FAA, or its metabolites by way of the circulating blood. The transport certainly accounted for the induction of atrophy and cancer at many sites outside the alimentary canal in the animals that ingested the 2,7-FAA. Furthermore, the induction of gastric adenocarcinoma by the intraperitoneal injection of 2,7-FAA demonstrated the lack of necessity for initial direct contact between the gastric mucosa and the 2,7-FAA in the gastric contents, unless it was regurgitated with the duodenal contents following excretion in the bile or resecreted into the stomach.

The gastric precancerous lesions induced by 2,7-FAA when injected intra-peritoneally were less numerous and individually less extensive, and the atrophy and gastritis less severe than in the experiment in which the compound was fed to rats, but they nevertheless were of the same general nature and the percentage of rats developing gastric adenocarcinoma was the same in the two experiments.

There have been three attempts, by experimentation with rats, to delineate the mechanism of action of 2,7-FAA on the glandular stomach. In brief these experiments purport to show that the gastric glandular mucosa can both absorb 2,7-FAA (RAY et al., 1961) and excrete it or its metabolites (RAY et al., 1965) and that these compounds may regurgitate with the duodenal contents into the stomach following their excretion in the bile (DYER and MORRIS, 1964). RAY and collaborators (1961) injected tritiated 2,7-FAA into the peritoneal cavity of rats which previously had tight ligatures placed just below the pylorus of the stomach. Four hours later the stomach and its contents were removed and separated. Measurable amounts of radioactivity were found in the stomach itself and in the gastric contents. The authors interpreted this to mean that the 2,7-FAA was absorbed from the peritoneal cavity into the circulating blood which subsequently transported it to the stomach where it was excreted by the gastric mucosa into the lumen. Since these authors had not reported on the condition of the stomach of their experimental animals, we repeated the experiment in part to observe the effects of obstruction itself on the state of the stomach. As they had done, we too ligated the gastrointestinal tract of rats just below the pyloric stomach. We killed the rats four hours later and fixed and sectioned the stomach and prepared histologic slides. We found areas of severe acute inflammatory erosion and ulceration of the gastric mucous membrane. We felt that if the stomach of the rats that RAY and his collaborators used had the severe lesions that our rats had, there would be little doubt that some of the 2,7-FAA could have escaped from the blood through exudation and tran-sudation rather than by way of an excretory mechanism on the part of mucosal cells.

DYER and MORRIS (1964) fed a single dose of 2,7-FAA-9-C[14] to intact rats and to rats with a bile fistula that drained on to the outside of the body. Ninety-six hours later they found less radioactivity in the gastric contents of the rats with the bile fistula than in the intact rats. They interpreted this to mean that since the bile with its content of 2,7-FAA and metabolites drained outside of the body, there was progressively less available in the duodenum to regurgitate back through the pylorus into the glandular stomach, which they believed to be an important route by which these compounds reach the stomach. This may be so but nevertheless, since the 2,7-FAA-9-C[14] and its metabolites were lost by excretion through the bile fistula onto the outside of the body the entero-hepatic circulation was by-passed leaving progressively smaller amounts of these com-pounds for reabsorption into the blood to be carried subsequently to the stomach. This alternate possibility might explain their findings.

In the third experiment, RAY and collaborators (1965) incubated, *in vitro*, the fundic mucosa of the glandular stomach of rats with tritiated 2-FAA or tritiated 2,7-FAA and found, on subsequent examination, that both compounds adhered to the surface of the mucosal cells and deposited between the cells. With the 2,7-FAA, the silver dots were more numerous and were additionally found within the cytoplasm of the mucosal cells. The authors interpreted these findings to mean that the 2,7-FAA compound became bound to the protein of the cytoplasm of the gastric mucosal cells. While at present we cannot fully assess the significance of these experiments with respect to the mechanism of induction of gastric adenocarcinoma, nevertheless they are of the type that are likely to prove helpful in revealing pathways by which the 2,7-FAA when fed to rats or injected into the peritoneal cavity can exert a carcinogenic effect on the glandular mucosa of the stomach.

Rats receiving 2,7-FAA by oral or intraperitoneal administration do develop atrophy of their endocrine and sex organs and these changes undoubtedly lead to hormonal alterations and imbalances that might secondarily influence the development of atrophic gastritis and gastric cancer. Perhaps some sort of remote mechanism might operate in the induction of the proliferative hypertrophy of the gastric mucosa that progresses to gastric cancer in mice exposed to whole body irradiation (NOWELL *et al.*, 1958). But it is not clear why with the whole body irradiation the gastritis was of the hypertrophic type whereas that induced by the 2,7-FAA was of the atrophic type. As mentioned above, a number of pathologists have, over the years, supported the view that chronic gastritis is a frequent precancerous lesion in man whereas other pathologists have denied this. The chronic atrophic gastritis that regularly developed in the rats that were treated with 2,7-FAA was similar to that seen in man. In the rat, erosion-cancer or ulcero-cancer was a feature of the pathologic process of chronic gastritis. We also wondered if there is any relationship between the atrophic and neoplastic gastric lesions induced by 2,7-FAA in the rat and the lesions of gastric mucosal atrophy, polyps and carcinoma that occur in the stomach of patients with pernicious anemia. Neither complete studies of the blood nor gastric analyses of the 2,7-FAA treated rats were done, but examination of blood smears from a number of them showed poikilocytosis, anisocytosis, and hyperchromasia of the red blood cells indicating severe anemia.

In patients with pernicious anemia and achlorhydria, CRILE (1958) believes it possible that cancer of the stomach may result from unrestrained antral mucosal overactivity and subsequent hyperplasia that progresses to cancer. According to CRILE's (1958) "signal substance" theory, the antral mucosa in patients with pernicious anemia overworks to stimulate the fundic mucosa to secrete hydrochloric acid. However, since the target cells, i. e., the acid cells of the cardia, are unable to respond to this stimulus or to inhibit it by a feedback mechanism, the efforts of the antral mucosa continue unabated and progress through hyperplasia to carcinoma. The continued effect of this stimulus directed at the unresponsive fundic mucosa may, he also believes, lead to the development of carcinoma there. Some such mechanism as hypothecated by CRILE (1958) could be a factor in the production of the fundic and pyloric carcinomas of the rats treated with 2,7-FAA since atrophic gastritis and precancerous lesions are regular features of this experiment.

From time to time we have been confused about the exact cells from which the carcinomas at the pylorus originate in rats that received the 2,7-FAA in the diet or by intraperitoneal injections. We have stated that these pyloric carcinomas could have originated from the lining mucosa of the stomach or duodenum or from the Brunner's glands or from any two or all three of these sources, and we cannot be any more specific at the present time. The majority of the plaque-like precancerous lesions occurred in the fundus of the glandular stomach, whereas the majority of umbilicate lesions were in the antrum. The hyperplastic and neoplastic lesions at the pylorus were not always plaque-like or umbilicate. The ratio of the epithelial neoplasms of the pyloric and fundic portions of the glandular stomach of rats that were treated with the 2,7-FAA was about the same as the ratio of epithelial neoplasms of the fundic and antral sites in rats that received intramural injections of 3-MCA. Thus with these induced tumors in rats and the spontaneous gastric carcinomas of man the distal portion of the glandular stomach is more susceptible than the proximal portion.

Other Carcinogenic Chemicals

Since the successful induction of adenocarcinoma of the glandular stomach of rats by the administration of 2,7-FAA in the diet or by intraperitoneal injection, other chemical agents have been tested and found to induce this neoplasm when administered in the diet or in drinking water, by stomach tube, by instillation through a gastrostomy tube or by intravenous injection. These, as reported, include 4-nitroquinoline-N-oxide given through a gastrostomy tube to rats receiving percutaneous applications of 3-methylcholanthrene (BABA, 1962), the aflatoxins from *Aspergillus flavus* administered in a diet of contaminated ground nut meal (BUTLER and BARNES, 1963; 1966) and certain nitroso-compounds (SCHOENTAL, 1963; DRUCKREY et al., 1964; DRUCKREY, 1966).

The discovery of the carcinogenic action of dimethylnitrosamine on the liver (MAGEE and BARNES, 1956) has led to the synthesis of numerous related compounds that induce cancer at different sites in the alimentary tract and in other tissues and organs as well. Depending upon their chemical structure, various nitroso-compounds can induce neoplasms of the tongue and oral mucosa, pharynx, esophagus, forestomach, glandular stomach, and intestines of animals. SCHOENTAL (1963) found a carcinoma of the glandular stomach in a rat that received a single dose of N-nitroso-N-methylurethane by stomach tube. She also found a papillary growth, suggestive of neoplasia, in the glandular stomach of a mouse that had received by stomach tube a single dose of N-nitroso-N-ethylurethane. DRUCKREY and associates (1964) reported an experiment in which cancer developed at a number of different sites following a single intravenous dose of N-methyl-N-nitroso-urea into strain BD rats; one of the cancers was a sarcoma of the glandular stomach. Professor DRUCKREY (1966) has written me about unpublished experiments in which he obtained gastric adenocarcinomas in rats and guinea pigs. He sent me gross photographs of these lesions induced by methylnitrosourea and ethylbutylnitrosamine in rats and by methylnitrosourea and methylnitrosourethane in guinea pigs. The ethylbutylnitrosamine was administered intravenously once weekly and the other compounds were administered in the drinking water from 5 to 7 days a week. The treatment was stopped at varying periods of time before the animals were sacrificed. The ages of the animals at death varied between 300 and 878 days.

The chemically defined aflatoxins from *Aspergillus flavus* that contaminate mouldy food and, in particular, mouldy ground nuts (peanuts) must be classed among the most powerful of chemical carcinogens. BUTLER and BARNES (1963, 1966) have described the induction of adenocarcinoma of the glandular stomach in a series of experiments in which toxic ground nut meal containing aflatoxins was fed to rats. In the various experiments that they summarized (1966), 3 rats developed adenocarcinoma of the glandular stomach, another a carcinosarcoma, while a fourth had metastatic adenocarcinoma, the primary site of which was thought to be the glandular stomach. The incidence of carcinoma of the glandular stomach induced by feeding ground nut meal containing aflatoxin was therefore roughly the same as the incidence of this neoplasm induced by 2,7-FAA given orally or intraperitoneally to rats.

Mechanism of Action by Nitroso-Compounds

The nitrosamines are as a group powerful carcinogens that are widespread in their effects. They share with certain other classes of chemical carcinogens the ability to induce cancer after a single dose. An average single carcinogenic dose of the nitrosamines is rapidly metabolized and excreted over a period of hours or a few days at most, the excretion being more rapid in rats than in mice. Then after a more or less long latent period tumors arise in the treated animal. Much has been written about the possible mechanism of toxicity and carcinogenesis by these compounds (MAGEE and SCHOENTAL, 1964) since MAGEE and FARBER (1962) detected the alkylation of nucleic acids of the liver by dimethylnitrosamine. The nitrosamines themselves are not considered to be toxic but the toxic agents must be diazoalkanes, monoalkylnitrosamines or the carbonium ions formed from them. One of the earliest manifestations of the effect of dimethylnitrosamine on the liver of the rat is a defect in protein synthesis as exemplified by impairment of incorporation of amino acids into liver proteins and this suggests damage to the microsome structures. Dimethylnitrosamine methylates liver proteins and nucleic acids, the histidines and 7-methylguanine and this change has been demonstrated in many organs and tissues of the body, but the liver is the site most affected. Some have speculated that there may be a correlation between the distribution of methylation in organs and their susceptibility to tumor induction but no quantitative correlation has as yet been established. The nitroso-compounds can be roughly divided into two groups, one exemplified by N-methyl-N-nitrosourethane which under appropriate conditions interacts with sulphydryl groups, and the other exemplified by dimethylnitrosamine which does not. All alkylnitroso-compounds that possess activated carbonyl groups would be expected to react to sulphydryl compounds. On decomposition both types of compounds yield diazomethane or its corresponding methyl carbonium ions. Hence the biologic action of both groups of alkylnitroso-compounds might be related to that of diazomethane.

To explain the induction of cancer at remote sites following the subcutaneous injection of the asymmetrical nitroso-compounds it has been assumed by DRUCKREY and associates (1964) that the inactive compound is transported to the site where it exerts preferential action. Each such site they believe possesses enzyme systems that can perform dealkylation and so it is at that site that the chemical reactions that dealkylate the compound are set into operation. Thus a possible mechanism of the action of the nitrosamines is their enzymatic oxidation by different cells as well as by serum, with the ultimate formation of diazoalkanes which as alkylating agents are believed to be the responsible carcinogens. A certain metabolic state and an enzymatic cellular exchange are believed responsible for direct contact between the carcinogen and the body cells and for the action of the carcinogenic substances circulating in the blood. Thus the inactive transport form of glucuronic acid esters is believed to exert a carcinogenic effect when the enzyme action of the cell is able to split the inactive esters leading to the liberation of the carcinogenically active components, the diazoalkanes or their corresponding carbonium ions.

Another mechanism of action by certain nitroso-compounds, the denaturing effect on proteins, has been postulated by ARGUS et al. (1965). Their reasoning is based upon experiments that showed dioxane to be carcinogenic for the liver of the rat. The cyclic dioxane is a structural analogue of the three cycloalkyl nitrosamines, N-nitrosopiperidine, N-nitrosomorpholine and N-nitrosopiperazine which three nitroso-compounds are among the most potent carcinogens of this class. ARGUS et al. (1965) believe that the carcinogenicity of these nitrosamines cannot be accounted for by the mechanism of monodealkylation followed by condensation to the corresponding diazoalkane and subsequent alkylation of nucleic acids. Instead they believe that these carcinogens like dioxane may act by denaturation of cellular macromolecules involved in metabolic control. Because the nitrosamines and dioxane show potent hydrogen bonding and protein denaturing ability, ARGUS et al. (1965) believe that these agents may bring about alterations in the molecular morphology of endoplasmic membranes and other macromolecular aggregates and may cause changes in the conformation of individual enzymes which lead to the induction of cancer.

X-ray

Whole body irradiation of mice with fast neutrons and roentgen rays was reported by NOWELL *et al.* (1958) to induce an obstructive hyperplastic gastritis that sometimes eventuated in adenocarcinoma of the glandular stomach. UPTON and associates (1960) obtained 0.23 per cent of adenocarcinomas of the stomach in 2780 mice exposed to gamma rays and 1.42 per cent in 282 mice exposed to fast neutrons. SAXÉN (1952) applied X-irradiation directly to the region of both chambers (glandular portion and squamous portion) of the stomach of C57 brown mice and to some of these irradiated mice he fed 9,10-dimethyl-1,2-benzanthracene. Some mice of both groups developed squamous cell carcinoma of the forestomach. Although in the irradiated mice the glandular stomach underwent atrophy and fibrosis, no mouse of either group developed cancer of this chamber. Hence the results obtained by NOWELL and associates and UPTON and associates (1960) could hardly have been due to the direct effect of the radiation on the glandular stomach, but must in some way have been a response to constitutional changes in the animal's body brought about by the whole body radiation. Rats protected against lethal doses of whole body x-irradiation by parabiosis have developed adenocarcinoma of the duodenum, jejunum, ileum and colon (BRECHER *et al.*, 1953). One of the carcinomas located at the pylorus, may have arisen partly from the gastric mucosa and partly from duodenal mucosa.

Summary

This paper was prepared as the basis for discussion at the Panel on Histogenesis and Epidemiology of Gastric Cancer, to be held at the Ninth International Cancer Congress in Tokyo. It reviews some of the experimental regimens that have been employed to induce adenocarcinoma and associated lesions of the glandular stomach. The regimens considered are the injection of the carcinogenic polycyclic hydrocarbons and in particular 3-methylcholanthrene (3-MCA) intramurally into the pylorus or fundus of the glandular stomach of mice or rats; the oral or intraperitoneal administration of N,N'-2,7-fluorenylenebisacetamide (2,7-FAA) or a combination of feeding 2,7-FAA to rats that had already received intramural injections of 3-MCA; whole body irradiation to mice and rats; the oral, intragastric or intravenous administration of nitroso-compounds, aflatoxins, 4-nitroquinoline-N-oxide or other fluorenamine compounds to mice, rats or guinea pigs. Among the features considered in this report on experimental cancer of the glandular stomach are the pathologic types and incidence of the neoplasms and precancerous lesions, the influence of genetics, the relative susceptibility to carcinogens of the pyloric, antral and fundic mucosa, the effectiveness of different routes of administration, the pathways utilized by the chemical compounds or their metabolites, the character and significance of atrophic and hyperplastic gastritis and the possible influence of atrophic lesions of the exocrine and endocrine glands on the mechanism of gastric carcinogenesis.

References

ARGUS, M. F., ARCOS, J. C., and HOCH-LIGETI, C., Studies on the carcinogenic activity of protein-denaturing agents: Hepatocarcinogenicity of dioxane. *J. nat. Cancer Inst.* **35**, 949—958 (1965).

BABA, T., Induction of cancer of the glandular stomach in a rat: a new form of experiment. *Gann* **53**, 381—387 (1962).

BENKO, A., KOVACS, K., and TISZAI, A., An experimental contribution to the pathogenesis of gastric neoplasm in the rat. *Arch. Geschwulstforsch.* **12**, 160—174 (1957).

BRECHER, G., CRONKITE, E. P., and PEERS, J. H., Neoplasms in rats protected against lethal doses of irradiation by parabiosis or para-aminopropriophenone. *J. nat. Cancer Inst.* **14**, 159—175 (1953).

BUTLER, W. H., and BARNES, J. M., Toxic effects of groundnut meal containing aflatoxin to rats and guinea pigs. *Brit. J. Cancer* **17**, 699—710 (1963).

— — Carcinoma of the glandular stomach in rats given diets containing aflatoxin. *Nature (Lond.)* **209**, 90 (1966).

CRILE jr., G., A speculative review of the role of endocrine imbalances in the genesis of certain cancers and degenerative diseases. *J. nat. Cancer Inst.* **20**, 235—236 (1958).

DRUCKREY, H., Personal communication 1966.

— STEINHOFF, D., PREUSSMANN, R., and IVANKOVIC, S., The production of cancer with a single dose of methylnitrosourea and various dialkylnitrosamines in rats. *Z. Krebsforsch.* **66**, 1—10 (1964).

DYER, H. M., and MORRIS, H. P., Path of N,N'-2,7-fluorenylbisacetamide (2,7-FAA) and its metabolites in ther rat (Abstract). *Proc. Amer. Ass. Cancer Res.* **5**, 16 (1964).

GRANT, R., and IVY, A. C., The abnormal repair and invasive growths following the implantation of hydrocarbon carcinogens in the gastric submucosa of the rat. *Gastroenterology* **29**, 199—218 (1955).

HARE, W. V., STEWART, H. L., BENNETT, J. G., and LORENZ, E. Tumors of the glandular stomach induced in rats by intramural injection of 20-methylcholanthrene. *J. nat. Cancer Inst.* **12**, 1019—1055 (1952).

HOWES, E. L., and DE OLIVEIRA, J. R., Early changes in the experimentally produced adenomas and adenocarcinomas of the stomach. *Cancer Res.* **8**, 419—428 (1948).

JÄRVI, O., A review of the part played by gastro-intestinal heterotopias in neoplasmogenesis. *Proc. Finnish Acad. Sci.* 151—187 (1961).

—, and KEYRILÄINEN, O., On the cellular structures of the epithelial invasions in the glandular stomach of mice caused by intramural application of 20-methylcholanthrene. *Acta path. microbiol. scand.*, Suppl. **111**, 72—73 (1955).

—, and LAURÉN, P., On the role of heterotopias of the intestinal epithelium in the pathogenesis of gastric cancer. *Acta path. microbiol. scand.* **29**, 26—44 (1951).

LORENZ, E., SHIMKIN, M. B., and STEWART, H. L., Preparation of dispersions of carcinogenic hydrocarbons and hormones with the aid of dioctyl ester of sodium sulfosuccinate (aerosol O. T.). *J. nat. Cancer Inst.* **1**, 355—360 (1940).

MAGEE, P. N., and BARNES, J. M., The production of malignant primary hepatic tumours in the rat by feeding dimethylnitrosamine. *Brit. J. Cancer* **10**, 114—122 (1956).

—, and FARBER, E., Toxic liver injury and carcinogenesis. *Biochem. J.* **83**, 114—124 (1962).

—, and SCHOENTAL, R., Carcinogenesis by nitroso compounds. *Brit. med. Bull.* **20**, 102—106 (1964).

MILLER, E. C., MILLER, J. A., and ENOMOTO, M., The comparative carcinogenicities of 2-acetylaminofluorene and its N-hydroxy metabolite in mice, hamsters and guinea pigs. *Cancer Res.* **24**, 2018—2031 (1964).

MORRIS, H. P., VELAT, C. A., and WAGNER, B. P., Carcinogenicity of some ingested acetylated mono- and diaminobiphenylcompounds in the rat. *J. nat. Cancer Inst.* **18**, 101—115 (1957).

Morris, H. P., Velat, C. A., Wagner, B. P., Dahlgard, M., and Ray, F. E., Studies of carcinogenicity in the rat of derivatives of aromatic amines related to N-2-fluorenylacetamide. *J. nat. Cancer Inst.* 24, 149—180 (1960).
— Wagner, B. P., Ray, F. E., Snell, K. C., and Stewart, H. L., Comparative study of cancer and other lesions of rats fed N,N′-2,7-fluorenylenebisacetamide or N-2-fluorenylacetamide. *N. C. I. Monogr.* No 5, 1—53 (1961).
— — — Stewart, H. L., and Snell, K. C., Comparative carcinogenic effects of N,N′-2,7-fluorenylenebisacetamide by intraperitoneal and oral routes of administration to rats, with particular reference to gastric carcinoma. *J. nat. Cancer Inst.* 29, 977—1011 (1962).
— — — — — Carcinogenic effects of N,N′-2,7-fluorenylenebis-2,2,2-trifluoracetamide (2,7-FAA-F6) administered orally to Buffalo strain rats. *J. nat. Cancer Inst.* 30, 143—161 (1963).
Morson, B. C., Carcinoma arising from areas of intestinal metaplasia in the gastric mucosa. *Brit. J. Cancer* 9, 377—385 (1955).
Nagayo, T., Effect of oral administration of N,N′-2,7-fluorenylenebisacetamide combined with traumatic ulcers of the glandular stomach of Buffalo rats. *J. nat. Cancer Inst.* 35, 829—840 (1965).
Nowell, P. C., Cole, L. J., and Ellis, M. E., Neoplasms of the glandular stomach in mice irradiated with X-rays or fast neutrons. *Cancer Res.* 18, 257—260 (1958).
Planteydt, H. T., Leemhuis, M. P., and Willighagen, R. G. J., Enzyme histochemistry of gastric tumours in animals. *J. Path. Bact.* 83, 31—38 (1962).
Ray, F. E., Cromer, M. A., Aycock, A. C., and Pitzer, N., The selection of gastric carcinogens. *Brit. J. Cancer* 15, 816—820 (1961).
— Rivers, F. T., and Hoch-Ligeti, C., Uptake by rat stomach tissues of 2-aminofluorene-³H hydrochloride and 2,7-diaminofluorene-³H hydrochloride *in vitro*. *Brit. J. Cancer* 19, 560—564 (1965).
Richardson, L., Induction of adenocarcinoma of the glandular stomach in rats by alcohol gastric lavage and feeding acetylaminofluorene (abstract). *Proc. Amer. Ass. Cancer Res.* 2, 141—142 (1956).
Saxén, E. A., Squamous-cell carcinoma of the forestomach in X-irradiated mice fed

9,10-dimethyl-1,2-benzanthracene, with a note on failure to induce adenocarcinoma. *J. nat. Cancer Inst.* 13, 441—453 (1952).
Saxén, E. A., and Stewart, H. L., Histogenetic classification of induced gastric sarcomas in mice. *J. nat. Cancer Inst.* 13, 657—679 (1952).
Schoental, R., Induction of tumours of the stomach in rats and mice by N-nitroso-N-alkylurethanes. *Nature (Lond.)* 199, 190 (1963).
Setälä, K., and Ermala, P., Chylomicrons as carriers for carcinogenic hydrocarbons. *Science* 114, 151—153 (1951).
Skoryna, S. C., and Ritchie, A. C., The experimental production of adenocarcinoma of the stomach in rats. *Gastroenterology* 39, 737—746 (1960).
Snell, K. C., Stewart, H. L., Morris, H. P., Wagner, B. P., and Ray, F. E., Atrophy, proliferative lesions, and tumors of the salivary glands of rats ingesting N-2-fluorenylacetamide or N,N′-2,7-fluorenylenebisacetamide. *N. C. I. Monogr.* No 5, 55—83 (1961 a).
— — — — — Intracranial neurilemmoma and medulloblastoma induced in rats by the dietary administration of N,N′-2,7-fluorenylenebisacetamide. *N. C. I. Monogr.* No 5, 85—103 (1961 b).
Stewart, H. L., Experimental cancer of the alimentary tract. In: *The Physiopathology of cancer* (Homburger, F., and Fishman, W. H., eds.), p. 3—45. New York: Paul B. Hoeber, Inc. 1953.
—, and Hare, W. V., Variation in susceptibility of the fundic and pyloric portions of the glandular stomach of the rat to induction of neoplasia by 20-methylcholanthrene. *Acta Un. int. Cancr.* 7, 176—177 (1950).
— —, and Bennett, J. G., Tumors of the glandular stomach induced in mice of six strains by intramural injection of 20-methylcholanthrene. *J. nat. Cancer Inst.* 14, 105—125 (1953).
—, and Lorenz, E., Morbid anatomy, histopathology, and histopathogenesis of forestomach carcinoma in mice fed carcinogenic hydrocarbons in oil emulsions. *J. nat. Cancer Inst.* 10, 147—165 (1949).
— Snell, K. C., and Morris, H. P., The combined effect of 3-methylcholanthrene and N,N′-2,7-fluorenylenebisacetamide on the induction of cancer of the glandular stomach of the rat. *J. nat. Cancer Inst.* 34, 157—174 (1965).

STEWART, H. L., SNELL, K. C., MORRIS, H. P., WAGNER, B. P., and RAY, F. E., Carcinoma of the glandular stomach of rats ingesting N,N'-2,7-fluorenylenebisacetamide. *N. C. I. Monogr.* No 5, 105—139 (1961)

SUGIMACHI, R., Experimental study of carcinoma of the glandular stomach of mice. *Igaku Kenkyu* **29**, 2034 (1959).

UPTON, A. C., KIMBALL, A. W., FURTH, J., CHRISTENBERRY, K. W., and BENEDICT, W. H., Some delayed effects of atom-bomb radiations in mice. *Cancer Res.* **20**, 1—60 (1960).

WATTENBERG, L. W., Histochemical study of aminopeptidase in metaplasia and carcinoma of the stomach. *Arch. Path.* **67**, 281—286 (1959).

WILSON, R. H., DE EDS, F., and COX, A. J., The toxicity and carcinogenic activity of 2-acetylaminofluorene. *Cancer Res.* **1**, 595—608 (1941).

WONG, R. L., and GRANT, R., The response to intramural gastric implantation of 7,12-dimethylbenz(a)anthracene with Gelfoam in rats. *Lab. Invest.* **14**, 2110—2121 (1966).

WONG, T. W., DANUTE, S. J., and WISSLER, R. W., Effects of concurrent feeding of Tween 80 on the carcinogenicity of orally administered 3-methylcholanthrene. *J. nat. Cancer Inst.* **22**, 363—399 (1959).

Panel 2

Evaluation of Techniques in Cancer Detection

Chairmen:

L. C. Robbins (U.S.A.), R. A. Malmgren (U.S.A.)

Members:

H. K. Fidler (Canada), R. Gerard-Marchant (France),
H. Grunze (Germany), T. Kurokawa (Japan)

Chairmens' Summary

Cancer detection differs from cancer diagnosis in its goal. In diagnosis, disease is present and the goal is to identify the pathology of this present illness. The diagnosis is necessary to define the problem. With a diagnosis the physician may examine and interpret to his patient the prognosis and compare means for improving it.

Cancer detection, on the other hand, is concerned with the periodic examination of apparently well, asymptomatic individuals who are without a complaint or symptoms suggestive of cancer. The goal of cancer detection is to achieve long-term survival by early discovery of cancer at a stage of the disease when therapy is most successful.

The problem posed by the patient who is not sick can only be defined by knowing what threatens his survival and by how much. As in curative medicine, the physician must examine the mortality experience of people whose prognostic characteristics are like those of the patient to know what the actual hazards to the patient's life may be. To give his patient a better prognosis, the physician must identify his patient's high risks and he must know that what he does will improve the patient's chances of survival from these risks.

With the goal of long-term survival in mind cancer detection should be preceded by the following considerations:

1. Prognostic Characteristics of the "Not-Sick" Patient. Certain prognostic characteristics must be known if prognosis is to be made on the "not sick". The most important of these are the patient's age, sex, and the racial, economic or cultural group he is in.

2. Cohort Mortality Experience. What are the risks of an individual patient? These risks are those of the group of people having the same prognostic characteristics as the patient to the extent that the patient is like the group.

3. Potential for Improved Prognosis. How much protection is there for a population provided with a particular detection procedure? Are there other sites of cancer or other causes of death the detection of which will result in a greater reduction in the risk of death?

4. Survival Advantage or Reduction in Total Risk of Death. How much does each cancer detection procedure reduce the total risk of death?

Here the viewpoint of the patient who wants long term survival from any cause of death, and those physicians who are concerned beyond the present illness is supported by a quantification of this patient's risk and the potential for risk reduction.

The physician is trained to look for the greatest survival advantage in his sick patient. If he could compare different detection methods for their ability to give survival advantage to his well patient he would undoubtedly find this to be useful as a guide to preventive medicine.

A quantitative expression of survival advantage has been made by estimating the risk of death from a specific cause using the Geller Tables of Probability[1], which give the risks of death for the individual by 5-year age groups to the extent that the individual is like the general population. This method of calculating survival advantage is designed to answer a question such as the following: "For a 45 year old white female, in the United States, what per cent of her total risk of death in the next 10 years will be reduced by an annual Papanicolaou smear?"

If we may assume that all cancers of the cervix which occur in the population including carcinoma in-situ, have a 10 year survival of 43 per cent without the PAPANICOLAOU smear[2] and that 10 year survival of patients with cancer of the cervix who have had an annual Papanicolaou smear is 90 per cent, then the survival advantage can be calculated in the following way:[3]

"This 45 year old white female, U.S.A., is a member of a group whose mortality experience has been recorded by the National Office of Vital Statistics. Among 100,000 of her cohorts, 4,600 will die in the following ten years. Two hundred and two of these will die of cancer of the cervix (estimated). With a mortality rate of 57 per cent the 202 deaths come from a total of 354 cases, 152 of which survived. Of the 354/100,000 who have cervical cancer, 10 per cent or 35 will die even though the Papanicolaou smear is used. The difference between 202 and 35 is 167 or 3.6 per cent of 4,600. The 3.6 per cent represents the survival advantage, or the portion of the total mortality which

---

[1] "Probability Study of Deaths in the Next Ten Years from Specific Causes", by HARVEY GELLER, Chief, Operation Studies Section, Cancer Control Branch, Division of Chronic Diseases, Public Health Service, Department of Health Education and Welfare, Washington, D. C.

[2] End Results in Cancer, Report Number 2.

[3] This method is described in a brochure presented at the Tokyo meeting and will be available, after revisions of the Committee on Cancer Detection and Registries, by writing to the committee secretary.

will be reduced by annual performance of the PAPANICOLAOU smear in this age-sex-race group.

It would seem that the true test of the value of a cancer detection technique would be how it effects the survival advantage. Therefore, to obtain the necessary data to make estimates of survival advantage for the cancer detection techniques for difference cancer sites, the panel was asked to answer five questions: (1) Will detection improve control efforts? (2) What is the consensus today of the best methods of detection? (3) What is the five-year survival when the method is used? (4) What is the cost of the procedure? (5) What effect does detection have on life expectancy?

These questions were also intended to reveal the degree of acceptance of a detection procedure among authorities, and the extent to which a detection procedure is practised. This summary will present the panels opinion on the relative value of the detection procedure for reducing the risk of death from cancer of a particular site.

1. Cancer Site for which there is the Best Evidence that Detection will Favorably Influence the Survival Advantage

Cervical Cancer

Dr. H. K. FIDLER presented the problem of cancer of the cervix and opportunities for control through the Papanicolaou smear. Dr. FIDLER said "Carcinoma of the uterine cervix is the first of the major cancers to be successfully influenced by a screening program". He bases his conclusion that detection reduces the risk of death on two pieces of evidence from British Columbia experience. The incidence of clinical invasive carcinoma of the cervix has fallen. This incidence was 28 per 100,000 in 1955 and has gradually dropped to 14.7 in 1965.

The incidence of clinically invasive carcinoma cases among the unscreened is almost seven times as high as the incidence among those who have had at least one Pap smear. While the screened have run from 4.1 to 4.65 per hundred thousand invasive cases, over the past five years, the unscreened have run from 21 to 29.

The fact that the mortality rates have not yet shown a decline is disturbing to many people. Dr. FIDLER, whose study has been conducted at a significant level since 1955 said, "Despite the fact that mortality rates have not yet shown a decline due to early detection, we feel that this must surely follow because the incidence of invasive carcinoma has dropped 48 per cent in the overall population."

Dr. FIDLER pointed to the widespread use of cervical cancer detection. In the U.S.A. about 15 per cent of all women over 20 were examined in 1963;

and in Canada it is 16.9 per cent in 1965. In British Columbia 41 per cent of the women were examined in 1965. Many other countries are beginning to develop mass screening programs for cervical cancer detection.

2. Cancer Sites for which there is Growing Evidence that Cancer Detection will Favorably Influence the Survival Advantage

Cancer of the Stomach

Dr. TOSHIO KUROKAWA discussed the new Japanese studies of detection for cancer of the stomach. He described the combined use of fluoroscopy with endoscopy for those who had exhibited suspicious lesions. Use of fiberoptics has permitted a better application of the gastric camera which has been used in cancer detection since 1959.

Dr. KUROKAWA bases his evidence that detection reduces the risk of death from stomach cancer on the ability to find early stomach cancer in those screened. Early cancer, that is limited to the mucous membrane or submucosa, gives a survival rate from 93 to 100 per cent.

The practice of stomach cancer detection also is growing in Japan. There are 140 mobile units doing fluoroscopy now, and almost a million people have been examined. The Japanese government has ordered 46 mobile units, which places one unit in each prefecture.

Cancer of the Oral Cavity

Detection among the asymptomatic for cancer of the oral cavity is accomplished largely by inspection combined with biopsy or cytology, according to Dr. MALMGREN. Suggestive evidence that periodic examination of the asymptomatic for oral cancer will reduce the risk of death lies in the reported 50 per cent survival for localized disease as compared with 15 to 25 per cent for late, non-localized cancers. Available studies on periodic examination for cancer of the oral cavity show that as high as 20 per cent of the lesions are unsuspected clinically and detected by cytology. In several countries both physicians and dentists are beginning to add inspection and to a lesser extent cytology, as a part of their routine periodic examination.

Cancer of the Breast

Both annual examination by palpation and mammography are being used experimentally as means of cancer detection according to Dr. ROBBINS. Many believe that detection alone is not enough and that self-referral preceded by frequent self-examination must be added. Evidence that detection alone is of value comes from the 18 year study in Minnesota where up to 7,000 women are examined yearly by palpation. Of the women found to have breast cancer the five year survival is 90 per cent, and 13 women have been followed for 10 years, with 10 survivors giving 77 per cent survival. The HIP study in a preliminary report of the value of combined palpation and mammography reports that those mammogrammed and biopsied had only half the lymph node involvement of the controls. The addition of mammography was found to double the number of cancers detected.

Doubts of the efficacy of detection of breast cancer lie in the failure to improve survival figures in spite of widespread educational efforts. Secondly, survival only seems to be increased because detection permits recognition of the disease earlier in its natural history, but long term survival is unchanged.

3. Cancer Sites for which there is Limited Evidence that Cancer Detection will Favorably Influence the Survival Advantage

Cancer of the Colon and Rectum

Dr. KUROKAWA reported on new studies with the fiberscope and a colon camera. He indicated that there was little prospective data from Japan on the value of annual detection examinations for colon-rectum cancer. However, the detection of a number of early cancers of the colon and rectum with this equipment offers hope that this may prove effective in reducing the risk from colon-rectum cancer. In the U.S.A. where this is a more common form of cancer than in Japan, GILBERTSON has reported on detection of cancer of the colon and rectum on 40,000 recheck annual proctosigmoidoscopic examinations. Of the 9 cancer cases found, one has died, and the 8 survivors, five of whom have been followed for five years, are without sign of cancer[4].

Corpus Cancer

Although cancer of the corpus can be detected by cytology, Dr. FIDLER reports that less than 10 per cent of the cases discovered are among symptom-free women. This is in contrast to the cytologic detection of cervical carcinoma where more than 90 per cent are asymptomatic. While vaginal pool aspiration is capable of detecting about 70 per cent of cases of symptomatic corpus carcinoma, these cases are more reliably investigated by diagnostic curettage. The accuracy of vaginal pool specimens in detecting preclinical lesions is not known. High risk groups are, however, known and special methods of collecting intra-uterine specimens are under investigation.

Bladder Cancer

Dr. MALMGREN compared survival of localized cancer of the bladder, 70 per cent, with that of cancer with regional disease which is 25 per cent.

---

[4] National Cancer Institute Monograph on end results of cancer therapy.

Eighty to 100 per cent of advanced bladder cancers are detectable by cytologic examination of the urine. But what of early cancers? Several investigators have reported finding in-situ cancer and grade I papillary carcinoma with a high degree of reliability. Although the data for this are not very great when combined with the studies in a high risk population like the Beta-naphthylamine workers where early cancer has been detected in 80 per cent of the cases it would suggest that cytologic examination of the urine is a useful cancer detection method, particularly in a high risk population. Does a detection examination among the asymptomatic reduce the risk of death? Since bladder cancer is relatively uncommon except in a high risk population the data are lacking on the effect of detection efforts on the risk of death in the asymptomatic patient.

4. Cancer Site for which there is no Evidence that Cancer Detection will Favorably Influence the Survival Advantage

Lung Cancer

Dr. GRUNZE pointed out that presently there is no single technique or combination of techniques available for the detection of lung cancer that provide results comparable to those in the early detection of cervix, oral, colon-rectum, or breast cancer.

Panel 3

New Facts in Environmental Cancer
Qualitative and Quantitative Aspects

Chairman:

R. Truhaut (France)

Members:

W. Butler (U.K.), G. J. van Esch (Netherlands), W. C. Hueper (U.S.A.),
M. Miyake (Japan), U. Saffiotti (U.S.A.), L. M. Shabad (U.S.S.R.),
M. Spatz (U.S.A.)

Panel 4

Cancer Chemotherapy

Chairman:

C. C. Stock (U.S.A.)

Members:

B. R. Baker (U.S.A.), G. Brulé (France), T. A. Connors (U.K.), T. C. Hall
(U.S.A.), W. Rundles (U.S.A.), Y. Sakurai (Japan)

Panel 5

Structure and Biochemistry of Tumor Cells

Chairman:

R. Kinosita (U.S.A.)

Members:

G. Barski (France), P. Emmelot (Netherlands), H. Lettré (F.R.G.), H. V. Gelboin (U.S.A.), R. M. Love (U.S.A.), W. Nakahara (Japan), S. Ohno (U.S.A.), J. S. Sorof (U.S.A.), T. Yamamoto (Japan), H. Busch (U.S.A.)

Panel 6

Immunological Aspects of Cancer

Chairman:

P. Grabar (France)

Members:

V. Shevljaghyn (U.S.S.R.), P. Burtin (France), K. Habel (U.S.A.), H. Hirai (Japan), E. Klein (Sweden), J. L. Melnick (U.S.A.), F. Milgrom (U.S.A.), C. M. Southam (U.S.A.), D. E. H. Tee (U.K.)

Panel 7

Viruses and Cancer

Chairman:

M. G. P. STOKER (U.K.)

Members:

R. DULBECCO (U.S.A.), M. GREEN (U.S.A.), H. HANAFUSA (Japan),
Y. ITO (Japan), G. KLEIN (Sweden), F. RAPP (U.S.A.), P. VIGIER (France)

Panel 8

Pathology of Spread of Cancer
and Metastasis Formation

Chairman:

P. DENOIX (France)

Members:

M. ABERCROMBIE (U.K.), F. LACOUR (France), H. SATO (Japan),
C. M. SOUTHAM (U.S.A.), P. STRÄULI (Switzerland), S. WOOD, jr. (U.S.A.),
J. LEIGHTON (U.S.A.)

Panel 9

Biochemistry of Carcinogenesis

Chairman:

J. A. MILLER (U.S.A.)

Members:

P. BROOKES (U.K.), E. HECKER (F.R.G.), C. HEIDELBERGER (U.S.A.),
P. N. MAGEE (U.K.), H. TERAYAMA (Japan)

Panel 10

Biological Aspects of Carcinogenesis

Chairman:

H. S. KAPLAN (U.S.A.)

Members:

M. ABERCROMBIE (U.K.), K. DAN (Japan), G. KLEIN (Sweden),
R. T. PREHN (U.S.A.)

Panel 11

Cancer of the Nasopharynx

Chairman:

K. Shanmugaratnam (Singapore)

Members:

J. C. Bailar, III (U.S.A.), A. J. Ballantyne (U.S.A.), J. Clemmesen (Denmark), P. Clifford (Kenya), H. C. Ho (Hong Kong), R. Preussmann (West Germany), C. Sirtori (Italy)

Summary

Incidence

In most countries of the world, and in most human races, nasopharyngeal cancer is a rare neoplasm. On the other hand, this neoplasm occurs with extraordinarily high frequencies among Chinese and among some of the peoples of Southeast Asia. An elevated frequency has also been reported in some tribes of Kenya.

Dr. Clemmesen discussed the incidence of the neoplasm in Europe, a low incidence area, with particular reference to Scandinavian experience. It is probable that the largest population under registration for malignant neoplasms is represented by the Scandinavian countries (Denmark, Finland, Iceland, Norway, and Sweden) with a total of about 20 million inhabitants[1]. The incidence rates for nasopharyngeal cancer in Norway for the years 1959—1961 are 0.4 per 100,000 per annum for males and 0.1 for females. In Denmark the incidence rates for combined cancers of the pharynx (i. e. including pharynx, hypopharynx and pharynx unspecified) were 0.8 per 100,000 for males and 0.4 for females for the period 1943—1957, based on 259 and 123 cases respectively.

Dr. Ho reviewed the incidence in China, a high incidence area, with particular reference to Hongkong. In 1965 there were 661 "new" cases of nasopharyngeal cancer from the Hongkong population, 75 per cent of which were confirmed by nasopharyngeal biopsy, giving a crude incidence of 25.2 per 100,000 for males and 10.6 for females. In a series of 1,438 consecutive cases

---

[1] It should be noted in this context that Sweden so far restricts registration to patients visiting hospitals (out- and in-patients).

seen during 1956—61 the peak age specific incidence was in the 40—44 age group in both sexes. An analysis of a smaller series of 367 cases in 1961 (Census year) showed the peak incidence rate to be in the 40—44 group in males and in the 60—64 age group in females; the peak age specific incidence was, however, also in the 40—44 group in both sexes. In China the incidence is particularly high in the Southern Provinces. In Hongkong the crude and standardised incidence rates were significantly higher in Chinese originating from the Southern Chinese province of Kwantung than in Chinese from central coastal provinces; the incidence was particularly high among the so-called "Tan Ka" or boat people of Hongkong who traditionally lived in boats and seldom settled ashore. Dr. Ho also reported an incidence rate of 26.7 per 100,000 per annum among the Hongkong Macaonese; such a high incidence among persons of mixed Chinese-Portuguese descent is most interesting but it was noted that the rate was derived from a small number of cases — 4 cases seen during the period 1959—1963 in a small population, roughly estimated to be about 3,000 persons.

Dr. SHANMUGARATNAM reviewed the incidence of the disease in Southeast Asia where high relative frequencies have been reported in Indonesia, Malaya, Philippines, Singapore, Thailand and Vietnam. In these countries the highest frequencies are found in persons of the Chinese race, but the frequencies in Malays, Indonesians, Vietnamese, Thais and Filipinos are also higher than in Western populations. In Singapore there were 1019 histologically diagnosed primary carcinomas of the nasopharynx in the period 1950—1961. The age adjusted *minimum* incidence rate, using SEGI's (1960) standard population, was particularly high among the Chinese, being 14.4 per 100,000 per annum for males and 5.6 for females; it was also significantly raised in Malays, being 2.4 for males and 2.0 for females (the true incidence is probably much higher in view of the relative infrequency with which Malay patients report to hospital) but low in Indians, being only 0.7 for males (there were no cases among female Indians). Nasopharyngeal cancer is rare in other parts of Asia, viz. Japan, Ceylon and India.

Dr. CLIFFORD discussed the incidence of the disease in Kenya. Between the years 1961—1965, 177 Kenyan African patients with nasopharyngeal cancer were found at the Kenyatta National Hospital in Nairobi. In both the Bantu and the Nilo-Hamitic groups the highest incidences occurred in those tribes which occupy the higher and colder areas of Kenya, e. g. the Kikuyu (57 cases — incidence rates of 1.01 per 100,000 for males and 0.36 for females), and the Embu/Meru (15 cases — 0.83 for males and 0.29 for females) — both central Bantu, and the Kipsigis (13 cases — 1.05 for males and 0.47 for females) and the Nandi (12 cases — 2.40 for males and 0.46 for females) — both Nilo-Hamitic. The disease showed a significantly lower incidence among the coastal Bantu living in the hot coastal areas of Kenya and in the Nilo-Hamitic tribes who live in hot desert country.

Dr. BAILAR stated that approximately 0.5 to 2 per cent of cancers at cancer treatment centres and approximately 0.2 per cent of cancers at cancer registries were primary in the nasopharynx; in Chinese populations more than 10 per cent of neoplasms were primary in the nasopharynx. The high incidence among the Chinese persists among persons migrating to areas where they are surrounded by, and to some extent mingle with, persons of European origin e.g. in New York City, California, Havana, Hawaii and elsewhere. ZIPPIN and others found a higher frequency among immigrant Chinese males in the United States than among Chinese males born in U.S. However, both groups had rates substantially above those in white populations. Unfortunately, the number of cases was very small (31 Chinese male patients with place of birth known) and the possibility remains that there may have been errors in statements of birthplace either in patient records or in the census data. An elevated risk has also been reported in populations unrelated to the Chinese — in Kenya and perhaps in parts of North Africa.

Regarding the commonly stated observation that nasopharyngeal cancer occurs at relatively younger ages, Dr. BAILAR found that in four predominantly white populations covered by cancer registers (Connecticut, New York, Norway and Sweden), the proportion of young patients was indeed higher than for all forms of cancer (6 per cent of patients being below the age of 30 and 30 per cent below the age of 50), but this differences is not as large as might be expected from statements in the literature. The fact that the average age of Chinese patients with nasopharyngeal cancer is lower than that of European patients may result entirely from the fact that the average age of Chinese without the disease is also lower than that of Europeans.

Aetiology

Dr. Ho did not support the common belief that carcinogens of domestic origin, such as cooking smoke in ill-ventilated houses, were aetiologically involved in nasopharyngeal cancer; this view does not accord with the finding of significantly higher incidence rates among males and among the "Tan—Ka" who live practically all their lives in boats and cook in the open. He also stated that the rarity of the cancer in Buddhist monks, nuns and temple keepers, who spend most of their time in incense-laden atmospheres, did not support incense as an aetiological factor. He found that the neoplasm showed no relationship with ABO blood groups, birth order, occupation, socio-economic status, vitamin or other nutritional deficiencies, chronic vasomotor rhinitis and nasal or pharyngeal infections. On the other hand, in two separate series totalling 1180 cases of nasopharyngeal cancer he found 15 patients whose family histories were highly suggestive of this neoplasm: 8 male patients had a brother with the disease, 1 male patient — two brothers, 2 male patients — sister, 1 male patient — father, 1 male patient — aunt, 1 female patient — brother and 1 female patient had a family history with a clustering of cases extending over three generations. He therefore supported the view that there was a genetically determined tendency or predisposition to develop nasopharyngeal cancer.

Dr. CLIFFORD presented some data on the ABO blood distribution of a series of cases in Kenya which suggested that Group A persons are "protected" against nasopharyngeal cancer. It has also been noted that in some areas of Southeast Asia where the incidence of nasopharyngeal carcinoma is relatively high, the general pattern of blood group gene frequencies is characterised by a relatively low A and high B. On the other hand the high incidence of the cancer in the higher and colder areas of Kenya was unrelated to the ethnographical distribution of the population and hence supported an environmental aetiology. The population in these areas lives in poorly ventilated huts in which there is a fire burning most of the day and for many hours of the night; carcinogenic hydrocarbons were isolated from specimens of soot taken from the roofs of huts of 44 patients of nasopharyngeal cancer. Commenting on the internal factors that may have an aetiological relationship with nasopharyngeal cancer, Dr. CLIFFORD stated that nasopharyngeal carcinoma appears to have a high incidence in some population groups which have the following characteristics:— (1) high nasal index — platyrrhine: (2) high frequency of severe vasomotor rhinitis; (3) Vitamin A and other dietary deficiencies; (4) increased oestrogenisation in males. Studies on the Kenyan population have shown that the excretion of oestrone, oestradiol-17, and oestriol was higher than that of Caucasian males, and the difference was more marked in cancer patients. The excretion of 11-deoxy-17-oxosteroids was much lower in Kenya African males than in a comparable Caucasian group, and the difference was most noticeable in patients with nasopharyngeal cancer. While the effect of adrenocortical activity on the nasal mucosa and cavernous tissue is uncertain, it is known that these tissues are sensitive to oestrogens — an increase in the circulating level of these hormones producing a form of vasomotor rhinitis with swelling and vasodilatation of the nasal mucosa and increased secretion of mucus.

Dr. PREUSSMANN discussed the experimental induction of cancers of the nasal and pharyngeal regions in laboratory animals (BD strain rats) by several nitrosamines. He reviewed some of the relationships between chemical structure and carcinogenic activity of N-nitroso compounds. Several nitrosamine compounds produced carcinomas of the nasal cavity and pharynx even after parenteral administration. These results indicate that cancers of the nasal and pharyngeal regions are not necessarily due to direct contact but can originate from systemic acting carcinogens.

Summing up the discussion, Dr. SHANMUGARATNAM stated that there was insufficient data to determine whether genetic or environmental factors are more important in the aetiology of nasopharyngeal cancer. The genetic hypothesis is supported by (a) the high incidence in Chinese populations in several countries, (b) the high frequencies of the disease among races of Mongoloid stock in Southeast Asia, (c) the low incidence in persons of non-Mongoloid stock residing in high incidence areas, and (d) the essentially negative results obtained in a few retrospective questionnaire studies on several suspected carcinogens. On the other hand, an environmental hypothesis is supported by (a) the reported distribution of the disease among Kenyans who have no genetic relationship with the Chinese, (b) reports suggesting that the incidence of nasopharyngeal cancer in Chinese born and living in America, although higher than in Caucasian people there, is lower than in Chinese immigrants who were born in China, (c) reports of an increased risk among the poorer classes and among persons exposed to certain wood fuel fumes in Kenya, (d) the fact that most of the neoplasms are squamous cell carcinomas which are mostly associated with environmental carcinogens, and (e) the experimental production of cancers of the nasal cavity and pharynx in laboratory animals by several nitrosamines. The panelists agreed that the arguments favouring the genetic and environmental hypotheses are neither conclusive nor mutually exclusive and that it is reasonable to postulate that some environmental factor or factors may exert a triggering effect in genetically susceptible persons.

Histopathology

The nasopharynx is lined by respiratory, squamous and transitional epithelia and contains various glandular, lymphoid and connective tissue elements. Consequently a wide range of neoplasms has been identified in this area. However, in areas with a high incidence of nasopharyngeal cancer the overwhelming majority of neoplasms belongs to that much debated group which has been variously termed squamous cell carcinoma, lymphoepithelioma, transitional cell carcinoma, etc. The majority of neoplasms present a characteristic "undifferentiated" appearance; there is a syncytial appearance due to poorly defined cell membranes and the nuclei are pale and vesicular and have prominent nucleoli. Several histological types have been described, but there is now widespread agreement that all are variants of squamous cell carcinoma — a view supported by the electron microscopic demonstration of keratin fibrils in undifferentiated tumours, including those classified as "lymphoepithelioma" and "transitional cell carcinoma" by light microscopy.

Dr. SHANMUGARATNAM illustrated the various histological variants of nasopharyngeal carcinoma and stated that in Europe and America, where the incidence is low, the ratio of carcinoma to sarcoma ranges between 3:1 to 7:1. On the other hand, in China and Southeast Asia where the incidence is high, the ratio is approximately 99:1. This ratio, therefore, may give a good idea of the prevalence of nasopharyngeal cancer in any population.

Dr. SIRTORI stated that the peculiar histological features of the undifferentiated variant of nasopharyngeal carcinoma (that he calls "nasopharyngioma") could enable histopathologists to suggest a nasopharyngeal primary after the examination of lymph node metastases. Dr. SIRTORI also presented the results of his electron microscopic studies on this neoplasm. The ciliated cells of the normal mucosa showed active pinocytosis, numerous cilia often united in groups and surrounded by common plasma membranes, numerous mitochondria, ribosomes, polysomes, rough surfaced endoplasmic reticulum and a distinct Golgi apparatus situated over the nucleus. Dr. SIRTORI found that electron microscopy of nasopharyngeal carcinomas revealed the presence of "introverted cilia" i. e. cilia incorporated in the cytoplasm like tubules instead of fluctuating on the surface.

Clinical features

Dr. BALLANTYNE reviewed the clinical features of nasopharyngeal cancer. The symptomatology of the disease, which may well be predicted by a knowledge of the anatomy or site of origin and manner of spread, may be divided into those dependent on blockage of nares or Eustachian tubes, bleeding, neurological symptoms and symptoms due to the presence of metastatic cervical nodes. Of all cancers of the head and neck region, those of epithelial origin in the nasopharynx have the highest incidence of regional lymph node metastasis and of extension into the cranial cavity. Frequently, the metastasis to the cervical nodes forms the dominant part of the disease and it is not at all unusual to find relatively massive cervical adenopathy from a primary tumour which is insignificant or poorly detectable. The second characteristic, that of intracranial spread is occasioned by the anatomical location of the tumor and its biological behaviour. Dr. BALLANTYNE mentioned the value of diagnostic X-ray studies and recommended laminography of the nasopharyngeal region both as a baseline prior to treatment and as a method of evaluating the extension of the tumor into bony structures which would not be recognised clinically.

Treatment

Most neoplasms are radiosensitive and radiation therapy is the treatment of choice. Some chemotherapeutic agents may be tried, but surgery has little place in the curative management of nasopharyngeal cancer.

Dr. Ho outlined the problems of radiation therapy. The irradiated volume in the treatment of nasopharyngeal carcinoma contains bones and gas-containing cavities in addition to soft tissue. For such a heterogenous medium 4—8 MeV X-rays or gamma rays from a kilocurie telecobalt unit are preferable to high energy electrons and orthovolt X-rays, because there will be less differential absorption of radiation and as a result the dose delivered to the target volume will be nearer homogeneity. The target volume which contains the tumor and the parts of head and neck which are considered to be potentially involved by the spread of the tumor would depend on the size and shape of the head and neck, and the stage of the disease. The decision to offer radical or palliative treatment is influenced by (a) age, general condition and concurrent disease, and (b) stage of the disease. Age is only a contra-indication to radical treatment if the patient is debilitated and is not expected to live much longer. As to the stage of the disease, radical treatment may be given as long as there is absence of haematogenous metastasis, or involvement of lymph nodes in the supraclavicular fossa or beyond, or involvement of lower cervical nodes in addition to extensive local disease, or involvement of several cranial nerves due to multi-directional spread, or extensive destruction of the base of the skull. The 5-year apparent cure rate following a radical course of radiotherapy is at least 50 per cent, in Stage I cases (cases with tumor confined to nasopharynx) and the over-all 5-year survival is about 20 per cent. Dr. Ho discussed briefly the radio-therapeutic technique, dosage, treatment results and the complications of radio-therapy and their prevention.

Dr. CLIFFORD accepted that radiotherapy is the most effective form of treatment for nasopharyngeal cancer, but as this form of therapy is not yet available in East Africa, he relied on cancer chemotherapy. Without treatment, the late stages of this disease can cause acute pain and severe misery to the patients most whom arrive in hospital when the disease is far advanced.

Panel 12

Chorioepithelioma

Chairman:

J. F. HOLLAND (U.S.A.)

Members:

K. D. BAGSHAWE (U.K.), T. HASEGAWA (Japan), P. HENDRICKSE (Nigeria),
R. HERTZ (U.S.A.), N. ISHIZUKA (Japan), W. W. PARK (U.K.)

Panel 13

Radiation as a Cancer Hazard in Man

Chairman:

S. WATANABE (Japan)

Members:

R. DOLL (U.K.), H. KAPLAN (U.S.A.), W. C. HUEPER (U.S.A.),
J. W. PIFER (U.S.A.), R. L. SWARM (U.S.A.), S. TAKAHASHI (Japan),
K. TSUKAMOTO (Japan), M. MIYAKAWA (Japan)

Chairman's remarks at the opening of the Panel Discussion on "Radiation as a cancer hazard in man".

Ladies and Gentlemen:

At the opening this session, I would like to make a few brief introductory remarks. It is now well established in experimental animals that every sort of radiation can induce various types of neoplasia. Whether this apparent carcinogenic property of radiation in animals can (how far and how much) be applied to the human is an important question. So far, the available data in the human are rather limited. Therefore, it is quite important to make an effort to accumulate such cases in the human. And the data should be carefully analysed in order to make the correct interpretation. Furthermore, it should be stressed that the potential hazard of radiation in our daily life may become a serious problem by increasing use of various types of radiation in industrial and medical fields. In this connection, I believe that we are fortunate in having an opportunity to hear and discuss the problems of radiation carcinogenesis in man which will be presented by experts in this field.

To open our discussion, Dr. DOLL will present extensive data on the development of leukemia and other neoplasms among patients with ankylosing spondylitis or metropathia haemorrhagica treated with x-rays in Britain. Then, Dr. PIFER will present data on the induction of thyroid tumors among people who had been treated by X-rays for an enlarged thymus during childhood. Dr.

Tsukamoto will discuss the incidence of leukemia among the A-bomb survivors in Japan. Dr. Hueper will present the development of lung cancers in the uranium miners in U.S.A. Dr. Takahashi and Dr. Miyakawa will report the appearance of various types of liver tumors as a result of internal irradiation with thorotrast. Finally, Dr. Egawa will make a brief comment on the induction of tumors in various tissues after radiation therapy in his clinic.

Now, I call Dr. Doll as the first speaker.

Neoplasia in Patients Treated with X-rays for Ankylosing Spondylitis or Metropathia Haemorrhagica

W. M. Court Brown[1], Richard Doll[2], and P. Smith[1]

[1] Medical Research Council, Clinical Effects of Radiation Research Unit,
Western General Hospital, Edinburgh
and
[2] Medical Research Council, Statistical Research Unit, University College
Hospital Medical School, London

When, in 1955, Court Brown and Abbatt, and van Swaay independently reported that patients with ankylosing spondylitis who had been treated by X-ray therapy developed an unusually high incidence of leukaemia, it was evident that they might form a particularly suitable group for studying the long-term effects of irradiation. A large number of patients had been treated over the preceding 20 years, the dose of radiation varied over a wide range, the patients were kept under prolonged medical observation, the general mortality rate among them was not high, and there were not thought to be any complications of the disease that would mask the diagnosis of leukaemia or other cancers. The principal disadvantage was that they were likely to be given drugs, some of which might conceivably have an independent carcinogenic effect.

In Britain a large-scale investigation was initiated under the auspices of the Medical Research Council and with the co-operation of all the leading radiotherapists. The preliminary results were reported by Court Brown and Doll in 1957, by which time it was evident that the early suspicions of an increased mortality from leukaemia were confirmed and that the experience of the patients was similar to that of the survivors of the atomic bomb explosions in Hiroshima and Nagasaki. Over an average of $6^{1}/_{2}$ years from the time of first irradiation, the leukaemia mortality was about 10 times what would have been expected in the absence of irradiation, the excess mortality was confined to acute leukaemia and chronic myeloid leukaemia, and the incidence was approximately proportional to the mean marrow dose summed over all areas and all treatment periods. When the results were extrapolated to low doses it was calculated that one rad to the whole marrow produced approximately 1 to 2 cases of leukaemia per million persons per year for the first few years after irradiation (COURT BROWN and DOLL, 1959).

This study has now been continued for more than 10 years and COURT BROWN and DOLL (1965) have recently shown that the mortality from cancer of many parts of the body that were directly irradiated was also increased

Table I. *Characteristics of study series.*

Characteristic	Patients irradiated for:	
	ankylosing spondylitis	metropathia haemorrhagica
No. of patients, men	12,161	0
women	2,393	2,068
Date of first treatment	1935—54	1940—60
Date of follow-up	Jan. 1st, 1960	Jan. 1st, 1964
Mean period of observations (years)	11.3	13.6
Per cent traced	98.3	99.3
Typical skin dose (rads)	900—2,000	550—1,050
Typical site of irradiation	whole spine and sacro-iliac joints	anterior and posterior pelvis
Repeat treatments per cent	48	0

— though to a much less extent than occurred with leukaemia. In round figures the excess mortality from all other cancers was approximately equal to that from leukaemia; it began to appear 6 years after irradiation and was still present — and possibly still increasing — 15 years after.

In the present paper, we report briefly some of the main observations on leukaemia and cancer mortality in the spondylitic patients, compare them with similar observations on a group of women who had received pelvic irradiation to produce an artificial menopause (COURT BROWN, DOLL and SMITH, 1967), and examine in greater detail the duration of the latent period before the appearance of disease. No attempt will be made to relate the observations to the dose of radiation, as we are in the process of re-examining the dose by a more accurate method.

The main characteristics of the two series are shown in Table I. From these it would appear that the women who were irradiated for uterine haemorrhage received a dose to the irradiated marrow of the same order as that received by the patients with spondylitis. They received, however, a substantially lower total dose as the amount of marrow directly irradiated was smaller and the treatment was not repeated. The periods of observations are also approximately the same, ranging from 5 to 25 years with a mean of 11.3 in the case of the spondylitics and from 3 to 24 years with a mean of 13.6 in the case of the women with uterine haemorrhage.

Mortality after Irradiation

The total mortality experiences of the two groups of patients are shown in Table II for three main categories — (i) those due to leukaemia, (ii) those due to cancers of directly and heavily irradiated sites, and (iii) those due to cancers

Table II. *Deaths by cause, showing number observed and number observed as proportion of expected.*

Cause of death	Deaths among patients irradiated for:			
	ankylosing spondylitis		metropathia haemorrhagica	
	No. observed	Observed as proportion of expected	No. observed	Observed as proportion of expected
Leukaemia	52	9.5	6	4.6
Cancer of heavily irradiated sites	200	1.6	33	1.3
Cancer of lightly-, or un-irradiated sites	60	1.1	29	1.1
Cancer of colon	25	1.7	—	—
Cancer of breast	—	—	9	0.6
Cancer generalized, primary unknown	—	—	3	(4.1)
Aplastic anaemia	15	29.4	2	(16.7)
Other causes	1,230	1.8	163	1.0
All causes	1,582	1.8	245	1.0

of lightly or unirradiated sites. Deaths from cancer of the colon are also shown separately in the spondylitic group, because colon cancer is associated with ulcerative colitis which is associated with ankylosing spondylitis irrespective of irradiation; and cancer of the breast is shown separately in the metropathia group because any form of artificial menopause is believed to reduce its incidence. Deaths due to generalized cancer of unknown primary sites are classified under heavily irradiated sites in the spondylitis group, because most of the important types of cancer that present in this way arise from sites that would have been heavily irradiated. This is not true for metropathia and, in this group, they have been shown separately.

For both groups of patients the results show a substantial and statistically significant increase in the mortality from leukaemia — greater in the case of the spondylitics than of the women with metropathia. Both also show a significant, but relatively small, increase in the mortality from cancers in heavily irradiated sites. Neither show any appreciable increase in mortality from cancers of lightly or unirradiated sites. Both groups, it may be noted, also show an excess mortality from aplastic anaemia. A few of these deaths occurred in patients who developed symptoms shortly after irradiation, and may be attributed directly to the treatment. Most occurred a few years later and may well represent cases of unrecognized aleukaemic leukaemia.

In contrast to these similarities the two groups of patients differ markedly in their mortality from all other causes combined. In the spondylitis group this is substantially raised; in the metropathia group it is almost identical with that of other women of the same ages over the same period in the same country. This difference is not unexpected, as spondylitis is a disease with an appreciable morbidity and numerous complications — including, for example, amyloid disease, aortic regurgitation, ulcerative colitis and pulmonary tuberculosis.

Taken by itself, the increase in mortality from all other causes among the spondylitics could, however, suggest the possibility that they suffered a generally increased mortality from a non-specific cause — possibly associated with the spondylitis itself, or possibly due to an "ageing" effect of radiation. Taken in conjunction with the evidence of the metropathia group, this hypothesis is not attractive. It seems more likely that the increase in mortality from leukaemia, cancer of heavily irradiated sites and aplastic anaemia is, in both groups, attributable to the irradiation, whereas the increase in mortality from other causes in the spondylitis group is due to a multiplicity of separate causes associated with the underlying disease.

Distribution of Latent Periods

This conclusion is supported by an analysis of the time relations between the date of first treatment and the date of death. Figs. 1 and 2 show the trend in the ratio of the observed to the expected deaths in the spondylitis group. For these data all observations have been included that have been made before 1st January, 1963. The proportion of patients traced to this date is lower, but the numbers of deaths recorded is known to be practically complete, and the longer follow-up provides more useful information about longer periods after treatment. For leukaemia and aplastic anaemia the ratio rises rapidly and reaches a peak 3 to 8 years after first treatment, and then falls. For cancers of heavily irradiated sites it begins high, due clearly to the inclusion of a few patients who presented with pain in the back from secondary deposits which was thought to be due to a recrudescence of their spondylitis; it then falls, to rise again steadily 6 and more years after first irradiation. For these diseases, the trends accord with the distribution of latent periods after irradiation expected from other observations. For cancers of lightly irradiated sites and for other diseases, no trend in the ratio with time is observed at all — which accords with the hypothesis that they are unrelated to the treatment.

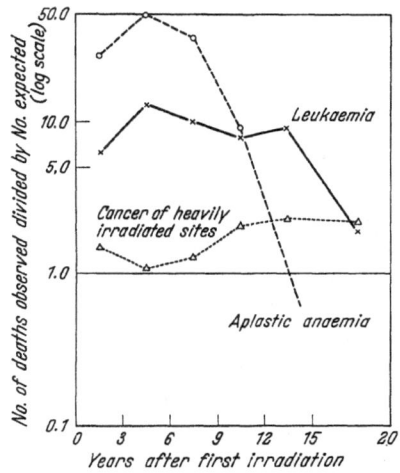

Fig. 1. Trend in the ratio of observed to expected deaths with the passage of time after first irradiation: aplastic anaemia, leukaemia and other cancer of heavily irradiated sites in patients treated for ankylosing spondylitis

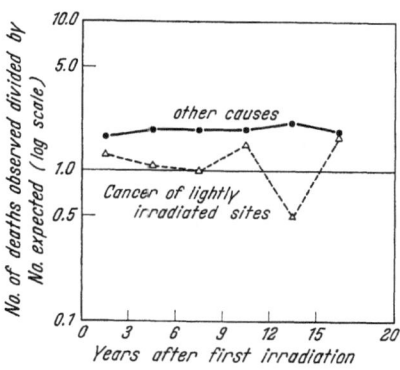

Fig. 2. Trend in the ratio of observed to expected deaths with the passage of time after first irradiation: cancer of lightly irradiated sites and "other causes" in patients observed for ankylosing spondylitis

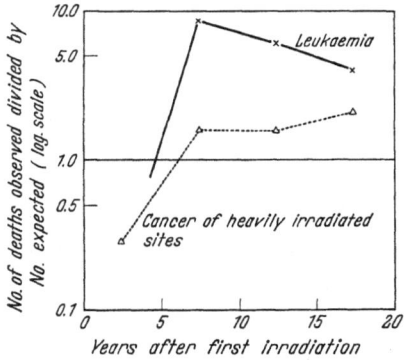

Fig. 3. Trend in the ratio of observed to expected deaths with the passage of time after first irradiation: leukaemia and cancer of heavily irradiated sites in patients treated for metropathia haemorrhagica

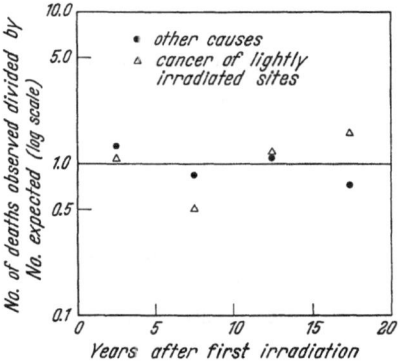

Fig. 4. Trend in the ratio of observed to expected deaths with the passage of time after first irradiation: cancer of lightly irradiated sites and "other causes" in patients treated for metropathia haemorrhagica

Observations on the women with metropathia are shown in Figs. 3 and 4. For each disease group the trend is similar to that in the spondylitics, but the numbers are less and the variation is correspondingly less regular.

But if the data provide good evidence of the qualitative effect of irradiation, they are only a weak foundation for estimating it quantitatively. The metropathia series is small and the results are subject to large sampling errors, while half the patients in the larger spondylitis series were given repeated courses of treatment at intervals ranging from a few months to over 10 years. More accurate information can be obtained, however, by limiting the observations to patients who had had only one course of treatment[1] and taking a weighted average of the data for both series.

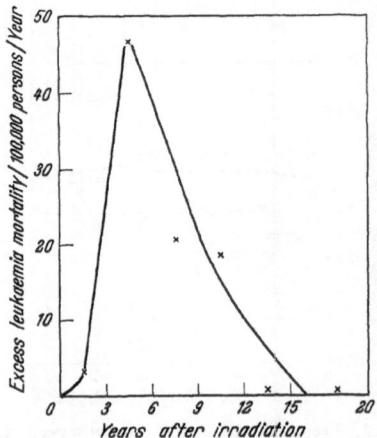

Fig. 5. Death rate from leukaemia attributable to irradiation at different periods after treatment: patients with ankylosing spondylitis or metropathia haemorrhagica treated once only

The results obtained in this way are shown for leukaemia in Fig. 5. In this case, observations are included up to the end of 1965, as information is available about all deaths attributed to leukaemia before this date. The excess mortality attributed to irradiation is obtained by subtracting the expected number of deaths from the observed number in each period and dividing by the number of person-years at risk. The results suggest that the risk rises rapidly to a maximum 3 to 5 years after irradiation and then falls more slowly to disappear about 15 years after irradiation. The numbers of deaths on which the points are based are not large (2, 14, 6, 5, 1 and 1 respectively), but the regularity of their arrangement justifies some confidence in the general conclusion. This conclusion will, however, need to be reviewed if the trend of the results differs from that observed in Hiroshima and Nagasaki.

Type of Leukaemia

Evidence of the type of leukaemia induced can be obtained from the total material, including patients who have been treated on more than one occasion. Altogether there are 84 patients in both series who have been diagnosed as having leukaemia after review of the clinical and haematological evidence, and 70 were certified as dying of the disease. One other patient was also certified as dying of leukaemia; but, on review, the diagnosis was not sustained. Of the remaining 14 patients accepted as having leukaemia, 2 are still alive, 8 were certified as dying of aplastic anaemia and in 4 others the cause of death was attributed to some other cause. The distribution of the various clinical and

---

[1] Including in the observations that part of the life history of patients who had repeated treatments, that occurred between their first and their second courses.

cytological types is shown in Table III. About 10 cases would have been expected in all, in the absence of irradiation, and the major risk is clearly limited to the myeloid series. It is, however, possible that there may also be a slight increase in the risk of inducing lymphatic leukaemia — proportionally comparable, perhaps, to the increased risk of inducing cancer in tissues other than the marrow.

Table III. *Types of leukaemia.*

Diagnosis	Number according to death certificates	Number after review of evidence
Myeloid leukaemia:		
acute	24	35
chronic	6	15
type uncertain	7	2
Lymphatic leukaemia:		
acute	6	4
chronic	2	3
type uncertain	4	0
Unspecified leukaemia:		
acute	14	14
chronic	1	0
type uncertain	7	11*
Unknown:		
still alive	2	0
Other causes:		
aplastic anaemia	8	0
other disease	4	1
Total	85	85

* including 9 not yet fully reviewed

Summary

Patients irradiated for ankylosing spondylitis or metropathia haemorrhagica have been followed-up from the time of irradiation and the mortality among them compared with the national experience.

Both groups of patients show an excess mortalitiy from leukaemia and from cancer in heavily irradiated sites.

The temporal distribution of leukaemia deaths suggests that the peak mortality attributable to irradiation occurs 3 to 5 years after exposure and that the risk may be largely over, 15 years after.

Cytological examination suggests that the leukaemia risk is largely limited to acute and chronic leukaemias of the myeloid type.

References

COURT BROWN, W. M., and ABBATT, J. D.,
The incidence of leukaemia in ankylosing
spondylitics treated with X-rays. *Lancet*
I, 1283 (1955).
—, and DOLL, R., Leukaemia and aplastic
anaemia in patients irradiated for ankylosing spondylitis. *Spec. Rep. Ser. med.
Res. Counc. (Lond.)* No. 295 (1957).
— — The study of delayed radiation effects
among individual spondylitics. *Report to
I. C. R. P.*, Munich Conference 1959.

COURT BROWN, W. M., and ABBATT, J. D.,
Mortality from cancer and other causes
after radiotherapy for ankylosing spondylitis. *Brit. med. J.* II, 1327 (1965).
— —, and SMITH, P., The long-term effects
of X-irradiation for metropathia haemorrhagica. *To be published* 1967.
SWAAY, H. VAN, Aplastic anaemia and
myeloid leukaemia after irradiation of
the vertebral column. *Lancet* II, 225
(1955).

Neoplasms in Man after Irradiation in Infancy *

L. H. HEMPELMANN and J. W. PIFER

*Division of Experimental Radiology, University of Rochester School
of Medicine and Dentistry, Rochester, New York, U. S. A.*

In this paper, we present the results of the third follow-up survey of a
series of approximately 3,000 persons treated with X-rays in infancy for
thymic enlargement. This epidemiologic study of the relationship between
radiation exposure and the subsequent development of neoplastic disease has
been conducted at the University of Rochester School of Medicine and Dentistry
during the past 12 years (SIMPSON et al., 1955; SIMPSON and HEMPELMANN,
1957; PIFER et al., 1963; TOYOOKA et al., 1963 a, b). The names of the irradiated
subjects were abstracted from the records of all hospitals and radiologists' offices
in Rochester, New York; X-ray treatments were given during the period,
1926—1957. During this time, it was common medical practice in the United
States to treat infants with X-rays for enlargement of the thymus gland. The
majority of the subjects were irradiated during the first six months of life —
many, a few days after birth. The data on tumor incidence in this irradiated
population was collected in 1963 by mail questionnaire sent to the subjects, or
to their parents. Eighty-four per cent of the total group responded to the
questionnaire. All indications of neoplastic disease or other serious illness were
verified by consulting medical records. Histological sections of all excised
tumors were reviewed, when possible, by one of the University pathologists
(ROGER TERRY, M. D.).

Table I summarizes the characteristics of the study population and the
radiation factors used in their treatment. More detailed data may be found in

* Supported in part, by a grant from the National Institutes of Health (RH 00210).

a previous publication (PIFER *et al.*, 1963). The study population consists of 2,878 irradiated subjects and their 5,006 untreated siblings who were used as non-irradiated controls. The average age of the irradiated subjects was

Table I. *Summary of characteristics of population and treatment factors*

	Treated subjects	Untreated siblings
Number	2,878	5,006
Mean age (yrs.)	17.4	16.4
Mean air dose (r)	222	
Mean port size (cm²)	43.9	
Port arrangement (per cent):		
Anterior only	75	
Posterior only	3	
A and P	17	
Not ascertained	5	

Table II. *Observed and expected number of selected types of neoplasms*

Type of neoplasm	Treated patients		Untreated patients	
	Observed	Expected	Observed	Expected
Malignant	33	8.1	14	14.6
Benign	62		32	
Total	95		46	
Malignant neoplasms:				
Thyroid	19	0.1	0	0.3
Leukemia	6	2.0	2	3.2
Salivary gland	4	0.1	1	0.2
Other	4	5.8	11	10.9
Benign neoplasms:				
Thyroid	22	1.6	3	3.1
Osteochondroma	15	—	0	—
Ratio: Thyroid Carcinoma				
$\dfrac{\text{Observed}}{\text{Expected}}$	$\dfrac{19}{0.14} = 136$		$\dfrac{0}{0.31}$	

approximately 17 years in 1963, and that of the controls, 16 years. The mean air dose used in treatment was 222 roentgens of orthovoltage X-rays (range, 25—1,250 r) and the average port size was slightly less than 6×8 cm². Almost all X-ray treatments were given to the anterior chest, however, 17 per cent were administered to the anterior and posterior chest.

Table II presents the observed and expected numbers of selected types of neoplasms for the treated and sibling populations. The expected numbers were calculated using the person-years-at-risk in five-year age categories for each group and the age-specific cancer rates for the general population of this geographic area. A total of 95 neoplasms was reported in the irradiated group, compared with 46 in almost twice as many untreated siblings. Thirty-three of the neoplasms in the irradiated population were malignant, whereas about eight cases were expected — a fourfold increase over expectation. In contrast, the number of malignancies in the untreated brothers and sisters was not excessive — 14 cases vs. 14.6 expected. The majority of the 25 excess cancers in the treated group are accounted for by the 19 cases of thyroid cancer. As can be seen in Table II, only one-tenth of a case of thyroid carcinoma was expected, resulting in a 136-fold increase over expectation. The other excess cases of malignant disease in the treated group are accounted for by the six cases of leukemia and the four cases of salivary gland tumors.

Table II shows that the number of benign neoplastic lesions in the irradiated and non-irradiated populations was 62 and 32, respectively. Although a little more than half the size of the sibling group, the irradiated population reported almost twice the number of benign tumors. Twenty-two of the 62 benign neoplasms in the exposed group arose in the thyroid gland, compared with three in the controls. Because valid age-specific incidence rates for benign tumors are unavailable, we cannot give accurate values for the expected numbers of such neoplasms. Using the ratio of malignant-to-benign tumors obtained from tumor registries, it is possible to approximate the expected numbers of selected types of tumors. As can be seen in Table II, comparisons of observed and expected numbers of thyroid adenomas in the treated group indicates an excess of 20 cases or a 14-fold increase over expectation.

Since we are interested not only in the types of neoplastic disease induced by radiation exposure, but also in the risks of such neoplastic transformation after exposure to specific doses of radiation, we have considered the incidence of neoplasms in the irradiated group as a function of radiation dose. This has been done for two categories of tumors, namely, thyroid tumors, and all tumors arising outside the thyroid gland. In the case of extra-thyroid tumors, the number of lesions of specific cell types per dose category is not sufficient to allow us to evaluate quantitative relationships; therefore, we have pooled extra-thyroid tumors of all cell types into two groups — all extra-thyroid tumors and only extra-thyroid tumors arising within irradiated tissues. The incidence of pooled tumors per 1,000 person-years at risk vs. cumulative air dose is shown in Figure 1. Since the tumor incidence is known to be strongly age dependent, we have excluded the younger individuals. The circles refer to individuals born between 1926 and 1940, and the crosses to persons born between 1926 and 1950. It is clear that the rates for both types of extra-thyroid tumors increase with increasing dose. We do not attempt to fit a dose-response curve to the data, however, as we believe this might be misleading for two reason: first, the small number of tumors per point introduces considerable uncertainty as to the exact values; and second, there are theoretical problems associated with the quantitative response of "pooled" neoplasms of different cell types.

Figure 2 shows the incidence of thyroid neoplasms per 1,000 person-years at risk plotted as a function of the estimated dose in rads to the thyroid gland.

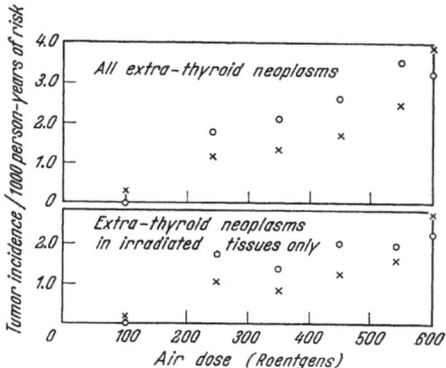

Fig. 1. Incidence of neoplasms per 1,000 person-years at risk *vs.* cumulative air dose for all extra-thyroid neoplasms and for extra-thyroid neoplasms in irradiated tissues. Circles (0) refer to persons born between 1926 and 1940 and crosses (x) to persons born between 1926 and 1950

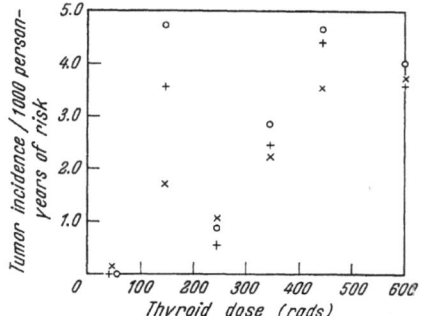

Fig. 2. Incidence of thyroid neoplasms per 1,000 person-years at risk *vs.* estimated thyroid dose. Plus signs (+) refer to persons born between 1926 and 1940 and crosses (x) refer to persons born between 1926 and 1950. Open circles (0) refer to "high risk" subgroup (see text)

(The detail of the dose calculations will be given in another publication (HEM-PELMANN *et al.*, 1967)). The plus signs (+) refer to persons born before 1940 and the crosses (×) to persons born before 1950. The open circles represent the tumor incidence in a special "high risk" subgroup mentioned later in this paper. Again, we do not attempt to construct a dose-response curve. Not only do the reasons given above apply to this situation, but there is evidence that the mail survey technique identifies only gross thyroid lesions. The values given in this figure, therefore, represent minimum incidence rates. Two conclusions may be drawn from these data. First, there is an increased incidence of thyroid neoplasms with increasing dose to the thyroid gland, and, second, there is a substantial incidence of neoplasms in persons receiving 100—300 rads of X-rays to the thyroid gland. However, with these data, it is not possible to determine whether or not there is a threshold dose for tumor induction.

Besides our interest in the types and numbers of neoplasms induced by radiation exposure, we are also concerned with the pathogenesis of these tumors. In the case of the thyroid tumors, further analysis of our data provides some evidence about the mechanisms involved in the neoplastic transformation. Figure 3 shows the distribution of the 41 persons with thyroid neoplasms in the irradiated series according to age at the time of histologic diagnosis. The

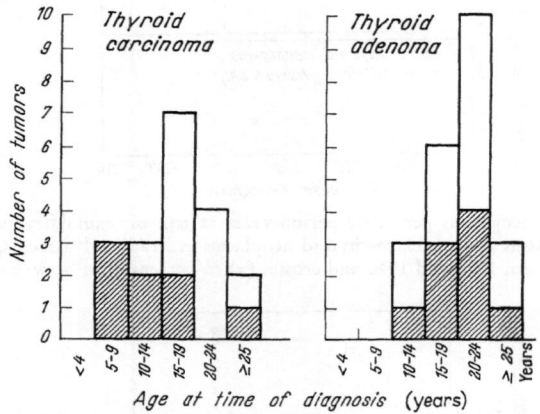

Fig. 3. Distribution of persons with thyroid neoplasms by age at diagnosis and by sex. Shaded bars refer to males and clear bars to females

abrupt increase in incidence of both thyroid carcinomas and adenomas in the 15—19 age category appears to be real. Because many of the subjects in the irradiated population were still in their twenties, the apparent decrease in incidence suggested by these data cannot be considered definitive. Nevertheless, it is apparent that the thyroid carcinomas tend to occur earlier in life than the adenomas. Studies subsequent to the 1963 survey suggest that the curve of incidence of thyroid neoplasms *vs.* age does, indeed, level off after age 20, and in the case of carcinomas actually seems to decrease (PINCUS *et al.*, 1967).

Because the period of rapid increase in the incidence of thyroid neoplasms corresponds to adolescence, which is known to place an increased demand on thyroid function, we have speculated that adolescence may play a rôle in the pathogenesis of neoplastic transformation. Further analysis of the data reveals three additional pieces of evidence that support this hypothesis. The first is that the interval between X-ray exposure and appearance of the tumor appears to be independent of the dose to the gland (Fig. 4). The second is that there is a poor correlation between the magnitude of the dose and whether a given lesion is malignant or benign. Thus, the ratio between thyroid carcinomas and adenomas shows little change in various dose categories. Lastly, the age of appearance of thyroid cancers in persons irradiated in childhood (age: 2—9 years) appears to coincide with that in persons irradiated in infancy (age: less than two years) DODGE et al., 1967). These observations suggest that factors other than radiation exposure *per se* play a rôle in the neoplastic transformation of the irradiated cells. It seems likely, therefore, that radiation damage to the thyroid cell is the primary event in the induction of the neoplastic process, and that thyroid stress during adolescence plays a secondary or promoting rôle.

In closing, we would like to mention a recent study of one so-called "high risk" subgroup of the irradiated population. The mail survey revealed that

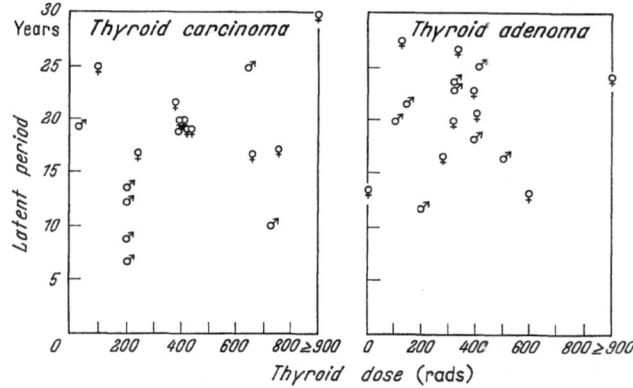

Fig. 4. Thyroid neoplasms distributed according to thyroid dose, latent period, and sex

Table III. *Cross tabulation showing thyroid nodularity as a function of age and thyroid dose*

Thyroid dose (rads)	Age at initial examination (yrs.)							
	<20		20—29		≥30		Total	
	No.	per cent	No.	per cent	No.	per cent	No.	per cent.
<400	2/12	17	2/31	6	1/10	10	5/53	9
400—599	1/6	17	6/25	24	2/4	50	9/35	26
>600	—	—	6/13	46	2/2	100	8/15	53
Total	3/18	17	14/69	20	5/16	30	22*/103	21

* Four cases, including one with a tumor, were omitted because the thyroid dose could not be calculated.

21 of the 268 persons in this subgroup reported surgical excision of thyroid nodules, indicating a high risk of developing thyroid neoplasms. Since it seemed likely that the mail survey technique identified only gross thyroid lesions, 107 persons in this subgroup who reported no thyroid disease on the questionnaires were examined by thyroid specialists (RALPH PINCUS, M.D., and

SEYMOUR REICHLIN, M. D.). In 23 of these individuals, solitary thyroid nodules or multinodular goiters were noted. Adding the known cases of thyroid neoplasms to these cases, and assuming the same incidence rate in examined and non-examined subjects, the projected incidence is approximately one in three or 30 per cent thyroid nodularity in this subgroup.

Table III shows a cross tabulation of the incidence of thyroid nodularity *vs.* age at examination and thyroid dose in this subgroup. Gross examination of these data suggests a stronger dose response than age response, and this is confirmed by analysis using the non-parametric Mann-Whitney test (PINCUS *et al.,* 1967). Five of the lesions which were surgically excised because they were suspected of being malignant on clinical grounds proved to be benign on histological examination. These observations support the hypothesis mentioned above that the incidence curve of thyroid neoplasms *vs. age* levels off after age 20, and that the incidence of thyroid cancer seems to decline.

In summary, this epidemiologic study shows a great excess of neoplastic disease in a population irradiated in infancy for thymic enlargement. Almost one-half of the neoplasms arose in the thyroid gland. Both thyroid neoplasms and "pooled" extra-thyroid tumors showed an increasing incidence with increasing dose. There is circumstantial evidence that thyroid stress during adolescence may play a secondary rôle in inducing neoplastic transformation of the irradiated gland. Our experience indicates that induced thyroid carcinomas respond well to therapy. All 19 persons with such malignancies were living in 1963, including nine with regional metastases and one with pulmonary metastases first reported in 1952.

References

DODGE, H. J., HODGES, F. J., PIFER, J. W., and HEMPELMANN, L. H., in preparation (1967).

HEMPELMANN L. H., PIFER, J. W., BURKE, G. J., TERRY, R., and AMES, W. R., *J. nat. Cancer Inst.* in press (1967).

PIFER, J. W., TOYOOKA, E. T., MURRAY, R. W., AMES, W. R., and HEMPELMANN, L. H., *J. nat. Cancer Inst.* 31, 1333 (1963).

PINCUS, R. A., REICHLIN, S., and HEMPELMANN, L. H., *New Engl. J. Med.* submitted for publication 1967.

SIMPSON, C. L., and HEMPELMANN, L. H., *Cancer (Philad.)* 10, 42 (1957).

— —, and FULLER, L. M., *Radiology* 64, 840 (1955).

TOYOOKA, E. T., PIFER, J. W., CRUMP, L., DUTTON, A. M., and HEMPELMANN, L. H., *J. nat. Cancer Inst.* 31, 1357 (1963 a).

— —, and HEMPELMANN, L. H., *J. nat. Cancer Inst.* 31, 1379 (1963 b).

Carcinogenic Effects of Atomic Bomb in the Survivors in Hiroshima and Nagasaki

KEMPO TSUKAMOTO

National Institute of Radiological Sciences, Chiba, Japan

I. Introduction

Although more than twenty years have already elapsed since the atomic bombing of Hiroshima and Nagasaki, there still remain to-day many unsolved, puzzling problems on the effect of radiation. Acute, or late, effects on the invidual survivors are not always consistent with that expected from the physically estimated dose. Such differences are probably due in part to limited knowledge of biological effects as between neutrons and gamma rays and also in part due to the difficulty in assessing the effects of shielding of individuals against radiation during the explosions.

To determine biological effects on survivors such as carcinogenic effects in the later years, it is vitally important to know the exact radiation dose received by each individual; however, as experiences of past accidents indicate, it is not easy to know this in each case. In many cases it has been necessary to make dose determinations long after the irradiation, and since it is impossible to reproduce the conditions which existed at the time of original exposure, many of these estimates inevitably have a wide margin of uncertainty. This is especially true for the atomic bomb survivors in Hiroshima and Nagasaki. Furthermore, all biological effects in the survivors are not necessarily attributable simply to radiation alone. Injuries from the enormous heat and blast are also involved, besides that, survivors were living under a very poor state of nutrition at the time of exposure, as it was near the end of the war. They have been heavily selected also by the lethal effect of radiation of the bomb itself so that the survivors may not necessarily be representative of the ordinary irradiated Japanese population with respect to the late effects such as radiation carcinogenesis. In any case, in order to clarify the radiation effects on the atomic bomb survivors more precisely, it seems necessary to review the radiation dose released by the bomb and to study the relation between the dose received by exposed individuals and the distance from the hypocenter of the explosions, by using most up-to-date technics of dosimetry.

II. Attempt of the Japanese National Institute of Radiological Science to Review the Radiation Dose Delivered during the Explosion

a) Neutron Dose Estimation

In our institute neutron dose estimation was made by using samples of iron rods which were the frame of concrete buildings exposed to the detonations at various distances from the hypocenters in Hiroshima and Nagasaki. In these samples a small quantity of Co^{59} is contained as an impurity, and this was activated into Co^{60} by fast neutrons released during the atomic bombs explosions and which thermalized to a maximum at a certain depth (about 8 cm) in the concrete. The iron was chemically extracted from the sample and finally electrodeposited with Pt plate. It was then counted in a coincidence-type beta-ray scintillation spectrometer with very low background, developed by TANAKA and HIRAMOTO (1963) in our institute.

b) Gamma Ray Dose Estimation

Another experiment in determining gamma ray dose from the two A-bomb explosions was made by HASHIZUME (1965) in measuring the thermoluminescence of ceramic materials caused by gamma radiation at the time of the explosions. The luminescence should not have faded even to-day if the exposed ceramic samples were neither heated by thermal energy released by the bomb during the explosion nor by the fire after the explosion. So they used ceramic

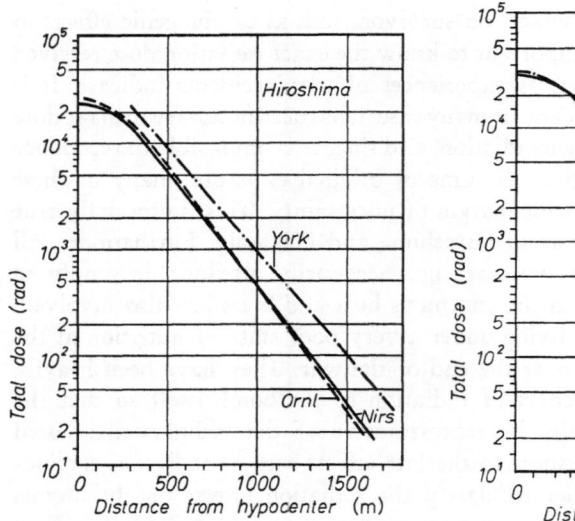

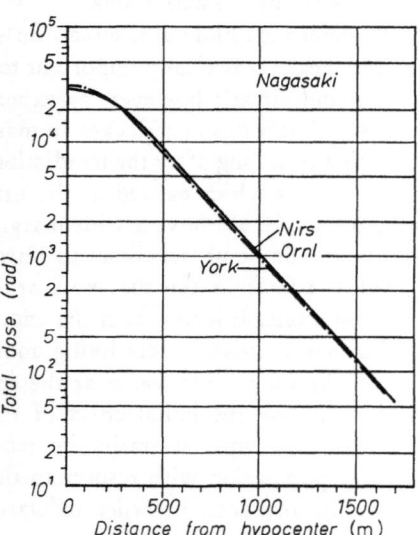

Fig. 1. Total air dose in Hiroshima as a function of horizontal distance from ground zero

Fig. 2. Total air dose in Nagasaki as a function of horizontal distance from ground zero

pipes which was buried within a certain depth in the ground at various distances from the hypocenter so that they were not heated at the time and after the explosions.

Figs. 1 and 2 show the comparison of the dose estimates in Hiroshima and Nagasaki made by York's group, Oak Ridge health physicists (ORNL) and a recent study in our institute (NIRS).

For the neutron dose in Hiroshima, the estimate of Oak Ridge is a little higher than ours but both these values are about a half or less than that of

York's estimate. However, in Nagasaki there is no difference between York's estimate and ours but the estimate of Oak Ridge is a little lower than the former two. For gamma ray dose in Nagasaki, there are not many discrepancies in the estimated doses by these 3 groups, but in Hiroshima the estimates of Oak Ridge and ours are about the same and the York's estimate is more than double the former two estimates. From these results the total dose from the neutrons and gamma rays in both cities at 1000 meters from the hypocenter are 970, 960 and 1000 rads in Nagasaki, which is a fair coincidence. However, in Hiroshima as shown in the Figs. 1 and 2 they are 1000, 450 and 430 rads by York, Oak Ridge and NIRS respectively.

It can be said that our method of dosimetry is superior to that of others in the following respects. As actually exposed materials were used for the objects of dosimetry and the same method was utilized for both cities, for the two different types of atomic bombs, any errors which may be involved in our methods for neutrons and gamma rays must be the same. This is important for the comparison of dose distribution and biological effects of radiation in Hiroshima and Nagasaki.

From the results obtained, it is felt that the evaluation of biological effects of the atomic bomb in Hiroshima, based on York's dose estimate up to present, might have been under-estimated to be less than a half of what it should have been as far as per unit dose is concerned. In other words, for instance, the incidence of leukemia in survivors with an estimate of 1—2 per million per year per rad should be revised to 2—4 at least in Hiroshima by Oak Ridge physicists and our recent estimate.

III. Leukemia among the Survivors

a) One of the most remarkable late effects attributable to radiation is the induction of leukemia among survivors of the atomic bomb. There are two kinds of separate study concerning its incidence. One was made by Dr. WATANABE, Chairman of this panel discussion, and his colleagues (WATANABE, et al., 1960; WATANABE, 1961) based on an assessment of the population of Hiroshima, using figures from the Japanese National Census of 1950, 1955 and 1960 as a denominator for the incidence. The other study was made by ABCC, based on a closed population Master Sample. The former study suffers from the disadvantage that little account was taken of population migration during the period of study, while the latter study has the limitation that only a limited number of persons exposed to the explosion were used. Fig. 3 gives WATANABE's findings regarding the incidence of leukemia among Hiroshima survivors, including all leukemia cases in the Hiroshima area for the 19 years between 1946 and 1964.

b) BRILL, TOMONAGA and HEYSELL (1962) summarized and compared previous findings on leukemia in atomic bomb survivors in Hiroshima and Nagasaki, as obtained from the ABCC Master Sample up to 1958 and reported in 1962. Based on these studies, a linear relationship between the dose and the incidence of leukemia could be confirmed and an estimate made of the absolute risk of an increasing incidence of leukemia in this group between 1 and 2 cases per rad per year per million of the exposed population within the dose range from about 100—900 rads. This dose range should also be changed to 50 to 450 rads by our estimates.

c) Another interesting but puzzling problem is the incidence of leukemia among the early post-detonation entrants to Hiroshima studied by WATANABE (1965). The number of leukemia cases developing between 1950 and 1964 (15 years) in this group is about 3 times as high as was expected from information on non-exposed populations in this country covering these 15 years. The majority of these cases were chronic myeloid leukemia. It developed in persons who entered within 3 days of the detonation (Table I). If this fact has some relation to the radiation, it must be due to residual radiation following the explosion owing to high near fall-out or neutron-induced radioactivity. Dosimetry with activation analysis of soil samples was made by BORG and CONARD (1961). From their study the dose which might be received by the entrants was said to be about 100 rads if they were within 300 m from the hypocenter one hour after the explosion to infinity in time. In the Institute recently, SAIKI and TANAKA (1966) measured the Sr^{90} content of the bone in 8 autopsy cases of leukemia in Hiroshima which included early post-detonation entrants. In some cases a relatively high value was obtained, compared to the upper limit of Sr^{90}

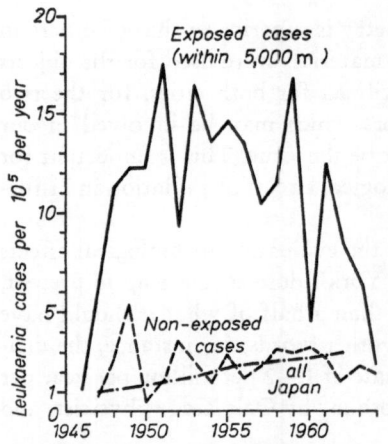

Fig. 3. Leukaemia cases in Hiroshima, 1946—1964 (modified from Watanabe). (From 1964 Report of UNSCEAR)

Table I. *Incidence of leukaemia developed among the early entrants in relation to entrance date* (1964 report of UNSCEAR, modified by Watanabe)

	Cases entered within 3 days	Cases entered between 4—7 days	Cases entered between 8—14 days	Cases exact date unknown	Cases entered within 2 weeks
Population	25,799	11,001	7,326	—	44,126
No. of leukaemia developed	33	7	1	8	49
Incidence per 100,000 per year	8.52	4.24	0.91	—	7.40

(1950—1964)

content in bone in the Japanese control during the corresponding years (Table II). However, from the results of this study alone, the existence of high near fall-out in Hiroshima at that time can neither be proved nor disproved; more samples are needed for the proof. Even with this study, therefore, it is difficult to explain the occurrence of leukemia in early entrants on the basis of the dose of radiation they might have received.

There seems to be no correlation between the length of latent period for induction of leukemia after the explosion and the doses received by the directly

Table II. *Strontium-90 content in bone of leukaemia cases in Hiroshima*

No.	Sex	Age (Year)	Date of death	Death certification	Type of exposure	Weight of Bone ash (humerus)	S. U. (^{90}Sr pc/g Ca)
1.	Male	25	Dec. 1951	Acute myeloid leukaemia	Early entrant (7. Aug. '45)	5.15 g	0.06 ± 0.02
2.	Male	32	Feb. 1953	Acute myeloid leukaemia	Directly Exposed	5.18 g	0.14 ± 0.12
3.	Male	54	Jun. 1954	Chronic myeloid leukaemia	Early entrant (8. Aug. '45)	4.76 g	0.20 ± 0.05
4.	Female	15	Oct. 1955	Acute myeloid leukaemia	Directly Exposed	5.17 g	0.35 ± 0.04
5.	Female	20	Nov. 1955	Chronic myeloid leukaemia	Directly Exposed	5.26 g	0.26 ± 0.05
6.	Female	56	Apr. 1958	Chronic myeloid leukaemia	Early entrant (8. Aug. '45)	5.02 g	0.12 ± 0.03
7.	Male	66	Oct. 1958	Acute myeloid leukaemia	Early entrant (9. Aug. '45)	3.88 g	0.42 ± 0.06
8.	Male	32	Aug. 1962	Acute lymphatic. leukaemia	Early entrant (6. Aug. '45)	5.09 g	0.10 ± 0.03

exposed individuals, although the incidence of leukemia is falling rather rapidly within a recent few years. This decrease may be due mainly to an absolute decrease in number of inductions of leukemia, but partly due to the shift in age distribution of the exposed to older age.

d) Among the survivors, 22 cases of polycythemia vera were reported by YAMAZAKI, KURITO and HOSHINO (1960). This is a rare disease in Japan and these cases comprise 22 per cent of all those reported in Japan since 1951. Also, 12 cases of myelofibrosis were reported by ANDERSON, HOSHINO and YAMAMOTO (1963) as a disease allied to leukemia. The more close to the hypocenter, the greater the incidence of this disease, indicating the greater dose received.

e) Recently HOSHINO, ITOGA and KATO (1965) made a study of leukemia in the offspring of parents exposed to the atomic bombs at Hiroshima or in Nagasaki. A total of 84 children born after June 1946 with leukemia were resident in either city but only 8 children among them were found that had been born within 2,000 m. Therefore, no statistically significant difference between dose and incidence could be detected in this group. In addition to this fact, no leukemia has to date been reported among children exposed *in utero* at the time of the explosion.

IV. Thyroid and Other Malignancies among the Survivors

Recently analyses were made by SHIMIZU, IDE, SHELDON and ISIDA (1965) in the Tumor Registries based on accumulated registered cases during 1957—1961 of the Hiroshima and Nagasaki City Medical Associations. This study was conducted jointly by the ABCC and the Japanese National Institute of

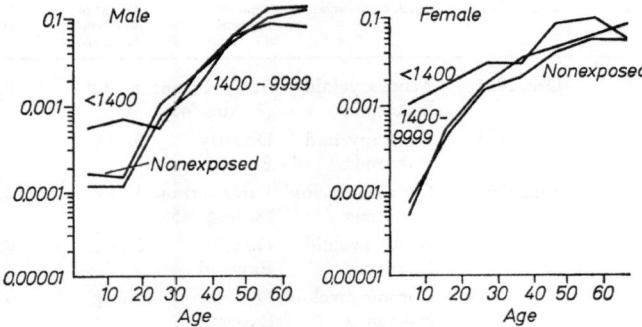

Fig. 4. Incidence rates from all malignant neoplasms excluding leukaemia and lymphoma, 1957—1961. Hiroshima and Nagasaki combined

Health using the JNIH-ABCC Life Span Study sample as a denominator. It totalled 75,100 in Hiroshima and 24,700 in Nagasaki. The sample consisted of all persons found to have been within 2,000 m of the hypocenters, as well as control groups obtained by random sampling among residents from both cities who were more than 2,000 m and migrants after the bombing, matching the sample by age and sex. Distance from the hypocenter was used as an index of the size of the radiation dose. In addition, trying to estimate accurately the individual radiation dose, intensive efforts were made by ABCC to obtain information on the precise state of shielding of each individual at the time of explosions within 2,000 m of the hypocenter.

a) Comparison was attempted between 2 groups, the first being the survivors within 1,400 m of the hypocenter (at this point those unshielded are assumed to have received about 100 rads) and the second group comprising the survivors further than 1,400 m. Fig. 4 shows the incidence curves of all malignant neoplasms excluding leukemia and lymphoma from the Life Span Study sample. An excess incidence among the male survivors within 1,400 m can be observed only in the under 20-age-group. For the female survivors within 1,400 m, however, an excess can be observed in all age-groups except 30—39 and 60 years and over.

b) Fig. 5 shows the incidence rates of leukemia in the sample divided into sex and age groups. The most striking finding is that the highest incidence of leukemia occurred in all age-groups of survivors from within 1,400 m of the hypocenter. The ABCC report of leukemia by HEYSSELL et al. (1959) stated that leukemia apparently reached its peak between the years 1950 and 1952, and thereafter, its incidence started diminishing. However, the tumor registry

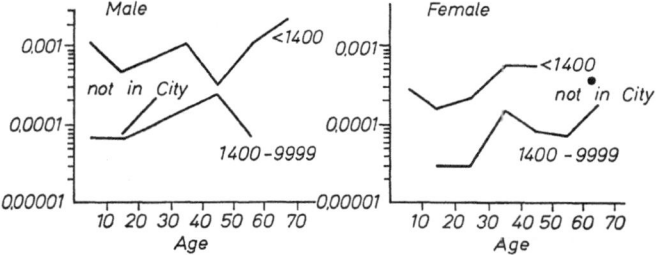

Fig. 5. Incidence rates from leukaemia; life span study sample, 1957—1961. Hiroshima and Nagasaki combined

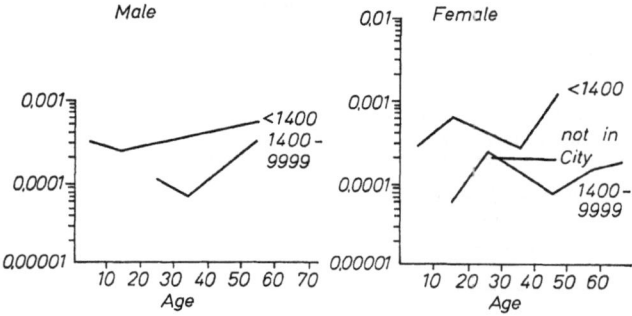

Fig. 6. Incidence rates from cancer of thyroid (940); life span study sample, 1957—1961. Hiroshima and Nagasaki combined

material of this time reveals a still higher incidence among the survivors from near the hypocenter (between 1957—1961) which corresponds to 12—16 years after the explosion.

c) Regarding the incidence of thyroid cancer, the present analysis reveals a significantly higher incidence among the survivors from within 1,400 m for females of both cities and males in Hiroshima but not among the male survivors of Nagasaki (Fig. 6). In another report (SOCOLOW, NERIISHI, NIITANI and HASHIZUME, 1963), on Adult Health Study, 21 cases of thyroid cancer (5 men and 16 women) were observed in the exposed group. Among those cases occurring in the under-30 age-group, over 80 per cent had been exposed within 1,400 m while in the over-30 age-group, only less than 50 per cent had been similarly exposed. These workers therefore concluded that the thyroid cancer in these heavily-exposed younger subjects might have developed 10 or 20 years later if the stimulus of additional radiation had not been superimposed.

V. Comparison of Radiation Dose for the Induction of Leukemia and Thyroid Cancer

In statistical studies of atomic bomb survivors such as the epidemiology of cancer induction or Life Span studies long after their original exposure, it must be remembered that other factors, like the socio-economic conditions of the

Table III. *Incidence of leukemia after the exposure to various radiation sources*
Estimation by Lewis (/10⁶ /rad /year)

Source of estimate	Radiation	Region irradiated	Types	Probability (/10⁶/rad/year)		best estimate
				estimated range		
				lower Limit	upper Limit	
Atom-bomb surv.	γ-rays + neutron	whole body	all	0.7	3	2
Ankylosing spondylitis	X-rays	spine	granulocytic (only?)	0.6	2	1
Thymic enlargement	X-rays	chest	lymphocytic (only?)	0.4	6	1
Radiologist (U. S.)	X-rays, radium, etc.	partial to whole body	all (?)	0.4	11	2

Incidence of thyroid carcinoma after the exposure to various radiation sources
Estimation by Pochin (/10⁶ /rad /year)

Report		Cases	Patient years	Dose	(/10⁶/rad/year)
Simpson *et al.*	C	10	ca 19,500	620	0.9 ± 0.3
Conti *et al.*	C	0	19,600	168	0.0 ± (0.5)
Saenger *et al.*	C	11	30,254	330	1.1 ± 0.3
Hanford *et al.*	A	8	5,711	845	1.6 ± 0.6
Hempelmann	C	1.8	ca 26,100	329	0.9 ± 0.3
Hempelmann	C	11.1	ca 10,300	126	0.8 ± 0.8
Socolow *et al.*	A	1 (7.5)	15,000	250	2.0 ± 1.0
Socolow *et al.*	A	1+11 (5.5)	15,000	170	2.2 ± 0.9

A: Adult, C: Children

population following irradiation, may influence the results of these studies. It is therefore difficult to reach any definite conclusion that these effects are due solely to the irradiation.

Table III is a comparison of cases collected by various authors indicating the dose required to induce 2 different types of malignancy, leukemia and carcinoma of the thyroid, with various types of radiation source, as well as under different conditions of irradiation. This is in spite of the fact that haematopoietic and thyroid tissues show great differences in radiosensitivity, at least in the radiotherapeutic responses of both types of malignancies. It is interesting that the dose required to produce cancer in both tissues is about the same, in the sense of what is known as "man-year risk per rad". This fact cannot be satisfactorily elucidated without assuming that the cancer cell-killing effects of radiation differ in some way or other from carcinogenic effects. Whether or not this assumption is right, cannot be clarified until the mechanism of radiation carcinogenesis is understood in the future.

VI. Chromosome Abnormalities Found in the Atomic Bomb Survivors

ISHIHARA and KUMATORI (1965) of our Institute studied chromosomal abnormalities found in persons exposed to various kinds of radiation (Table IV). In every case the incidence of chromosomal aberration was higher in the irradiated individual than in the normal individual. Also, chromosomal ab-

Table IV. *Comparative chart of chromosome abnormalities*
(by T. ISHIHARA and T. KUMATORI, 1965)

Case	Age	No. of samples	No. of cells examined	Aneu-ploid cells (%)	Acentric fragments (%)	Dicentrics and tricentrics (%)	Rings (%)	Others (%)	Total chromosome abnormalities (%)
Normal	28—35 ♂	8	1,174	1.50	0.13	0	0	0	1.63
Normal	42—53 ♂	7	1,200	2.57	0.21	0	0	0	2.79
Normal	24—34 ♀	5	500	2.20	0	0	0	0	2.20
Thorotrast		15	3,425	2.75	2.60	1.39	0.31	1.22	8.27
I131		6	800	3.00	1.00	1.00	0.25	0.67	5.92
Bikini		14	2,700	3.18	0.46	0.29	0.036	1.32	5.29
Atomic bomb		6	1,100	3.67	0.25	0.33	0.08	0.42	4.75
Occupational exposure		5	1,000	3.30	1.50	0.10	0	0.80	5.70
Accidental exposure		2	280	2.85	1.35	0.55	0	0	4.75

normalities such as dicentrics, rings, and other exchanged chromosomes which are not normally present were more frequently observed in the majority of cases. The frequency of acentric fragments was very high in the cases of thorotrast injection, and I131 treatment. It is of particular interest that in the case of the Bikini fishermen chromosomal abnormalities such as the karyotype with a monocentric abnormal chromosome, which will not disturb cell division, had remained present until today, long after the radiation exposure.

Another study was made by Iseki and Inokuchi (1965) of Nagasaki University School of Medicine. They also studied chromosomal abnormalities, especially on the atomic bomb survivors (Table V). From their results it can be concluded that chromosomal abnormalities in exposed persons are higher than in non-exposed persons; also that victims near the hypocenter (group 1) with acute radiation symptoms such as a haemorragic diathesis and/or epilation show more chromosomal abnormalities than those further away from the hypocenter (Group 2).

From these studies it can be said chromosomal abnormalities such as dicentrics and rings which cannot live through the cell division existed more fre-

Table V. *Chromosome abnormalities of leukocyte cultures from thorotrast-injected persons*

Case	No. of cases	Age (sex)	Injected amounts (cc)	No. of cells examined	Aneuploid cells (%)	Acentric fragments (%)	Dicentrics (%)	Rings (%)	Others (%)	Total chromosome abnormalities (%)	Cells with chromosome abnormalities (%)
Normal	5	42—53 (5 male)	0	1200	2.57 (2.0—4.5)	0.21 (0—0.5)	0	0	0	2.79 (2.0—5.0)	2.79 (2.0—5.0)
Thorotrast	12	47—65 (11 male) (1 female)	8—45	3425	2.75 (1.4—5.6)	2.60 (1.0—6.0)	1.39 (0—3.0)	0.31 (0—2.0)	1.22 (0—5.0)	8.27 (4.5—15.0)	5.65 (3.0—9.5)

quently in thorotrast and I^{131} injected patients in whom radioactivity still exists within their bodies. However, a clear-cut linear relationship between dose and the frequency of chromosome aberrations is difficult to demonstrate by these studies. Further study is needed to establish this correlation. It is not known yet whether or not an exposed individual with chromosome abnormality is more susceptible to malignancy than the ordinary individual.

In closing my talk to-day, I wish to thank to all those scientists who supplied me with valuable data from their works, and I also hope that the scientists who are here will realize that the research on atomic bomb survivors is still of actual importance and should be continued, overcoming the difficulties which are involved in the task, for the better understanding of possible hazards in man from the peaceful use of atomic radiation in future for the benefit of mankind.

References

ANDERSON, R. E., HOSHINO, T., and YAMA-MOTO, T., Myelofibrosis with myeloid metaplasia in survivors of the atomic bomb in Hiroshima. The ABCC Technical Report Series, 10—63, 1—25 (1963) and *Ann. intern. Med.* 60, 1 (1964).

BORG, D. C., and CONARD, R. A., Activation analysis of Hiroshima soil samples with estimations of residual activity following atom bomb detonation in August 1945. Report BNL-7676 (1961).

BRILL, A. B., TOMONAGA, M., and HEYSSEL, R. M., Leukemia in man following exposure to ionizing radiation. A summary of the findings in Hiroshima and Nagasaki, and a comparison with other human experience. *Ann. intern. Med.* 56, 590 (1962).

HASHIZUME, M., Study on neutron and gamma dose estimation of atomic bombs in Hiroshima and Nagasaki. *Hlth. Phys.* **12**, (1965).

HEYSSEL, R., BRILL, A., LOWELL, A., NISHIMURA, E., GHOSE, T., HOSHINO, T., and YAMASAKI, M., Leukemia in Hiroshima atomic bomb survivors. The ABCC Technical Report Series, 02—59, 1—72 (1959).

HOSHINO, T., ITOGA, T., and KATO, H., Leukemia in the offspring of the parents exposed to the atomic bombs in Hiroshima and Nagasaki. *Acta haemat. jap.* **28**, 450—451 (1965).

ISEKI, T., and INOKUCHI, H., Chromosome aberrations of the circulating leukocytes in atomic bomb survivors. *Acta haemat. jap.* **28**, 451—452 (1965).

ISHIHARA, T., and KUMATORI, T., Chromosome aberrations in human leukocytes irradiated *in vivo* and *in vitro*. *Acta haemat. jap.* **28**, 291—307 (1965).

SAIKI, M., and TANAKA, G., unpublished data (1966).

SHIMIZU, K., IDE, M., SHELDON, W. F., and ISHIDA, M., Malignant neoplasms among A-bomb survivors, Hiroshima and Nagasaki, 1957—1961. The ABCC Technical Report Series, 03—65 (1965).

SOCOLOW, E. L., NERIISHI, S., NIITANI, R., and HASHIZUME, A., ABCC—JNIH adult health study, Hiroshima and Nagasaki 1958—1961. Thyroid cancer. The ABCC Technical Report Series, 13—63 1 (1963).

TANAKA, E., and HIRAMOTO, T., Background of coincidence type beta-ray spectrometer. *Nucl. Inst. Meth.* **22**, 292 (1963).

WATANABE, S., On the incidence of leukemia in Hiroshima during the past fifteen years from 1946 to 1960. *Jap. J. Radiat. Res.* **2**, 131 (1961).

— Leukemia in early post-detonation entrants in Hiroshima. Personal communication 1965.

— ITO, T., and MATSUBAYASHI, Y., Statistical observations on leukemia in Hiroshima during the past fourteen years (1946—1959). *Jap. J. Radiat. Res.* **1**, 81 (1960).

YAMAZAKI, K., KURITA, S., and HOSHINO, A., Statistical observations on polycythemia vera in Japan. Abstracts, VIIIth Internat. Congr. of Haematology, Tokyo 1960, p. 80.

Occupational Cancers of the Lung in Radioactive Ore Miners in U.S.A.

W. C. HUEPER

*National Cancer Institute, N.I.H.
Bethesda, Md., U.S.A.*

The recently published data on the excessive liability of American radioactive ore miners to develop cancers of the lung are of distinct scientific and practical interest. The historical record of the studies leading to this discovery provides a deep insight into the astounding mentality of public health agencies toward such serious health hazards and of the peculiar policies adopted by them to cope with such threats from respiratory cancer hazards to special worker groups as well as to the general population. The information yielded by these investigations has reaffirmed even to the expediently and conveniently sceptic the unpleasant scientific fact that the prolonged inhalation of radioactive gases and dust induces under proper conditions of exposure cancers of the lung in an astonishingly high percentage of the exposed individuals. Because of the progressive contamination of the general human environment, including the air, with radioactive matter, although in much smaller concentrations than those encountered in American pitchblende mines and non-ferrous metal mines of the Colorado Plateau, these observations have distinct general implications.

It is an intriguing fact that cancers of the lung among radioactive ore miners represent the oldest known occupational cancers of this organ system, since they were first recognized for the radioactive cobalt ore miners employed at Schneeberg, Saxony, in 1879. Similar observations were made in 1926 among the uranium ore miners working in the nearby Joachimsthal, Bohemia. Despite a wide acceptance of the concept that these lung cancers had an occupational, radioactive etiology, serious doubts were raised in 1948 against my proposal to a Government agency for conducting a comprehensive epidemiologic study of the American uranium ore miners for possible lung cancer hazards. Both Government officials with medical background as well as some of their special advisors objected against such studies for various reasons. Among others, it was asserted that the degree of exposure to radioactive materials sustained by the miners for occupational reasons was minor when compared with that sustained to cosmic radiation. It was held by others that the European experiences and conclusions were not valid and applicable, since occupational exposure to other substances encountered in the mines, such as arsenic, or a prolonged "inbreeding" of the local population in Schneeberg might account for an excissive susceptibility to the development of lung cancers among the miners. The last mentioned concept seemed to have a special appeal, since it was proposed by a well known physicist of the National Cancer Institute, who neglected to consider the biologically embarassing fact that the city of Schneeberg had a population of about 25,000 and a railroad station for many years. Some objectors to an epidemiologic survey claimed that there could not be a lung cancer hazard for these miners, since the lungs were refractory to the carcinogenic action of radioactive matter. Perhaps the most candid objection was advanced by those who maintained that such studies were not in the "public interest" and that the proponent of such investigative schemes displayed "bad scientific judgement" and should best be dismissed from the Service.

After these initial difficulties had been overcome measurements of the radioactivity of the air in numerous uranium ore mines of the Colorado Plateau made by representatives of the U.S.P.H.A. Division of Occupational Health demonstrated readily that an appreciable number of these mines showed values of radioactivity well above acceptable level. Several mines indeed had a degree of radioactivity which was several fold that demonstrated in the worst mines at Schneeberg, the so-called "death-shaft". An inspection of a uranium ore mill demonstrated that in the early days of this survey, respiratory exposure to radioactive matter was not limited to miners but extended also to millers as well as to the population living or working near such establishments, since large heaps of the finely ground wastes containing radium were collected in the yards of such mills and were readily spread by wind and rain in their inhabited neighborhoods, where they polluted the air and the water of nearby rivers.

With the physical basis for respiratory radiation hazards thus firmly established, the population of miners consisting of over 5,000 workers was then subjected to periodic medical examinations which concentrated mainly on pulmonary reactions (X-ray examination, sputum examination, physical examinations), in addition to blood and urine studies. When finally in 1964 a report on the epidemiologic aspects of lung cancers among underground uranium miners was published, it appeared that miners with an underground experience of more than five years revealed a lung cancer liability 15 times the expected one. Because of the relatively large labor turnover among these miners and the comparatively short period of operation of the mines, it can be anticipated that the incidence rate of lung cancer among members of this occupational group will continue to rise and may equal that reported from Schneeberg, where about 70 per cent of all deaths among these miners were due to lung cancer for many years.

Since these extraordinary lung cancer hazards prevailed in non-uranium mines at Schneeberg, similar observations have recently been reported from a radioactive fluorspar mine in Newfoundland, where the miners exhibited a twenty-fold greater incidence of lung cancer than that of the general population of Newfoundland. It is remarkable that the fluorspar there is free from arsenic and that therefore arsenic cannot account for the lung cancers observed, as this has incorrectly been claimed for Schneeberg in past decades. This finding deserves moreover consideration, because the increased rate of lung cancers found by WAGONER et al. (1963, 1964) among the nonferrous metal ore miners who become exposed during their work to radioactive gases and dust as well as to arsenic still awaits final explanation, i.e. whether these cancers are induced by radioactive matter, or arsenic, or by both agents. Although the levels of radioactivity in these mines in the Rocky Mountains are much lower than those prevailing in the pitchblende mines of this region, the observation of increased lung cancer rates among the nonferrous metal miners is of importance, since it may indicate the existence of radiation lung cancer hazards for even these less exposed groups of workers. Such findings are of additional significance, because mines in other regions of the U.S.A. (New York, Arkansas) as well as of other countries (Germany, Egypt, South Africa) have been found to be radioactive. Thorough epidemiologic analyses of these specific worker populations appear to be particularly valuable because data concerning a minimal radioactive level of inhaled air creating a lung cancer hazard may thereby be attained. Such information may in turn prove to be of distinct value in assessing the safety level of radioactive air pollutants for the general population from all natural and man-made sources.

Because of the wide acceptance of the contention that cigarette smoking is the principal cause of lung cancer in males, that certain squamous cell metaplasias in the bronchial mucosa are specific for exposure to cigarettes, and in view of the present attempts to incriminate cigarette smoking as a significant contributory factor in the production of lung cancer in uranium ore miners, it must be pointed out that the epidemiologic-statistical analyses of WAGONER *et al.* (1963) on uranium and non-uranium ore miners of the Colorado Plateau as well as those by PARSONS *et al.* (1964) on radioactive fluorspar miners in New-foundland have conclusively shown that the highly excessive lung cancer rates among the workers involved cannot be attributed to cigarette smoking as the main factor. Such an explanation indeed appears to be ludicrous because some 200 Schneeberg miners succumbed to lung cancer between 1869 and 1900 i. e. during a period in which cigarette smoking was at best a negligible, if not absent, environmental factor. It should be of distinct value to cite in this connection the histologic findings of SCHMORL (1928) on a series of 21 lung cancers affecting Schneeberg miners: squamous cell carcinomas with cornification, 7; squamous cell carcinomas without cornifications, 5; small cell carcinomas of polymorphous structure, 6; small, lymphoid cell carcinomas, 3. Similar observations on other types of occupational cancers of the lung (chromates, asbestos, arsenic, nickel) as well as on some of the precancerous bronchial lesions have been described by HUEPER (1942, 1966), who considered such histologic reactions as etiologically nonspecific. They obviously reflect the polyetiology of lung cancers.

Because of the still growing incidence of lung cancers in most countries, there is an immediate need for exploring all channels of information on the causes of these neoplasms. Epidemiologic studies of miners and millers of all types of radioactive ores, of employees in nuclear power plants, of workers handling in industry various types of radioactive machinery, such as, for instance, electrostatic eliminators, might serve usefully in ascertaining foci of such hazards as well as the effective levels of radioactivity. While it is unlikely that the inhalation of radioactive matter represents at present a major cause of cancer of the lung, with an increasing military and non-military use of nuclear energy, especially in the field of power production, it may become so in the future, unless reasonable precautions are taken.

References

HUEPER, W. C., *Occupational tumors and allied diseases*, p. 896. Springfield (Ill.): Ch. C. THOMAS 1942.

— *Occupational and environmental cancers of the respiratory system*, p. 214. Berlin-Heidelberg-New York: Springer 1966.

PARSONS, W. D., VILLERS, A. J. DE, BART-LETT, L. S., and BECKLAKE, M. R., Lung cancer in a fluorspar mining community. *Brit. J. industr. Med.* 21, 110—116 (1964).

SCHMORL, G. Pathological study of Schnee-berg lung cancer. *Rept. Int. Conf. Cancer,* London, p. 272. John Wright & Sons, Ltd. Bristol 1928.

WAGONER, J. K., ARCHER, V. E., CARROLL, B. E., HOLADAY, D. A., and LAWRENCE, P. A. Cancer mortality patterns among U. S. uranium miners and millers, 1950 through 1962. *J. nat. Cancer Inst.* 32, 787—801 (1964).

— MILLER, R. W., LUNDIN, F. E., FRAUMENI, J. F., and HAIJ, M. E. Unusual cancer mortality among a group of underground metal miners. *New Engl. J. Med.* 269, 284—289 (1963).

Statistical Study on Thorotrast-induced Cancer of the Liver in Japan

Shinji Takahashi

Department of Radiology, Nagoya University School of Medicine, Nagoya, Japan

The study consists of the results of the following three independent surveys.

1. Prospective Study

The clinical records of the war-wounded in the Army Hospitals have been safely kept under the supervision of the Demobilization Bureau after the War. As the examination with thorotrast was carried out in some selected hospitals of these Army Hospitals, about 20,000 clinical records of these hospitals were subjected to this study, The war-wounded were Japanese males, and had been injured between 1935 and 1943. Out of 20,000, 147 were thorotrast maintainers confirmed by the clinical records. These patients had received thorotrast injection in amounts of 3 to 75 cc in their 20 to 36 years of age. Out of 147, 138 or 94 per cent were examined by angiography, 2 by hepatolienography and the remaining by other examinations.

By follow-up study the prognosis was ascertained: 112 were alive and healthy in 1964, 27 were dead, and no confirmation of life or death was obtained in 8. Among 27 deaths, there were 3 cases of cholangiocarcinoma of which diagnosis were established histopathologically, 2 liver cirrhosis, 1 leukemia, 15 inflammatory diseases including other non-malignant diseases, and 6 cases of unknown causes.

A similar survey was made on 1,678 control persons who were admitted to the same Army Hospitals during the same period as thorotrast patients but not examined radiologically using contrast media. Prognosis: 1,209 were alive in 1964 without need of medical treatment, 217 were dead before 1963, and 252 were unknown of life or death. Among the 217 dead, there were 1 leukemia, 5 liver cirrhosis, 12 cases of stomach cancer including that of other tumor, 144 cases of other non-malignant diseases, and 55 unknown cases. It is remarkable that no liver cancer was reported in controls.

In this survey, both in the patient and in the control group, there were too many unknown follow-up cases to make proper statistical excution. Thus some presumptive considerations became necessary to get conclusions.

First, the incidence of cancer in thorotrast and in the control group were compared with each other under the conditions of disregarding unknown causes of death. The statistical test showed that the rate of incidence of cholangiocarcinoma was higher in the thorotrast group with a statistically significant difference at the 1 per cent level.

Compared with the death rate under the same conditions as the above of death, a similar result was also obtained.

Next, the incidence of cancer in the thorotrast group was compared with that of general Japanese males over 30 years of age by the Vital Statistics, official periodical in 1951. Results indicated that the incidence of leukemia and cholangiocarcinoma in the thorotrast-injected patients was significantly higher than that of the general Japanese males.

2. Retrospective Survey

In this study the thorotrast maintaining rate in liver cancer patients and controls was surveyed and compared.

By sending questionnaires to big hospitals in Japan for the year of 1962, 466 cases of liver cancer were collected. Out of these, four cases (0.85 per cent) with thorotrast shadows in the hepatic and splenic region were found on the abdominal X-ray film. Histologically, these 4 cases were cholangiocarcinoma.

On the other hand, on the X-ray photos of the upper abdomen of 1,398 controls collected by matching the sex and age distribution to the patients group, thorotrast shadows were found only in 1 or 0.07 per cent. By chi-square test it was concluded that there was a positive relationship between an administration of thorotrast and incidence of the liver cancer.

3. Autopsy Cases Survey

Thirty-eight cases of autopsies of thorotrast-maintained patients were collected with the help of pathologists belonging to big hospitals in Japan. Of 38, 27 were primary liver malignancy, in which 5 hepatomas, 17 cholangiocarcinomas, and 5 endotheliomas were included. As compared with the distribution of cause of death of autopsied patients in general Japanese population obtained by reference to the Japanese Autopsy Annual Report, the expected number of hepatomas, cholangiocarcinomas and endotheliomas were 18, 8 and 1 respectively. Cholangiocarcinoma and endothelioma occurred more frequently in autopsied thorotrast-injected patients with a statistically significant difference.

From these three surveys the research group concluded that primary liver malignancy, particularly cholangiocarcinoma, tended to occur more frequently in thorotrast-injected persons.

Thorotrast and Primary Malignant Tumors of the Liver

MASASUMI MIYAKAWA

Nagoya University School of Medicine, Japan.

A total of 39 autopsy cases was collected by inquiry at main hospitals throughout Japan. Among these cases, primary malignant tumors of the liver were noticed in 25 cases. Table I shows a classification of these tumors according to histologic pattern. Hemangioendothelioma was observed in 5 out of the 25 cases (20 per cent). Since hemangioendothelioma is an extremely rare malignancy in Japan, its incidence is undoubtedly much less than one per cent of all the primary liver malignancies in general. This striking difference in the frequency of hemangioendothelioma between thorotrast and the general group is highly significant.

The proportion of either hepatic cell carcinoma or cholangiocarcinoma to primary liver malignancy of epithelial cell origin is shown in the Table II. In

Table I. *A histological classification of primary malignant tumors of the liver in thorotrast group*

	Number of cases	Per cent
Hemangioendothelioma	5	20
Cholangiocarcinoma	15	60
Hepatic cell carcinoma	5	20
Total	25	

Table II. *The ratio in incidence of cholangiocarcinoma to hepatic cell carcinoma*

	Thorotrast group		General group*	
	Number of cases	(per cent)	Number of cases	(per cent)
Cholangiocarcinoma	15	(75)	29	(7.1)
Hepatic cell carcinoma	5	(25)	373	(90.9)
Mixed type	0	(0)	8	(2.0)

* MIYAJI, T., *Trans. Soc. Path. Jap.*, **54**, 23 (1965)

thorotrast group, cholangiocarcinoma was noticed in 15 out of 20 cases (75 per cent), while in a general group it was observed much less frequently (7.1 per cent). This difference is again highly significant. Table III shows that the concentration of thorium deposits remained in the liver which was measured chemically. In two cases which received thorotrast for hepatolienography, it was 9.80 and 11.78 mg respectively per gram of tissue. In seven cases which were injected with thorotrast for angiography, it ranged from 1.01 to 4.04 mg per gram of tissue. In one case which received 18 ml of thorotrast 25 years before death, it was calculated that approximately 61 per cent of the injected dose still remained in the entire liver.

Table III. *Concentration of thorium deposits in the liver*

Purpose	Years after injection	Amount of thorium deposits mg/gm tissue
Hepatolienography	25	9.80
Hepatolienography	18	11.78
Angiography	29	1.01
Angiography	21	1.75
Angiography	25	1.88
Angiography	28	1.91
Angiography	31	2.93
Angiography	32	2.50
Angiography	21	4.04

In cases with hemangioendothelioma, multiple nodules colored darkly red were frequently observed at the surface of the liver. Histologically, the neoplastic cells resembling Kupffer cells were contained. Some liver cells were found scattered among the neoplastic cells in some cases.

In cases with cholangiocarcinoma, a very large mass of dense fibrous tissue was a general finding. Microscopically, foci of neoplastic cells were usually found within the scarred tissue. They often showed ductular structures containing mucinous substance. The tumors with such a histologic pattern (adenocarcinoma) have generally been diagnosed as cholangiocarcinoma. Remarkable deposition of thorotrast was present in the scarred tissue especially striking at the area adjacent to a tumor mass.

Panel 14

Techniques and Evaluation of Anti-Smoking Campaigns

Chairman:

JOHN WAKEFIELD (U.K.)

Members:

J. CLEMMESEN (Denmark), D. HORN (U.S.A.), A. C. MCKENNELL (U.K.),
A. J. PHILLIPS (Canada), EVA J. SALBER (U.S.A.)

Education of Key Groups

EVA J. SALBER

Department of Epidemiology, Harvard University School of Public Health

This paper is concerned with some of the people to whom anti-smoking education should be directed, since my studies have to a certain extent been concerned both with the factors involved in the initiation of smoking and with the continuation of smoking.

Students give many reasons for starting to smoke, but behaving as the crowd does is the commonest reason given. That is, students say they want to do as their friends do; they want to be part of the gang, they don't want to be the oddball, and they are afraid to be called "chicken". They give other reasons also, such as wanting to be adult, wanting to appear sophisticated and wanting to impress others. Some students start smoking because they are curious to see what it is like.

This is what they say. In my own and other studies there has been a search for some of the factors that contributed to smoking behaviour. Most investigators agree that in general students who smoke come from families who smoke. Twice as many students smoke if both parents are regular smokers than if neither parent smokes. The most striking differences are seen amongst students who are heavy smokers. Seven times as many girls smoke heavily when the parents are regular smokers. It is also interesting that one parent smoking has almost as much influence as both parents smoking, and it does not seem to matter whether the parent who smokes is the mother or the father. A child is also influenced by the smoking habits of his older siblings and he himself influences the smoking patterns of the younger children. In other words there is a family pattern of smoking.

Student smoking increases as the socio-economic status goes down. This applies to both boys and girls, and particularly to heavy smokers.

Children who smoke differ in many respects from children who do not smoke. Non-smokers achieve better at school than smokers, and light smokers achieve better than heavy smokers. More non-smokers take upper academic curricula at school and more take honours courses. Smokers spend more time watching television and less time reading books than non-smokers. Smokers attend dances and movies more frequently and are car owners more often than non-smokers. On the other hand, smokers belong to fewer clubs and organizations than non-smokers. Smokers, and particularly heavy smokers, have less satisfactory relationships with authority in general and parental authority in particular than non-smokers.

Since an important social drive in this age-group is the need for status and prestige, it seems to me that children who do not adjust well to family relationships and adult authority are more likely to seek security with their peers and to use a cigarette as a symbol of companionship, adulthood, superiority and defiance.

The foregoing remarks are based on the results of a survey carried out in 1959 on 7,000 junior high and high school children in the public schools of Newton, Massachusetts. In 1965 we followed a sample of students who were 15 years old in 1959, to see if we could discover any characteristics which might have predicted later smoking behaviour.

We found, in general, that only 12 per cent of the students who were smokers had stopped smoking, whereas 36 per cent of the non-smokers and 71 per cent of the discontinued smokers had become smokers. The trend, therefore, is towards new recruits to smoking as the students get older. In fact, twice as many of the students smoked at 21 years old as had done at 15.

Predictive Variables

There are several variables which are predictive of non-smokers taking up smoking and discontinued smokers relapsing, but few which diminish this risk and reduce smoking. Young students who do not smoke seem well aware of whether they will remain non-smokers or whether they are merely delaying the onset of smoking. We asked the non-smokers in 1959 whether they anticipated smoking in 5 years: their own anticipation is a powerful predictor of future smoking. Students who find smoking distasteful on moral or aesthetic grounds are more likely to remain non-smokers.

I have reported previously that a majority of 16-year-old discontinued smokers became smokers within a year. Our present study confirms the instability of the discontinued smoking status. Relapses are more likely to occur among a non-college population of lower academic achievement who do not participate in honour courses in high school. The amount of tobacco consumed influences the amount smoked by those who relapsed, and this is in the expected direction. Belief in the causative effect of smoking and lung cancer has a slight deterrent effect, and those who earlier in life express an unfavourable attitude towards smoking are less likely to relapse later on. A belief in the causative effect of smoking in lung cancer also has some influence in stopping some smokers from continuing to smoke.

Reasons Given for Stopping Smoking

Students who said they had stopped smoking originally because others had told them to relapsed more often than those who did not give this reason, but students are more likely to remain discontinued smokers if "no enjoyment of, or dislike for smoking" was the initial reason that they had stopped.

Parental Smoking Habits

Parental smoking has been shown repeatedly to be of the utmost importance in the initiation of smoking. It is no longer of such importance at this older age-level. Nevertheless, if neither parent smokes, students are less likely to relapse than if one or both parent smokes, and if neither or one parent smokes they are more likely to discontinue smoking than if both parents smoke.

Social Class

We showed in our original study that young children whose parents belong to upper socio-economic groups smoke less frequently than the others. Social class, however, does not predict later smoking behaviour. Possibly in this age-group education is a better predictor of social status than father's occupation.

Health Education — Acceptability to girls and boys

MORISON (1961) in Canada, and HORNER (1962) in Britain, suggest that girls exposed to health education campaigns are less concerned about the adverse effects of cigarette smoking and alter their smoking habits less favourably than boys. In the present study we find that the smoking habits of boys can be predicted more often than those of girls. New recruits to smoking come mainly from non-smokers in girls and from discontinued smokers in boys.

Implications of the Study

Between 15 and 21 the influence of the home is diminishing, though parental smoking habits do still have some effect. Since not smoking at school may mean only delayed smoking, and since discontinued smokers relapse readily, all categories of students must be included in anti-smoking programmes. Special attention, however, should be lavished on the academically disadvantaged child of smoking parents, on the young, discontinued smoker, and on the young non-smoker who anticipates smoking in the future. It seems that only a comprehensive and continuing programme beginning with elementary schools and including parents, teachers, and other adults who guide the young child has any hope of succeeding in counteracting the forces created by adults who smoke, the power of the cigarette manufacturers, and the insidious effects of the cigarette itself.

References

HORNER, S. J., *Med. Officer* 108, 305 (1962).   MORISON, J. B., and MEDOVY, H., *Canad. med. Ass. J.* 84, 1006 (1961).

Anti-Smoking Campaigns in Denmark

JOHANNES CLEMMESEN

Finsen Institute, Copenhagen, Denmark

The anti-smoking campaign in Denmark has developed gradually in a way which makes it difficult to say when deliberate considered campaigns were introduced. This has been caused by the steady accumulation of evidence which, since about 1952, has been brought to the attention of the public through the press gradually as fresh information became available.

One rather important factor in this development was that in 1942 the Danish Cancer League established its Cancer Registry, which as one of its immediate tests set out to find whether the increase reported in lung cancer cases was only apparent, perhaps due to improvements in diagnostic technique, or whether it was real. As soon as evidence was available, the Symposium on the Endemiology of Bronchial Carcinoma was called at Louvain in 1952, and immediately results were communicated to the Danish public at the annual meeting of the Anti-Cancer League.

This was, of course, only the beginning, since there was a tacit reluctance on various sides to accept the evidence as decisive, although no objections were raised. However in 1959, the Danish Cancer Registry, after consultations with the Health Service, the Medical Association, and the Danish Cancer League, undertook a joint project together with the heads of the services for thoracic surgery and the Dispensary for Chest Diseases, and immediately afterwards a joint committee was established by the three organizations.

After a period of 18 months, this committee issued its report in October 1961, almost exactly simultaneously with the publication of the British report. Although this was entirely fortuitous, there can hardly be any doubt that the impact on public opinion of two independent reports at one time was heavier than had they appeared with some interval.

Another 18 months passed before the Ministry of the Interior established a new committee, charged with making proposals to reduce the dangers involved in cigarette smoking. Not unexpectedly this committee was unable to make recommendations very different from those already put forward by the first commission.

The major proposals were:

1. Information campaigns against cigarette smoking must be conducted over long periods, and should aim first of all at school children and young adults, although they should not be restricted to these younger persons.

2. Information should also be distributed particularly in youth clubs and at military establishments.

3. Radio, television, short films in cinemas, posters, advertisements in newspapers and pamphlets by mail, should also be used. Persons appearing in television, in films, etc., particularly doctors, teachers and persons in positions of responsibility, should be made aware of the importance of not smoking in public.

4. Finally a commission was proposed, established by the Ministry for the Interior to supervise a continuous information service on the subject.

As direct measures the following steps were urged:

a) A law prohibiting advertisements of cigarettes and window displays of the same. (This has not been carried out.)

b) Taxation should be shifted to cigarettes from less harmful kinds of tobacco. (Some trend in this direction is now discernible.)

c) The prohibition on the sale of single cigarettes already in existence should be enforced more vigorously.

d) Cigarettes should not be offered at meetings and negotiations in ministries and other public authorities.

e) Cigarettes should not be sold outside ordinary shopping hours, at kiosks, railway stations, etc., nor at restaurants. (This has not been enforced.)

f) Smoking in public transportation used for shorter journeys should not be permitted. (This is now being carried out as tramcars are abolished.)

g) Cigarettes should not be offered as prizes in lotteries.

It may be noted that although the general impression is that there is a trend among the younger generation to turn to smoking pipes, and among physicians — at least at professional meetings — to turn to cigars, there is not at the moment much to report by way of results. One unexpected result of a campaign in Danish schools, described by CRAMER (1966), was that although there was no significant change in the smoking habits of the children, a significant number of parents had stopped — even though the educational campaign had not been specifically directed at them.

References

CRAMER, T., State measures against cigarette smoking in Denmark, *Bulletin, U.I.C.C.* 4, No. 1 (1966).

The Canadian Smoking and Health Programme

A. J. PHILLIPS

National Cancer Institute of Canada, Toronto, Canada

and

MICHAEL E. PALKO

Health Education Consultant, Department of National Health and Welfare, Ottawa, Canada

Of Canada's 20,000,000 population there are 8,000,000 under the age of 20. Each of the ten provinces is responsible for the health of its people; hence the development of a programme in smoking and health must be in collaboration with provincial governments. Except for a short pamphlet on smoking published in 1940, provincial governments had not been inclined to mount an active anti-smoking programme during the period 1940—1950. In 1951, however, the Canadian Cancer Society, a voluntary agency, published a lead article in its quarterly *Newsletter* drawing attention to the increase in Canada in deaths from lung cancer and to the experimental evidence which incriminated cigarettes. Unfortunately, little action resulted until the period 1958—1960, when the National Cancer Institute, the Canadian Medical Association, the Canadian Heart Foundation, the Canadian Public Health Association, the Canadian Thoracic Society, and the Canadian Tuberculosis Association came forward with a statement to the effect that cigarette smoking was an important factor in the causation of lung cancer and was largely responsible for the increase in lung cancer death rates in Canada. The Canadian Cancer Society then appointed a committee to promote a broad programme of public education on the problem of lung cancer and smoking. Studies of the smoking habits of Canadian school children indicated that smoking began at an early age and the greatest increase occurred in the 11—16 year age group. The Canadian Cancer Society programme, therefore, is directed mainly to school ages.

The content of this programme is made up of:

A. Films. A filmstrip "To Smoke or Not to Smoke" originally produced by the American Cancer Society has been adapted for use in Canadian secondary schools (ages 15—19 years). For those between the ages of 10 and 14 years a filmstrip "I'll Take the High Road" has been adapted. In addition, a movie "The Huffless Puffless Dragon" is used in the elementary school programme.

B. Posters and Essays. The idea of posters and/or essays on the general topic of smoking is considered an important aspect of the smoking and health programme in Canadian schools. There are 23,700 elementary and secondary schools in Canada and approximately 35 per cent of these participate annually in the poster and essay competitions.

C. Literature. The Canadian Cancer Society has produced numerous pieces of literature dealing with smoking and health for distribution in schools. At the secondary school level a manual entitled *A Clear Look at Cancer* has been popular and at the elementary school level, a comic booklet *Smoking and Cancer* has met with favourable response. In addition, coloured posters have been prepared for display in schools, public transportation, etc. Each poster shows a well-known Canadian athlete and gives an explanation in a few words of why he does not smoke.

D. Curriculum. The Canadian Cancer Society has discussed with the provincial departments of education the content of the health courses and the most recent data on smoking are now included. It must be admitted that in secondary schools of Canada the subject of health remains secondary to mathematics, languages, history, etc.

In addition to the programme in schools, the Canadian Cancer Society has promoted an anti-smoking programme among adults. This programme includes exhibits, which are shown at spring and fall fairs in local communities, displays which are generally attached to the tops of automobiles, films which are shown at some function or meeting of the Canadian Cancer Society.

E. Clinics. Recently smoking withdrawal clinics have been organized but these have not been in operation long enough to discuss their value.

In 1963 the Minister of National Health and Welfare issued a statement to the House of Commons of Canada pointing out the scientific evidence "that cigarette smoking is a contributory cause of lung cancer". The Minister's statement pointed out further the need for information on this potential health hazard to children and young adults and urged the Department of National

Health and Welfare to work in close cooperation with the provincial health and other departments, voluntary agencies and professional associations concerned with this problem. In November of the same year, the first national conference on smoking and health was called in Ottawa, to which were invited representatives of the provinces, voluntary health agencies, professional associations and tobacco industry and growers. The most significant achievement of this conference was the unanimous acceptance of the medical evidence linking cigarette smoking with lung cancer and other conditions, and general agreement on the need of a nation-wide programme. Through the efforts of the Federal government a Canadian *Reference Book on Smoking and Health* has been prepared and distributed to all physicians, medical students, public health workers and school libraries. In addition an information kit on smoking and health has been put together for distribution by the provinces to teachers and other interested individuals. This kit contains several publications and a bibliography of studies and papers on the general subject of smoking and health. Finally, a *Resource Guide* for Canadian teachers of Grades 5—12 has been prepared and universally accepted by the provinces. This guide was prepared in cooperation with the Canadian Teachers' Federation and the Canadian Education Association.

Probably one of the most significant events sponsored by the Department of National Health and Welfare was the holding of the Canadian Youth Conference on Smoking and Health in May of 1965. This was designed to serve as a model which would assist the provincial and local health and education authorities to sponsor similar conferences in the future in the hope that the young people who attended would encourage their colleagues to remain, or become, non-smokers.

The promotion of research into the extent and nature of the smoking habit was also considered to be one of the National Department of Health and Welfare's roles in the general Canadian programme. Several research projects have been completed to date, such as studies related to instruction about tobacco in Canadian schools, attitudes towards smoking, prevalence of smoking, evaluation of some of the health education techniques and surveys of cigarette advertising.

Evaluation

Any programme which aims to change the smoking habits of the population of a country can be assessed in various ways. An attempt has been made in Canada to assess the efforts of the Canadian Cancer Society at the secondary school level in an attempt to determine to what extent the filmstrip "To Smoke or Not to Smoke" has affected the smoking habits of those who have seen it. In one province in which 47,000 students participated it was found that 33 per cent of all boys and 15 per cent of all girls smoked cigarettes, but of those who smoked, 35 per cent reduced their daily cigarette consumption or had stopped the use of cigarettes altogether. Of this group, approximately one-third indicated that they had changed their smoking habits because of seeing the filmstrip "To Smoke or Not to Smoke". In another province a control study was undertaken between schools in a test area which were exposed for three years to a concentrated programme in smoking and health and control schools in which no such programme was undertaken. It was found that:

(a) there was a significant reduction in the smoking habits of students in the schools in the test areas;

(b) students in the test area were more aware of the hazards of smoking;

(c) the belief that smoking cigarettes caused lung cancer was more common among students in the test area;

(d) a large number of students smoke in spite of admission of the harmful effects of the habit.

With respect to the evaluation of the programme of the Federal government, it is somewhat premature to make any pronouncement since this programme is only in its third year. However, a series of evaluative devices was incorporated in the early planning of the programme to evaluate its main objective, namely the reduction of the incidence of lung cancer and other diseases attributable to cigarette smoking. It is planned to obtain periodic data on the prevalence of smoking in the Canadian population, regular reports on cigarette consumption and reliable data on the level of public awareness of the hazards of cigarette smoking.

In conclusion, the programme in Canada in smoking and health may be expected to expand as new facets of the problem are revealed. A sudden change in the smoking habits of Canadians is not anticipated, but it is felt that an active programme will be effective in the control of lung cancer from cigarette smoking.

Research in the Anti-Smoking Programme in the United Kingdom*

A. C. McKennell

Social Survey Division, Central Office of Information, London

The work described is part of a programme of research designed to aid the British Government's anti-smoking campaign. We have conducted two national surveys, one in 1963 and one in 1964, with the object of (1) providing a base-line against which future changes in smoking behaviour and attitudes can be

---

* presented, in the author's absence, by the Chairman.

assessed and (2) studying the attitudes that govern the reaction to anti-smoking appeals.

In both studies we followed the general principle of organisation and technique of surveys conducted by the Government Social Survey. We have a permanent field force consisting of mainly part-time interviewers who are carefully selected and go through a standard training procedure. For any particular survey there is a further short period of training consisting of special briefing on the questionnaire schedule to be used. This questionnaire is then applied to a sample of informants who have been randomly selected by methods that ensure their representativeness.

In the 1963 survey, which was in the nature of a dipstick or try-out, just over 1200 people aged 15 upwards were interviewed. In the 1964 survey, contact was made with nearly 3000 people, but only 1 in 2 adult non-smokers, and 1 in 3 adolescent non-smokers were interviewed. Analysis of the 1964 survey is still continuing, but more limited analysis of both the 1963 and 1964 data is reported here.

Beginning of Regular Smoking

It has been observed that many children nowadays are becoming regular smokers while still at school, and to a much greater extent than in the past. The current smokers among our informants were asked at what age they began smoking regularly, and whether they were still at school or working at the time. Regular smoking was defined as one cigarette a day for at least a month. Only 5 per cent of the smokers in the adult sample said they began at school, compared with 43 per cent of the adolescents; the difference is not due to the raising of the school-leaving age. Half the young people aged 16 to 20 who are smoking today had begun their smoking career by the time they were 15. The rate of increase of regular smoking in the school period accelerates sharply year by year, the sharpest increase being at the age of 15, the final year at school. Taking the smokers who begin in their 12th, 13th, 14th and 15th years the percentages beginning to smoke regularly are 2, 5, 12 and 31, respectively. Thus, 31 per cent or nearly one third begin in their 15th year. Of these we find only 7 per cent had left school at the time they began, leaving 24 per cent who started in their final year at school. The importance of this final year at school can be seen another way. Of the 43 per cent of adolescents who began regular smoking at school, the majority, 24 per cent, did so in their final year. The figures quoted are for the 1963 data. The results for 1964 were very similar, give or take one or two per cent.

These figures provide justification, if any were needed, for health education in the schools to prevent smoking. They could also be interpreted as supporting action at an earlier age than 15. However, we need to know more about the attitudes and motivation of children and the factors influencing their smoking as they approach this critical age. We have embarked recently on a study of this kind.

It is more convenient to carry out anti-smoking work in schools than elsewhere, and though our figures support this view, they do not justify an exclusive concentration of effort in the schools. Just as many adolescents began their regular smoking in their first job — 43 per cent — exactly the same proportion as said they began at school. This indicates the importance of contact with the adult world, together with the money which becomes available on entry into that world. We expect to be able to confirm nationally what several workers have found in local samples, that the incidence of smoking in children depends markedly on whether or not the parents or older siblings smoke.

Our data show that, by the time the adolescent reaches the age of 18, the decision to become a regular smoker or not is largely over for all but a few. But most tend to be very light smokers when they start, smoking less than five a day, though a year later only one third are smoking as little as this. More than half the adult smokers said it took them four years or more from the time they started to reach their present rate of smoking. Just under half the adults smoke 15 or more cigarettes per day; whereas only 15 per cent of the adolescents smoke this amount. What these figures illuminate is the simple but important fact that adolescent smokers are still only in the process of developing the habit.

Giving Up Smoking

The health educator must also persuade or help smokers to give it up. We were able to confirm a finding by Martin in his Edinburgh study that 2 out of 5 smokers say they would like to give up smoking if they could do so easily. The proportion of adolescent smokers who say this is about the same as for adults.

Surprisingly, too, adolescents do not differ much from adults in the reasons they produce for wanting to give up. Money considerations predominate, accounting for half the replies. The remaining reasons concern health, with lung cancer fears being referred to by about 20 per cent and concern with minor health matters by about half of those replying.

In my view all these three elements should be stressed in anti-smoking persuasion. Campaigns that neglect the expense argument are missing a consideration that weighs heavily with potential converts from smoking. Although money considerations alone may not be enough to sway many smokers, it would seem good strategy to start from grounds on which there is general agreement, and to link other appeals with the expense argument to which smokers are already so predisposed. The lung cancer hazard accounted in 1963 for a substantial proportion (20 per cent) of the reasons for wishing to give up smoking, and the 1964 survey showed that there had been a small but significant increase, most marked among adolescents, under this heading.

The importance of the minor health hazards is seen in smokers who have actually tried to give up, if only for a short time. In all, over half the adolescents and just under two-thirds of the adult smokers said they had at some time stopped smoking for a week or more. By far the most important single reason, accounting for 40 per cent of these temporary cessations, was an actual illness; it was mentioned twice as often as money, and more than twice as often as any other single reason, such as influence by other people, test of will power or fear of possible health effects. The 1964 results were much the same as those of 1963, except that with adolescents money considerations were found to weigh more heavily in 1964.

It might be held that these short-term cessations due mainly to minor illnesses are no more than a reaction to the temporary discomfort of smoking at these times. But further evidence suggests that this is a good time to persuade them to stop more permanently. About half the ex-smokers mention the occasion of an actual illness as the main reason for their stopping. The main difference in the replies given by ex-smokers and those stopping temporarily was the stress placed by the former on money considerations. This received heavier weight among the ex-smokers, but actual illness was still the predominant reason given.

Nevertheless, there is additional evidence in support of the view that the cessations caused by minor illnesses, reinforced by money considerations might lead to more permanent stoppages if the social circumstances were right. This is seen in the reasons given for resuming smoking. The category "Recovered from illness" which includes all those who returned to smoking merely because their health conditions improved (20 per cent) is not the most important. The category "Social pressure/influences", on the other hand, includes more than three times this proportion of adolescents and double this proportion of adult smokers.

The next main category of reasons covered replies where some positive benefit from cigarettes was claimed, e.g. "Helped relax from worry/tension/pressure at work/responsibility", "Was becoming irritable". They presumably indicate something like an addiction factor, physiological or psychological, in cigarette smoking. Twice as many adults as adolescents gave this reason for resuming. But whatever the factors may be that influence some heavy smokers, among that large section of the population of smokers who from time to time free themselves of the habit, it is the chains of social influence rather than the chains of addiction that prevent their complete escape.

This important finding has its encouraging and discouraging aspects. It is discouraging because it is now well attested by research that behaviour and attitudes are more resistant to change when they are anchored in the existing behaviour patterns of social groups. These studies (reviewed in KLAPPER, 1960; KATZ and LAZARSFELD, 1955) show also that the effects of personal influence in every day face-to-face relations is many times more effective than persuasive mass communication. The propagandist is in a favourable position when attempting to create opinion on an entirely new issue, and even more so if his message is consistent with existing opinion. His disadvantage is greatest when his message conflicts with the norms of groups to which the individuals he is addressing belong or wish to belong. As the same time the health educator can gain some encouragement from the fact that a large proportion of smokers can give it up, if only for a short time, and the findings that it is social influence rather than fixation of the habit by addiction which makes them start again. If the popular fashion could be made to change, social influence would work in favour of the health educator instead of against him.

Social influence does count already among the factors causing some smokers to stop both, temporarily and permanently. Among the reasons given for stopping smoking was a category of replies such as "my husband/boy friend stopped", "pressure from my wife to stop", "I stopped when my friend stopped", which accounted for 17 per cent of temporary stoppages among adolescents, 13 per cent among adults and 20 per cent among ex-smokers. Ex-smokers and people stopping temporarily are likely to have fewer friends who are smokers. Thus social influence is not altogether a one-way force.

Opinion on the Health Hazards of Smoking

We found in 1963 that about a third of adolescents and adult smokers considered, in reply to a direct question, that smoking currently affected their health. In 1964 an even greater proportion of adolescents, but not adults, admitted this.

By asking about the effects of smoking on the health of smokers we could compare the answers of smokers and non-smokers, and we obtained much evidence of the defensiveness of smokers. To a much greater degree than non-smokers they would enter qualifications after admitting the possibility of undesirable effects on health. These would only occur if they smoked too much, or only happened to people who were predisposed. Non-smokers were much more ready to admit the long-term causal effects of smoking than were smokers, who tend to be relatively more taken up with the minor effects which accompany smoking, or are aggravated by smoking. However, even among smokers the greater willingness to admit lung cancer as a possible causal effect of smoking was more pronounced among adolescents than among adults.

Smokers who accept that a risk exists assess it as beginning at what for most of them is a safe level of smoking in terms of the number of cigarettes per day.

An experiment to measure the effects of an anti-smoking film showed how vigorous are the defences which smokers maintain against acceptance of the risk of lung cancer. The film did convince them that smoking can cause lung cancer, but they did not alter and were even hardened in their opinion that the pleasures of smoking are worth the risk to health. An explanation of these results would seem to lie in the 'boomerang effect'. Smokers were even *more* convinced *after* seeing the film than *before* that "human lungs are strong and not easily damaged by smoking". Apparently these smokers had been able to see the lung cancer and bronchitis patients in the film as suffering the fate of rare clinical specimens with atypically weak lungs. They were able to retain the comfortable belief that lung cancer, as far as they were concerned, was a remote and unlikely event.

It should be stressed that there is no lack of information about lung cancer and smoking among the public. All but three per cent of informants said that they had heard or read about the connection. This level of information is near the limit that can be expected on any topic. The need is to convince the majority of smokers who remain sceptical, or who contrive to believe that it does not apply to them.

In conclusion, one finding emerged from our investigation, which could be of great value. The general public is almost completely ignorant of the incidence of lung cancer. The great majority believe, for example, that there are more deaths from road accidents than from lung cancer. This is one belief about lung cancer that does not appear to be motivated, since there is little difference between the opinion of smokers and non-smokers. The data reflect rather a state of straightforward and widespread public ignorance that might be put right by an adequate information campaign.

References

KATZ, E., and LAZARSFELD, P. F., *Personal influence*. Glencoe (Ill.): Free Press 1955.

KLAPPER, J. T., *The effects of mass communication*. Glencoe (Ill.): Free Press 1960.

An Analysis of the Educational Problems of Controlling Cigarette Smoking

DANIEL HORN

Director, National Clearinghouse for Smoking and Health, U. S. Public Health Service, 4040 North Fairfax Drive, Arlington, Virginia

Basically the aim of our programme is to help people achieve insight into their own behaviour — why they continue, or why they might decide to try to stop, to develop an understanding of the gratifications derived from smoking and, accordingly, how best to cope with them; and to work towards an environment in which the social forces support and reinforce non-smoking behaviour.

The view is often expressed that it is too late to do very much about adults who are continuing smokers. I disagree, because unless we can make serious inroads into adult smoking, we shall fail in our efforts to reduce the rate at which children take up smoking. The climate of social acceptability, which is a strong influence in the taking up of smoking by children, stems largely from the adult practices which are so pervasive.

Furthermore, it would be unforgivable to write off the millions of adults (48 million in the United States alone) who are now cigarette smokers. These are the people in whom the extra hundreds of thousands of premature deaths will be occuring each year for the next 20 or 30 years, who suffer from the premature disability of heart disease and chronic respiratory disease. We have much to indicate that the potential for change is good. Changing smoking habits in adults is neither as simple as some would have us believe, nor as complex as others seem to think. It is a manageable problem, but needs systematic analysis and research to diagnose the problem and prescribe the treatment.

Two-thirds of the adult cigarette smokers in the United States have never discussed their cigarette smoking with a physician. Yet we know that the proportion of smokers who have given up smoking is significantly higher in those who report that the physician has clearly indicated that smoking is harmful. Obviously we need to encourage physicians to initiate a dialogue with their smoking patients in which they make clear the potential for harm in continued cigarette smoking.

There are four basic questions which need to be asked about any aspect of smoking behaviour:

1. Why consider engaging in this behaviour (motivation)?

2. What conditions are necessary for the decision to behave this way (perception)?

3. What are the inner satisfactions that must be handled (psychological factors)?

4. What are the external conditions for reinforcement (social and cultural factors)?

To elaborate on these, according to the model presented by HORN and WAINGROW (1966):

1. The Motivation For Change. In the light of current knowledge of the effects of cigarette smoking on death and disability, we think of health as the *only* factor in determining whether or not an individual tries to give up smoking. At least four other broad classes of reasons are important in the motivation to change smoking: a. *The Exemplar Role* (typified by the parent who gives up cigarettes in order to set a good example for his children); b. *Economics* (the threat of death or disability to economic security may serve as a more powerful motivation than the direct cost); c. *Aesthetics* (the unpleasant aspects of smoking can also become factors for change; the pleasures of good health can also be a part of this underlying motivation for change); d. *Mastery* (the inability to exert intellectual control can be more threatening than the danger of death and disability which led to the attempt to give up smoking in the first place).

Nevertheless, it is the information on the effects on health of cigarette smoking that makes the problem of giving up smoking different from what it was in the past.

2. The Perception of the Threat. Whatever the stated reasons for anyone's trying to give up smoking at the present time, it would be difficult to ignore the health-threat component. There appear to be at least four necessary conditions for engaging in self-protective health behaviour as a part of the perception of the threat. These conditions are: a. An awareness of the threat; b. the acceptance of the importance of the threat; c. the relevance of the threat; d. the susceptibility of the threat to intervention. All of these appear to be necessary conditions for self-protective action, but the absence of any one can serve to inhibit action. Our data indicate that it is the latter two conditions — personal relevance, and susceptibility to intervention that represent the primary needs in public education.

3. The Development and Use of Alternative Psychological Mechanisms. This dimension has been discussed from a theoretical point of view by TOMKINS (1966) who distinguished four types of smokers — smoking with no affect or emotional feeling, smoking to increase positive emotional feelings, smoking to reduce negative emotional feelings, and psychologically addictive forms of smoking behaviour.

Basically, people who smoke derive different types of gratification from their smoking, and TOMKIN's analysis distinguishes these on the basis of the use of the cigarette in managing emotional feelings. The smoker who uses the cigarette to increase positive emotional feelings (whether stimulation, relaxation, or the satisfaction of muscular and sensory involvement) has a different problem from the person who uses the cigarette to reduce negative feelings (whether irritability, nervousness, anxiety, guilt, etc.). The difference is between the person who smokes "to feel better" and the person who smokes in order "not to feel so bad". I am sure you are familiar with people who use or over-use food, alcohol, and other forms of gratification in these ways. The person who smokes with no affect, no emotional feeling, may have originally smoked to increase positive affect or to reduce negative affect, but at the present time his smoking is a pure habit pattern and has no affective component. This is the person who smokes automatically, almost as reflexive behaviour, lighting a cigarette when he already has several burning in an ashtray, but not really missing the cigarette when he puts it down. The addictive smoker, on the other hand, shows an alternation between positive affect increase and negative affect reduction. He is characterized as always being acutely aware of the fact he is not smoking when this is the case, and his desire for a cigarette grows with each minute that passes since his last one.

The important point from all this is that different smokers gain different kinds of benefits from their smoking. These gratifications are learned and reinforced by experience. For the adult who wishes to give up smoking, the type of smoker he is has important implications for the kind of procedure which will be successful for him.

4. Factors Facilitating or Inhibiting Continuing Reinforcement. Giving up smoking is best thought of as a process, rather than as an event. If so, the primary role of *social forces* (including action by official and voluntary agencies, whether in the health field or not, and legislative bodies at various levels of government), of *interpersonal influences* (including the behaviour and attitudes of family, friends, acquaintances, and people at work) and of activity by, and exposure to, the *mass media,* particularly television, is seen as facilitating or inhibiting the change process and modifying the strength of any health threat influence, and these facilitators and inhibitors should be considered when constructing any model of behaviour change.

The behaviour and attitudes of key groups such as health workers in general and physicians in particular are important factors as is the general level of acceptability of smoking behaviour that exists at a given time. The *current* climate of acceptability of smoking is probably one of the strong counter-influences to those factors which would otherwise facilitate the cessation of smoking. Restrictions on the places and conditions in which smoking is permitted, and reduction in the influence of cigarette advertising might be two mechanisms for changing this climate. Acceptability, being a social phenomenon, *is* subject to social change. With the sharp reduction in physician smoking that has taken place in the past 15 years in the United States, the acceptability of smoking in physician groups has also diminished. A similar reduction in the general population might lead to the same kind of self-generating reinforcement, or bandwagon effect. On a smaller scale, the same kind of process can take place within small social units such as families, circles of friends, clubs, or work groups.

The Taking up of Smoking. What happens when we try to apply this same model of behavioural change to the process whereby a young person takes up smoking? Asking the four questions we asked of adults, in some cases we get quite different answers.

1. Why consider initiating this behaviour? The reasons include *exploration and curiosity, adult emulation, peer conformity, rebellion against authority, identity searching,* and *immediate gratification.* The educational implications are clear that it is important to reduce each of these as a motivating force, either by reducing its importance or by increasing the attractiveness of being a non-smoker in each case.

Non-smoking becomes more attractive when such factors as adult emulation and peer conformity lead to the decision not to start smoking. In other words, if the adults which are admired or the peers to which one conforms are non-smokers, the action is in the direction we would prefer.

Perhaps the two most difficult problems are to provide the proper perceptions to deal with *identity searching* and with *immediate gratification*.

2. Our perceptual question was what conditions are necessary for the decision to behave this way. In the case of *identity searching* we must help to create an image of the non-smoker that comes closer to filling the young person's aims than his image of the smoker. At this point we do not know how children perceive the smoker in all its varieties. How can we minimize the chances of a child being guided into smoking behaviour by stereotypes he accepts?

In the case of immediate gratification, we need to counter-balance the gratification provided by smoking. These include both short-term and long-term negative effects. We have known for some time that the long-term health effects of smoking can reduce the taking up of smoking in high school students, but presumably this is effective primarily in those youths to whom long-term considerations are already important. We need to know more about the immediate consequences of smoking both in terms of its physiological effects and the image it creates for other youth.

Long-term health effects certainly play a role even with youth, but probably have a more indirect effect on their behaviour than on adult behaviour. These indirect effects operate largely through their potential effect on adult behaviour and adult views of youths' behaviour. In any event, the same characteristics of awareness, acceptance, relevance, and susceptibility to intervention apply as with the adult. Clearly, personal relevance of the health threat to a 17 year-old boy thinking about taking up smoking is different from that of a 57 year-old man who has been smoking for 40 years. Similarly, the inexperienced smoker views smoking as something completely susceptible to his control.

3. The management of affect applies both to the beginner and the confirmed smoker, but the new smoker has yet to learn that this form of behaviour may help him in his management problems. Learning to handle these efficiently would preclude the necessity for leaning on such a weak and dangerous crutch as the cigarette for such an important function.

4. For the new smoker the external conditions that reinforce the continuation of smoking are very like those already described for the smoking adult, although the emphasis may be different.

The same four dimensions, then, play a significant role in the taking up of smoking. If one is to attempt to intervene, the potential utility of that intervention can be evaluated in terms of the extent to which it can modify one or more aspects of these dimensions. As with the adult smoker, a well-rounded program of intervention would attempt to deal with all four of these, not just with the long-term health effects.

References

HORN, D., and WAINGROW, S., Some dimensions of a model for smoking behavior change *Amer. J. publ. Hlth* (Suppl.) (in press) (1966).

TOMKINS, S. S., A psychological model of smoking behavior. *Amer. J. publ. Hlth* (Suppl.) (in press) (1966).

Summary of Discussion by the Chairman

Supporting the speakers, delegates from New Zealand, Norway and the U.S.A. agreed that anti-smoking campaigns should be directed at much younger children than has hitherto been the case. Mr. O. JACOBSEN (Norway) spoke of a new programme being directed at children from the age of eight — not dwelling on disease, but making the point in songs and humorous poems (featuring a character based on Norwegian folk-tales, Troll Nikotin) that smoking is bad for a number of reasons. Studies in most countries confirm that children begin to experiment with cigarettes well before the age of eleven.

In a discussion of smokers' withdrawal clinics, the general opinion was that, although they could scarcely be justified on economic grounds in view of the poor permanent success rates, they might well be justified as a public demonstration that there was official care and concern for those who seek help for a problem which they find beyond solution by themselves. The importance of such official stances was also stressed in consideration of other measures: banning of smoking on public transport, in theatres and other places; the warning inscription now compulsorily printed on cigarette packets in the U.S.A.; the banning of advertising on radio and television; and the differential taxation on cigarettes (and in favour of cigars and pipe tobacco) as has been used with notable success in the Netherlands. There was widespread concern about the patent disparity between the official precepts of health ministries on the one hand and the heavy dependence of most governments on massive revenue either from the manufacture of cigarettes or from taxation on tobacco, a situation which fosters public cynicism regarding the true intentions of those in authority.

There was also concern that in some instances, anti-smoking propaganda had been too exclusively linked with the threat of lung cancer, ignoring the other major and minor health hazards which have been shown to be closely related to heavy cigarette smoking. The formation of inter-agency councils (e. g. in the U.S.A. and Canada) involving *all* health agencies interested in the effects of smoking was seen as the logical solution to this problem. Dr. HORN (U.S.A.) made the point that their research had made it clear that to young adults premature disability was much more threatening than premature death, whereas the converse was true for older people. To stress the risk of fatal lung cancer to the young is therefore to weaken the effect of propaganda by emphasizing the matters of least immediate importance.

The strongest point to emerge from the discussion was the paramount importance of personal example, particularly by parents, teachers, and all those standing *in loco parentis* to young people. Above all, doctors have a special responsibility for demonstrating by personal example their conviction that cigarette smoking is a serious health hazard. Since their patients and the public at large rightly regard them as persons with special knowledge and authority in this matter, doctors cannot absolve themselves of their responsibility for supporting by their public behaviour the uncompromising declarations of expert bodies appointed by their own profession.

Panel 15

Chemotherapy as an Adjuvant to Surgery and Radiation Therapy

Chairman:

G. H. FLETCHER (U.S.A.)

Members:

V. DRAGON (Roumania), H. IMANAGA (Japan), K. KARRER (Austria),
T. KONDO (Japan), H. VERMUND (U.S.A.)

Chemotherapy as an Adjuvant of Radiation Therapy in Cancer Disease

VASILE DRAGON

Oncological Institute of Bucharest, Bucharest, Roumania

Until the last two decades the treatment of various localizations of the cancer disease were based almost exclusively on the utilization of divers techniques of surgery and radiation therapy. Over the last period the anti-cancer therapeutic assembly has been enriched by larger and larger use of cytostatic chemotherapy, either as a unique therapeutic act, or, more often, in association with the other forms of therapy. As a unique therapeutic act — with palliative character — chemotherapy is applied especially to advanced cases (stages III, IV or recurrent cases after previous treatments). In other conditions, chemotherapy has a prophylactic character being associated with radical surgical or radiological therapeutic acts in view of reducing the number of local recurrences or distant metastases (KARNOFSKY, 1965).

Medical literature of the last years is rich in various experimental or clinical researches meant to demonstrate the efficacy or the lack of efficacy of chemotherapy associated with radiation therapy. The purpose of this therapy is to obtain a synergistic effect, a reciprocal potentation or a summing up of favourable individual effects, while avoiding as much as possible the summing up of toxic effects (AGATI and STOPPA, 1965; BRULÉ, 1964; SVOBODA, 1964).

The two methods of therapy complement each other, since irradiation represents a localized treatment applying only to known — clinically detected — tumor foci, while chemotherapy, can also influence occult foci (KARNOFSKY, 1965; KUNSTADT et al., 1965). There are many conflicting opinions as to the mode of biological action of this association: it is possible that cytostatics increase tumor radiosensitivity, or that there is only a summing up of the effects of these two forms of therapy (AGATI and STOPPA, 1965; BRULÉ, 1964; KUNSTADT et al., 1965). For this reason even the authors supporting chemo-radiological therapy do not hold a unanimous point of view concerning the technique of the mixed treatment employed: chemotherapy before or after irradiation, or simultaneous treatment? It appears though, that in spite of the danger of side-effects, the simultaneous chemo-radiologic treatment is the most indicated and many authors recommend it (COOK et al., 1959; DRAGON, 1963; DRAGON et al., 1965; GOLLIN et al., 1964; KLVANA, 1959; KUNSTADT et al., 1965).

When utilizing massive-dose chemotherapy before irradiation, one can sometimes come across the risk of a partial resistance towards irradiation, induced by previous chemotherapy (KUNSTADT et al., 1965). On the other hand, when applying an intensive irradiation followed by cytostatic chemotherapy, the latter is generally lacking in efficiency because of the locally altered field in the irradiated area where there occur radiofibrosis and devascularization phenomena (KLVANA, 1959; KUNSTADT et al., 1965). Simultaneous chemo-radiologic therapy avoids the aforementioned risks, reduces the treatment time, as well as the total doses given in separate therapies and sensibly decreases the risk of an adaptation resistance (KLVANA, 1959).

Within the chemo-radiologic association, the cytostatics are almost always used as fractionated treatment, per os or parenterally. In general, three different antimitotic groups are used (BRULÉ, 1964):

— alkylating or radiomimetic agents which alter DNA molecules in cancer cells (nitrogen mustard, Endoxan, Sarcolysine, TEM, Thio-TEPA, E 39, Trenimon, Degranole, etc.);

— antimetabolites which inhibit tumor cell synthesis (methotrexate, aminopterin, 6-mercaptopurine, etc.);

— anticancer antibiotics (actinomycin, mitomycin, sarcomycin etc.)

Generally, a single cytostatic is associated with irradiation, trying as far as possible to apply that particular drug which has been clinically proved to have a degree of "specificity" for a certain tumor type or a certain cancer disease localization, such as TEM in retinoblastoma (REESE et al., 1957), sarcolysine in ovarian tumors (LARINOV, 1963; POMMATAU, 1964), 5—FU in lung tumors (BRULÉ, 1964; GOLLIN et al., 1964), actinomycin D in Wilms tumors (ANGIO, 1962; LIEBNER, 1962), methotrexate in chorioepithelioma (POMMATAU, 1964), etc.

Yet it appears that therapeutic results are imposed by the use of several cytostatic agents, either in exclusive chemotherapy or in chemo-radiologic associated treatment, the favourable effects being expressed by the decrease or disappearance of tumor formations, amelioration of subjective symptomatology and extension of survival period. This simultaneous polychemotherapy has been utilized in cancers of the testis (DARGENT et al., 1964; LI MIN CHIU et al., 1960), ovary (DARGENT et al., 1964), lung (ISRAEL et al., 1965), etc. Usually, in this type of polychemotherapy, the authors are concomitantly employing an alkylating agent, an antimetabolite and an anti-cancer antibiotic.

Table I. *Cytostatic drug used*

Cytostatic	Localisation				Total cases
	Lung	Breast	Lymph node sarcomas	Ovary	
Tem	22	8	20	1	51
Sarcolysine	19	3	8	8	38
Endoxan	11	5	7	3	26
E 39	4	4	5	1	14
Trenimon	4	—	2	—	6
Degranole	—	2	5	2	9
Total	60	22	47	15	144

At the Oncological Institute of Bucharest, over the period 1958—1965, 144 cancer cases in advanced stages (III and especially IV) but in a satisfactory general state, were subjected to the simultaneous chemo-radiologic treatment; 60 lung cancers, 22 mammary, 47 lymph node sarcomas and 15 ovary, have been treated.

Irradiation was given particularly by deep röntgentherapy, a smaller number of cases being subjected to telecobalt-therapy (especially in lung cancer); the partial and total doses were generally high, similar to the usual ones in exclusive irradiation. In the 4 localizations analyzed, 6 types of alkylating agents (Table I) were used in chemotherapy. Administration of cytostatics was concomitant with the radiologic treatment, the drugs being given as fractionated treatment, orally or parenterally, more seldom intracavitary in cases of pleural or peritoneal neoplastic exudates. The majority of cases were treated with TEM, Sarcolysine and Endoxan. In 67 of the 144 cases studied, a single type of cyto-static drug was used during radiotherapy, while in another 77, two or three types of cytostatics were used. The successive utilization of several types of cytostatics was done for those cases where no tumor sensitivity to drug is found during the mixed chemo-radiologic treatment, or for those cases where, throughout the treatment, the setting up of chemo-resistance to the first cyto-static given is noticed. Partial and total doses given in this fractionated treatment were generally lower (about 50—75 per cent) than those normally used in exclusive chemotherapy. After completion of irradiation, chemotherapy was continued as maintenance treatment in a reduced number of patients.

This energetic chemo-radiologic therapy was applied in most cases under hospital conditions. The treatment was generally well tolerated, the side-effects such as stomatitis, gastro-intestinal disorders, hematologic disorders, etc. being rather reduced. To maintain the general state and to avoid, or correct, the side-effects, blood perfusions, hepatic extracts, iron preparation, vitamins B_1, B_4, B_6, C, delta cortisone and antibiotics were given during hospitalization.

Table II. *Results of chemo-radiologic treatment. Single + associated cytostatics*

Localization	No. of cases	Ameliorated		Stationary		Uninfluenced	
		No.	%	No.	%	No.	%
Lung	60	22	36.7	12	20.0	26	43.3
Breast	22	17	77.3	3	13.6	2	9.1
Lymph node sarcomas	47	31	65.9	12	25.5	4	8.5
Ovary	15	6	40.0	6	40.0	3	20.0
Total	144	76	52.8	33	22.9	35	24.3

The *results* obtained in these 144 cancer cases in advanced stages were analyzed for the amelioration of objective and subjective symptoms and for the average survival period from the beginning of treatment. Those patients where the objective symptoms improved (decrease of tumor formations) with over 12 months survival were considered as *ameliorated;* there were considered as *stationary* those patients where only the subjective symptoms were ameliorated, with 6—12 months survival; *uninfluenced* were those cases showing neither subjective nor objective symptom amelioration, and survival under 6 months.

Out of the total of 144 patients, 52.8 per cent were ameliorated, 22.9 per cent were stationary, and 24.3 per cent remained uninfluenced by the treatment (Table II). The rate of improvement was higher when associations of cytostatics were used — 63.6 per cent — (Table III), than when only one cytostatic was given — 40.3 per cent — (Table IV). The same applies to the average survival duration (Table V) which was 27.4 months with multiple cytostatics and 20.8 months with a single cytostatic.

If the results obtained are analyzed for malignant tumor localization, then, as well, it is found that both the amelioration and the average survival duration are considerably higher in patients treated successively with several types of cytostatics. In lung cancer, ameliorations increased from 23.5 per cent with a single cytostatic to 53.9 per cent with multiple cytostatics, while average

Table III. *Results of chemo-radiologic treatment. Associated cytostatics*

Localization	No. of cases	Ameliorated		Stationary		Uninfluenced	
		No.	%	No.	%	No.	%
Lung	26	14	53.9	4	15.4	8	30.7
Breast	12	10	83.4	1	8.3	1	8.3
Lymph node sarcomas	30	23	76.7	6	20.0	1	3.3
Ovary	9	2	22.2	5	55.5	2	22.2
Total	77	49	63.6	16	20.8	12	15.6

Table IV. *Results of chemo-radiologic treatment. Single cytostatic*

Localization	No. of cases	Ameliorated		Stationary		Uninfluenced	
		No.	%	No.	%	No.	%
Lung	34	8	23.5	8	23.5	18	53.0
Breast	10	7	70.0	2	20.0	1	10.0
Lymph node sarcomas	17	8	47.0	6	35.3	3	17.7
Ovary	6	4	66.7	1	16.6	1	16.6
Total	67	27	40.3	17	25.3	23	34.4

Table V. *Average survival in 144 cancer cases in advanced stages treated chemo-radiologically*

Localization	Single cytostatic No. of cases	Average survival months	Associated cytostatics No of cases	Average survival months	Total cases	Average survival months
Lung	34	15.6	26	17.7	60	16.5
Breast	10	38.9	12	39.6	22	39.3
Lymph node sarcomas	17	18.6	30	35.9	47	29.6
Ovary	6	27.1	9	10.7	15	17.3
Total	67	20.8	77	27.4	144	24.3

survival increased from 15.6 to 17.7 months; in lymph node sarcomas, (lymphosarcoma, reticulosarcoma, Hodgkin's disease) the proportion of ameliorations increased from 47.0 per cent to 76.7 per cent and the average survival from 18.6 to 35.9 months (Tables III, IV, V).

In conclusion, we consider that simultaneous chemo-radiologic therapy in advanced cancer cases, judiciously selected and carefully supervised, may be followed by a high proportion of objective and subjective amelioration and by a considerable lengthening of the survival period.

Summary

144 cancer cases in advanced stages are presented (lung 60, mammary 22, ovary 15, lymph node sarcomas 47), treated at the Oncological Institute of Bucharest over the period 1958—1965 with concomitant chemo-radiologic association. The irradiation consisted of deep röntgentherapy or telecobalt-therapy, and chemotherapy with alkylating agents (TEM, Endoxan, Sarcolysine, E 39, Trenimon, Degranole). A single cytostatic was used during irradiation in 67 cases, 2 or 3 alkylating agents being successively used in another 77.

The proportion of objective ameliorations was 40.3 per cent with utilization of one cytostatic, and 63.6 per cent with multiple cytostatics; average survival in months from the beginning of treatment was 20.8 months with one cytostatic and 27.4 months with multiple cytostatics.

La Chimiotherapie Comme Adjuvant de la Radiotherapie dans la Maladie Cancereuse

Résumé

On présente 144 cas de cancers en stades avancés (60 pulmonaires, 22 mammaires, 15 ovariens et 47 sarcomes ganglionnaires) traités à l'Institut Oncologique de Bucarest entre 1958—1965 par association simultanée chimio-radiologique. L'irradiation a été effectuée à l'aide de la röntgenthérapie péné-trante ou de la télécobalt-thérapie, la chimiothérapie utilisant des agents alky-lants (TEM, Endoxan, Sarcolysine, E 39, Trénimon, Dégranole). Dans 67 cas pendant l'irradiation a été utilisé un seul cytostatique, et dans 77 cas successive-ment 2 ou 3 agents alkylants.

La proportion des améliorations objectives a été de 40,3 % lorsque a été utilisé un seul cytostatique et de 63,6 % dans le cas des cytostatiques multiples; la survie moyenne a été de 20,8 mois depuis la prise en traitement pour le cytostatique unique et de 27,4 mois pour les cytostatiques multiples.

References

AGATI, G., and STOPPA, I. M., Osservazioni cliniche sull'associazione chemio-radio-terapica nel trattamento dei tumori maligni. *Radiol. med. (Torino)* 51, 113—133 (1965).

ANGIO d' G. J., Clinical and biological studies of actinomycin D and röntgen irradiation. *Amer. J. Roentgenol.* 87, 106—109 (1962).

BRULÉ, G., Doit-on modifier le traitement du cancer du poumon? *Rev. Tuberc. (Paris)* 28, 642—645 (1964).

COOK, J. C., KRABBENHOFT, K. L., and LEU-CUTIA, T., Combined radiation and nitro-gen mustard therapy in Hodgkin's disease as compared with radiation therapy alone. *Amer. J. Roentgenol.* 82, 651—657 (1959).

DRAGON, V., Protraction of the survival period Action d'une chimiothérapie triple associée anti-cancéreuse. Etude portant sur 32 ma-lades. *Sem. Hôp. Paris* 40, 481—497 (1964).

DRAGON, V., Protraction of the survival period of broncho-pulmonary cancer patients in the advanced stages of the disease by chemo-radiologic treatment. *Acta Un. int. Cancr.* 19, 1004—1005 (1963).

— PINELES, S. et BUNESCU, U., Résultats du traitement chimio-radiologique des cancers broncho-pulmonaires inopérables. *XI Con-gr. Internat. de Radiologie*, Rome, Ab-stracts, 253—254 (1965).

GOLLIN, F. F., ANSFIELD, F. J., and VERMUND, H., Clinical studies of combined chemotherapy and irradiation in inoperable bronchogenic carcinoma. *Amer. J. Roentgenol.* 92, 88—95 (1964).

ISRAEL, L., SORS, C. et REBOUL, R., 91 cas de polychimiothérapie simultanée continue dans les cancers du poumon inopérables. *Presse méd.* 73, 701—704 (1965).

KARNOFSKY, D. A., Chemotherapy. *J. Amer. med Ass.* 191, 30—32 (1965).

KLVANA, M., Some remarks on the combined radiation and chemotherapy of solid tumors. *Neoplasma (Bratisl.)* 6, 183—189 (1959).

KUNSTADT, E., PIVONKA, M. et CICHÝ, Á., Traitement radiologique et chimiothérapique associé des hématoblastoses. *Ther. hung.* 13, 109—114 (1965).

LARIONOV, F. L., Chimioterapia tumorilor maligne, p. 418—420. Bucureşti: Edit. Medicală 1963.

LI MIN CHIU, WHITMORE, W. F., jr., GOLBREY, R., and GRANSTALD, H., Effects of combined drug therapy on metastatic cancer of the testis. *J. Amer. med. Ass.* 174, 1291—1299 (1960).

LIEBNER, E. J., Actinomycin D and radiation therapy. *Amer. J. Roentgenol.* 87, 94—105 (1962).

POMMATAU, E., Indications résumées de la chimiothérapie dans les épithéliomas. *Sem. Hôp. Paris* 40, 520—522 (1964).

REESE, A. B., HYMAN, G. A., MERRIAM jr. G. R., and FORREST, A. W., The treatment of retinoblastoma by radiation and triethylene melamine. *Amer. J. Ophthal.* 43, 865—872 (1951).

SVOBODA, V. Therapeutischer Synergismus als wahrscheinliche Erklärung für die kombinierte Wirkung von Röntgenbestrahlung und Myleran bei chronischen Myelosen. *Neoplasma (Bratisl.)* 11, 95—101 (1964).

Chemotherapy as an Adjuvant to Radiotherapy[1]

G. H. FLETCHER[2], H. D. SUIT[2], R. D. LINDBERG[2], C. D. HOWE[3], M. L. SAMUELS[3], R. H. JESSE[4], and J. P. SMITH[4]

The University of Texas
M. D. Anderson Hospital and Tumor Institute, Houston, Texas

The rationale of combining a chemotherapeutic agent with radiation therapy can be on one of two hypotheses:

1. Agents like 5-fluorouracil (5-FU) or 5-bromodeoxyuridine (5-BUdR) have been shown to be radiation sensitizers (BAGSHAW, 1961; BERRY and ANDREWS, 1962; BOSCH *et al.*, 1958; DJORDJEVIC and SZYBALSKI, 1960, KAPLAN *et al.*, 1961, 1962; VERMUND, 1961). The limiting factor in the effectiveness of such a sensitizing agent is the fraction of cells which can be affected by the agent. Furthermore, as the agent also sensitizes normal cells, clinical usefulness depends on the fraction of tumor cells which are sensitized versus the fraction of normal cells sensitized in the volume of tissue irradiated.

---

[1] This investigation was supported by Public Health Service Research Grant Nos. CA-06294 and CA-05654 from the National Cancer Institute.

[2] Department of Radiotherapy.

[3] Department of Medicine.

[4] Department of Surgery, Sections of Head and Neck Service and Gynecology.

2. Alkylating agents or antimetabolites like methotrexate are cytotoxic agents producing shrinkage of tumors but are not radiation sensitizers. The rationale of the combination of chemotherapy with such an agent prior to irradiation is based on the following radiobiological facts.

Survival fraction studies have shown that the dose necessary to control a tumor permanently is a function of the number of malignant cells. It has also been proven in tissue culture and solid animal tumor systems that a fraction of cells are hypoxic or anoxic and therefore more radioresistant. As normal oxygenation of a tumor depends on the vascularization of the tumor, it is likely that the larger the tumor the more areas of hypoxic cells are present therefore diminishing considerably the likelihood of permanent control (POWERS, 1965).

The preliminary administration of a cytotoxic agent producing shrinkage of a tumor would then have the double advantage, as the tumor would be of smaller size at the inception of radiation therapy, of lessening the number of cells to be sterilized and there ought to be fewer hypoxic cells.

Timing of the Combined Therapy

When one uses a cytotoxic agent which is not a radiation sensitizer, chemotherapy should be administered prior to radiation therapy which should not be initiated until maximum regression has been obtained.

With 5-FU which produces shrinkage of the tumor and is also a radiation sensitizer there is a rationale to use 5-FU either prior to, or concomitantly with, radiation therapy.

Clinical Material

The squamous cell carcinomas of the upper respiratory and digestive tracts provide suitable material for the evaluation of combined chemotherapy and radiotherapy because results on the primary lesion and on the metastatic nodes to the neck can be assessed accurately by inspection and palpation.

At the M. D. Anderson Hospital background information was available because, for years, both normal tissue reactions and regression rates had been plotted for lesions of the various anatomical sites of the oropharynx by stage of the primary lesion. This staging was not identical but along lines similar to those recommended by the International Union Against Cancer (Table I). The percentage of permanent control of the primary lesions was known for the various anatomical sites according to this T staging. The best local control was obtained in the lesions of the tonsillar area and soft palate. Advanced lesions of the pharyngeal walls had the worst local control.

A pilot study was initiated giving a total of 60 mg/kg of 5-FU in five injections prior to radiation therapy. Radiation therapy was started on the day after the last injection. Originally additional biweekly injections of 10.5 mg/kg of 5-FU were done until toxicity developed, but were abandoned because the toxicity interfered with treatment, not so much because of increased local reactions but general toxicity producing complications such as pulmonary infection. In the first part of the study 5-FU was given five days prior to treatment, the treatment being initiated on the day of the last injection. Because of Bagshaw's findings (1961) that 5-FU acts *in vitro* as a radiation sensitizer to cells only if the drug is present in the culture medium when the radiation is given, the five injections of 5-FU were, later on, given during the second week of irradiation therapy.

Table I. *Staging of tumors and metastases*

Staging of primary tumor:

T_1 — < 3 cm in diameter
T_2 — 3—5 cm with minimal extension to adjacent structures
T_3 — > 5 cm with limited extension to adjacent structures
T_4 — massive

Staging of lymph node metastases:

N_0 — no nodes
N_1 — single small to moderate size (< 3 cm)
N_2 — large movable node (> 3 cm) or multiple unilateral
N_3 — fixed large unilateral node or bilateral nodes
M — distant metastases when first seen

Courtesy: FLETCHER, G. H., *et al.*, Clinicial method of testing radiation-sensitizing agents in squamous cell carcinoma. *Cancer* 16, 355—363 (1963).

Because of the known increased tissue reaction with 5-FU, originally 800 rads per week were given to a total of 5,000 rads. However, it was found that 1,000 rads per week to a total of 6,000 rads could be tolerated.

Plotting of regression rates during treatment had been done in a sufficient number of cases to establish base line data (Fig. 1). The regression rates of the lesions in the pilot study are shown compared with the base line data. Because of these apparently encouraging results a systematic study was initiated for the T_3 and T_4 oropharyngeal lesions.

The squamous cell carcinomas of the tonsillar area, soft palate, and lingual epiglottis shown in Table II include the original cases of the pilot study. There are only four control patients after the randomized study was started. Twenty-eight patients with pharyngeal wall lesions were entered in a double blind study. In the patients who randomized to 5-FU, 1,000 rads were given to a total dose of 6,000 rads in six weeks. Those patients who randomized to radiation alone, conventional treatment was used, i. e., an extra 1,000 rads were given through reduced portals after 6,000 rads making a total of 7,000 rads in seven weeks.

Lesions of the anterior oropharynx regress rapidly with radiation therapy (Fig. 2) and for some of the patients who did not receive 5-FU, the total dose was no more than 6,000 rads because regression had been complete at the end

of six weeks. For the pharyngeal wall lesions there is statistical significance in
the regression rates in favor of the patients who were treated with 5-FU (Fig. 3).
Actually in all patients treated with 5-FU no tumor was palpable at the end of
six weeks treatment whereas in most of the patients treated without 5-FU there

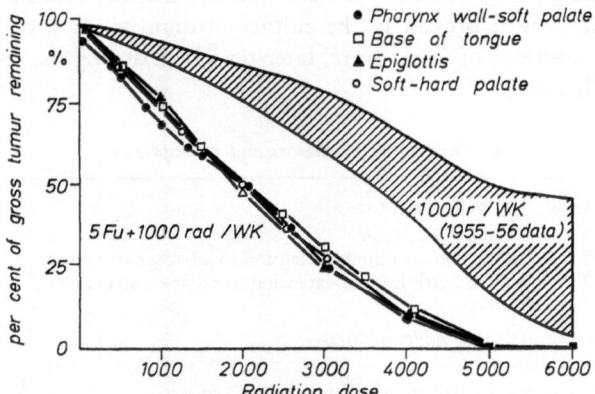

Fig. 1. Regression of advanced oropharyngeal carcinoma during Co⁶⁰ alone and Co⁶⁰ plus
5-FU therapy. Courtesy: FLETCHER, G. H. *et al.* Clinical testing of radiation-sensitizing agents.
Cancer 16, 355—363 (1963).

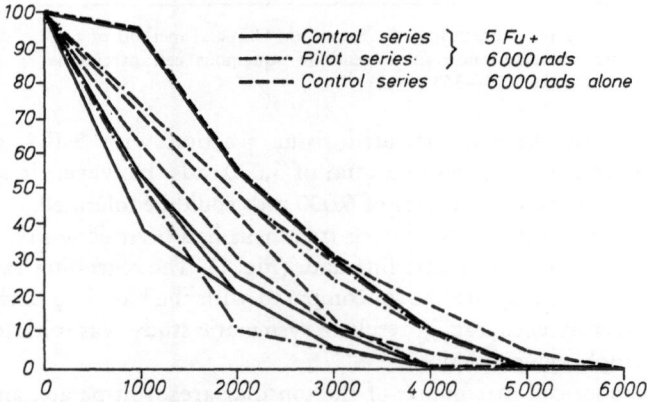

Fig. 2. Regression of T_3 and T_4 squamous carcinoma of the tonsil, pillar, palate, and epiglottis
(previously untreated). Courtesy: FLETCHER, G. H. *et al.* Clinical testing of radiation-sensitizing agents. *Cancer* 16, 355—363 (1963).

was clinically residual tumor at the end of six weeks (FLETCHER *et al.*, 1963;
HOWE *et al.*, 1964).

Eighty per cent of the patients receiving 5-FU developed bone marrow
toxicity. Leukopenia was the most frequently noted finding, and this was severe
in 30 per cent of the patients (below 1,000), noted on median nadir day 17.
Generally, leukopenia recovery was observed at about the end of the fourth
week. There were five associated severe pulmonary infections which were felt

to be related to the leukopenia. Although mild platelet depression was also common, severe thrombopenia (below 100,000) was observed in only three patients and was not associated with hemorrhagic phenomena. Severe gastro-intestinal reactions were seen in about 30 per cent of the patients, consisting of nausea, vomiting, diarrhea, and stomatitis. A generalized maculo-pappular skin eruption was seen in two patients, which responded promptly to treatment, and alopecia was observed in two patients.

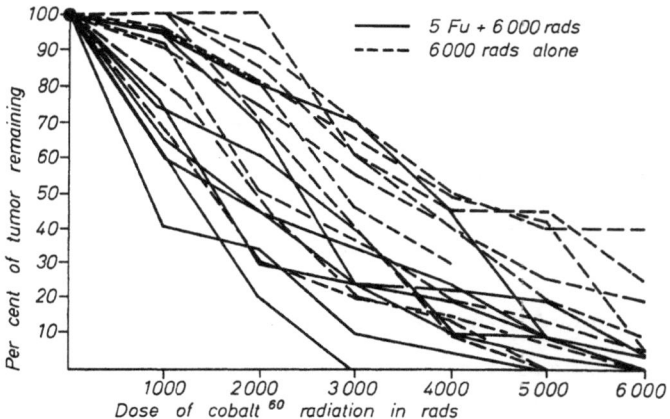

Fig. 3. Regression of T_3 and T_4 squamous carcinoma of the posterior and lateral pharyngeal wall (previously untreated). The null hypothesis (that there is no difference in the regression of the tumors in the two groups) is rejected at the levels of 0.03 for 1,000 rads, 0.06 for 2,000 rads, 0.08 for 3,000 rads, 0.07 for 4,000 rads, 0.11 for 5,000 rads, and 0.04 for 6,000 rads (Mann-Whitney rank test for nonparametric distribution). Courtesy: FLETCHER, G. H. et al. Clinical testing of radiation sensitizing agents in squamous cell carcinoma. *Cancer* 16, 355—363 (1963).

Table II. *Results at five years T_3 and T_4 lesions of the tonsillar area, soft palate, and lingual epiglottis (not randomized)*

Study	No. of cases	NED	Primary uncontrolled	DM	Un-known	ID	Compli-cations
5-FU * + Co⁶⁰ (6,000 rads)	13	3	2	2	2	3	1
Co⁶⁰ (6,000—7,000 rads **)	4	1	2	1	—	—	—

* 60 mg/kg 5-FU in five injections prior to radiation treatment.
** The total dose varied depending on the status of the disease at six weeks.

The long-term results for the anterior oropharynx lesions treated with 5-FU and radiation are not superior to radiation alone (Table II). In the 5-FU group there were several severe complications and marked tissue fibrosis. For the pharyngeal wall lesions there are fewer survivors and more local failures in the

5-FU plus 6,000 rads than with 7,000 rads alone (Table III). Furthermore, complications, primarily severe fibrosis, were more common in the patients with 5-FU plus radiation than in those with radiation alone.

Table III. *Results at five years in randomized series of pharyngeal walls lesions*

Treatment	Staging		No. of cases	NED	Primary uncontrolled	DM	Un-known	ID
	T_3	T_4						
5-FU * + Co⁶⁰ 6,000 rads	3	9	12	1	8	2	1	0
Co⁶⁰—7,000 rads	5	11	16 **	5 ***	4	1	1	2

    * 60 mg/kg of 5-FU intravenously in five days
      19 patients received radiation treatment after 5-FU
       9 patients received 5-FU during second week of radiation treatment.
  ** Three patients died from complications.
*** One patient salvaged by surgical excision of residual disease.

Intra-Arterial 5-FU and Radiation Therapy

A group of massive T_4 tumors of the oral cavity (anterior two-thirds of the tongue, floor of mouth, and gum) were chosen for intra-arterial 5-FU given concomitantly during the first 10 days of radiation therapy, the dose being 6 mg/kg/day/catheter. One thousand rads were given per week limited to a total of 5,000 rads in five weeks. Table IV shows that out of 24 patients so treated there was complete regression of these massive tumors in 12, seven patients being NED one year or more. This control rate is better than expected for only 5,000 rads in five weeks.

Table IV. *Intra-arterial* 5-FU and radiation therapy**, oral cavity T_4^+ lesions, 24 patients*

No benefit	10
Death from complications	2
Complete regression at end of treatment	12
NED 1 year or more	7

   * 6 mg/kg/day/catheter for first two weeks of treatment
  ** 5,000 rads in five weeks.

A similar study of combining 5-FU intra-arterially with radiation therapy has also been initiated for massive squamous cell carcinomas of the uterine cervix. With a laparotomy, catheters are introduced into the hypogastric arteries and 10 mg/kg/day are given for the first 15 days of radiation treatment. The total dose is 5,000 rads in five weeks.

Twenty-two patients were entered into the intra-arterial 5-FU study; nine were rejected because of positive para-aortic nodes and one because of omental metastases (Table V). This high percentage of disease beyond the conventionally irradiation area shows vividly the limitations of localized treatment.

Table IV shows the preliminary results in terms of primary disappearance of the disease for a minimum of six months. For a limited tumor dose of 5,000 rads in five weeks without additional intracavitary radium therapy it seems to be a better control than expected.

Table V. *Intra-arterial 5-FU (10 mg/kg/day for first 15 days of treatment)*
(5,000 rads TD/5 weeks)

Category	Total	Stage			
		II$_B$	III$_A$	III$_B$	IV
Explored	22	1	4	14	3
Accepted	12	0	2 (2)	7 (5)	3 (1)
Rejected*	10	1	2	7	0

* Nine for positive para-aortic nodes, one for omental metastases.
() NED six months or more.

Discussion and Summary

Despite faster and more complete initial regression of the tumor with systemic administration of 5-FU with radiation, there was no increased permanency of control of advanced squamous cell carcinomas and increased complications. The lack of correlation between regression rate and permanency of control has been confirmed in an animal tumor system and in oropharynx squamous cell carcinomas (SUIT et al., 1965).

Intra-arterial administration may have effectiveness although only pilot studies have been done so far. A high concentration of the chemotherapeutic agent is required to be effective. For an agent like 5-FU which is both radiation sensitizer and cytotoxic, the best timing of administration has not been determined. The lesions which are suitable for intra-arterial infusion are rare, making a very small fraction of the overall management of cancers. Therefore that combination therapy shows little promise practical ways.

Studies on tumor models have demonstrated, using mathematical calculations, that the present doses given in human radiotherapy are below the doses necessary to permanently control cancers (SUIT et al., 1966). This is in conflict with the well documented fact that there are in fact patients permanently cured of their cancers by radiotherapy, suggesting the presence of natural mechanisms which help radiation therapy. An investigation of natural immune host response mechanisms and studies of population kinetics might shed light on the subpopulations responsible for lack of control. These studies might be more promising than hoping to find a differentially cytotoxic agent.

References

BAGSHAW, M. A., Some experimental evidence for clinical enhancement of radiation response *in vitro*. In: *Research in radiotherapy; Approaches to chemical sensitization* p. 138—149 *(Kallman, R. F., ed.)*, Nuclear Science Series, Report No 35. Washington, D. C.: National Academy of Sciences; National Research Council; Publ. No 888 (1961).

BERRY, R. J., and ANDREWS, J. R., Modification of radiaton effect on reproductive capacity of tumor cells *in vivo* with pharmological agents. *Radiat. Res.* 16, 82—88 1962).

BOSCH, L., HARBERS, E., and HEIDELBERGER, C., Studies on fluorinated pyrimidines; V. Effects on nucleic acid metabolism *in vitro*. *Cancer Res.* 18, 335—343 (1958).

DJORDJEVIC, B., and SZYBALSKI, W., Genetics of human cell lines. III. Incorporation of 5-bromo- and 5-iododeoxyuridine into deoxyribonucleic acid of human cells and its effect on radiation sensitivity. *J. exp. med.* 112, 509—531 (1960).

FLETCHER, G. H., SUIT, H. D., HOWE, C. D., SAMUELS, M., JESSE jr. R. H., and VILLAREAL, R. U., Clinical method of testing radiation-sensitizing agents in squamous cell carcinoma. *Cancer (Philad.)* 16, 355—363 (1963).

HOWE, C. D., FLETCHER, G. H., SAMUELS, M. L., and SUIT, H. D., Combined 5-fluorouracil and cobalt irradiation evaluted by double blind technique. *Acta Un. int. Canc.* 20, 400—403 (1964).

KAPLAN, H. S., SMITH, K. C., and TOMLIN, P. A., Radiosensitization of *E. coli* by purine and pyrimidine analogues incorporated in deoxyribonucleic acid. *Nature (Lond.)* 190, 794—796 (1961).

— — — Effect of halogenated pyrimidines on radiosensitivity of *E. coli. Radiat. Res.* 16, 98—113 (1962).

POWERS, W. E., Radiation biologic considerations and practical investigations in preoperative radiation therapy. *J. Canad. Ass. Radiol.* 16, 217—225 (1965).

SUIT, H. D., LINDBERG, R. D., and FLETCHER, G. H., Prognostic significance of extent of tumor regression at completion of radiation therapy. *Radiology* 84, 1100—1107 (1965).

—, WETTE, R., and LINDBERG, R., Analysis of tumor recurrence time. Publication pending 1966.

VERMUND, H., Clinical experiences with 5-fluorouracil and related compounds in combination with radiotherapy. In: *Research in radiotherapy; Approaches to chemical sensitization*, p. 185—192 *(Kallman, R. F., ed.)* Nuclear Science Series, Report No 35. Washington, D. C.: National Academy of Sciences; National Research Council; Publ. No 888 (1961).

Chemotherapy as an Adjuvant to Surgery *

K. KARRER

*Institut für experimentelle Krebsforschung,
Universität Wien, Vienna, Austria*

WURNIG in Vienna in 1955 began a systematic study of chemotherapy as an adjuvant to radical surgery of patients with bronchial carcinoma stage II. In this initial study, one, two or three courses of Mitomen beginning 5 or 6 days after surgery were administered within a period of six months. Each course of treatment consisted of 10 daily i. v. injections of 50 to 75 mg of Mitomen at

* This study was supported by the Austrian Research Council

intervals of 6 weeks (DENK and KARRER, 1955, 1956). This treatment was ineffective in increasing the survival time and number of survivors (DENK, 1957; WURNIG et al., 1960), therefore a new study was undertaken using a different chemotherapeutic treatment (DENK and KARRER, 1959; WURNIG, 1958).

The second study included patients who received radical surgery for stage I, II and III bronchial carcinoma. All the operations were performed in either the II. University Clinic of Surgery, Director, Professor Dr. H. KUNZ or in the Vienna-Lainz-Hospital under the direction of Professor Dr. G. SALZER. The drug protocol called for 8 courses of drug treatment to be administered over a period of 2 years. Each course of treatment consisted of either 50 mg of Mitomen injected i.v. daily for ten days or 200 mg of Cytoxan administered i.v. in hospitalized patients and orally in out-patients. Mitomen treatment was discontinued in 1962 in favor of exclusive Cytoxan treatment.

Preliminary evaluations of this second study showed an improvement in survival time in the patients receiving chemotherapy as an adjuvant to surgery as compared to those receiving only surgery (DENK and KARRER, 1961 a, b; DENK et al., 1961, 1964; KARRER, 1962, 1964; KARRER and WURNIG, 1962; KARRER et al., 1965). Therefore, it was proposed to extend the drug treatment to 3 years after surgery. A new treatment protocol was initiated which required treatment with Cytoxan in courses of 30 daily doses of 200 mg per day for a total of 6,000 mg per course. Three courses of treatment were given in the first six months and 2 courses in each of the five succeeding 6-month periods for a total of 13 courses in three years. The results of this second study up to March 1966 are presented in Fig. 1. The curves show the survival rates of patients exclusive of postoperative mortality. Two operation control curves are presented. One curve (historical control) represents patients operated upon before 1955 (BUCHBERGER and JENNY, 1965; JENNY, 1961; JENNY and BUCHBERGER, 1962) and the second curve represents those operated upon during the period of this study. The difference between these two control curves is not significant. The shaded areas represent the areas in which there was a statistically significant difference between the number of surviving patients who received chemotherapy as an adjuvant to radical surgery and those who received only radical surgery in the period 1955 to 1963. The number of patients represented by each individual point on the curves in Fig. 1 and the statistical significance of the difference (calculated according to Fisher's direct method (1958) between these points are presented in Table I.

The drug-treated patients represented in Fig. 1 were divided into 2 groups: those which developed leucopenia (below 3,000 cells per cu. mm) and those which did not develop leucopenia (Fig. 2).

The number of survivors is greater in the leucopenic patients. The areas in which there was a significant statistical difference are shaded. The number of patients represented by each point and the statistical significance of the difference in these points are presented in Table II.

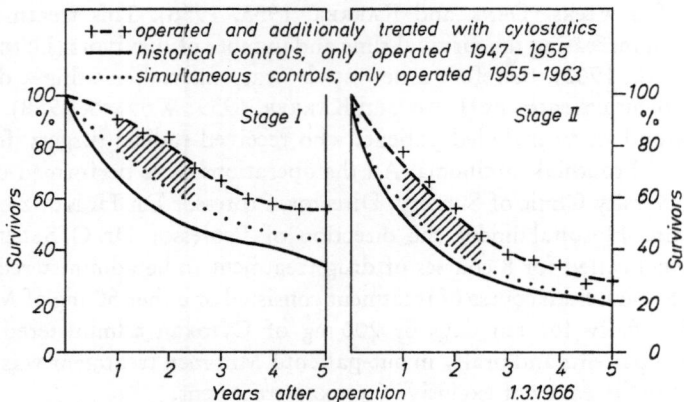

Fig. 1. Comparison of survival rates for patients after radical operation for bronchial carcinoma stage I and II with and without adjuvant chemotherapy

Table I. *Survival rates of patients after radical surgery for bronchial carcinoma Stage I and II
with and without adjuvant chemotherapy (postoperative mortality excluded)*

Chemotherapy treated				Operated controls			
Post operative years	Original Number	Survivors		Original Number	Survivors		
		Number	Percent		Numbers	Percent	p — value
Stage I:							
1	57	52	91	249	197	79	0.02
1.5	57	49	86	249	173	69	0.007
2	57	48	84	249	155	62	0.001
2.5	57	41	72	249	142	57	0.03
3	57	38	67	249	136	55	—
3.5	57	34	60	224	113	50	—
4	57	33	58	210	103	49	—
4.5	50	28	56	204	92	45	—
5	48	27	56	193	84	44	—
Stage II:							
1	89	69	78	125	76	61	0.007
1.5	89	59	66	125	55	44	0.001
2	89	50	56	125	49	39	0.01
2.5	89	40	45	125	41	33	0.048
3	89	34	38	125	37	30	—
3.5	89	32	36	118	31	26	—
4	89	30	34	113	27	24	—
4.5	70	19	27	110	25	23	—
5	61	17	28	106	23	22	—

A comprehensive statistical study was made of pooled data from the previously discussed patients plus additional data on patients who were operated on for bronchial carcinoma before March 1965 in other cooperating hospitals. The comparison of the life-table (method of SHEEHE, personal com-

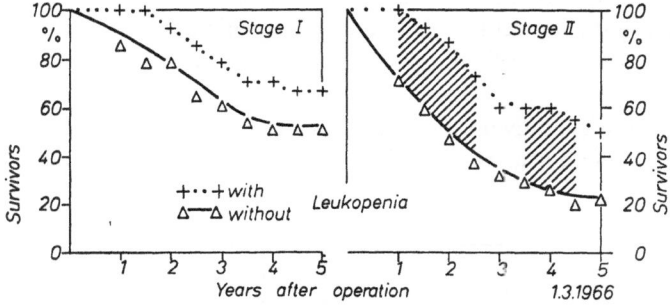

Fig. 2. Survival rates of patients with stage I and II bronchial carcinoma, with and without leucopenia

Table II. *Survival rates of patients with Stage I and II bronchial carcinoma with and without leucopenia as the result of adjuvant chemotherapy*

Patients with leucopenia				Patients without leucopenia			
Post operative years	Original Number	Survivors		Original Number	Survivors		
		Numbers	Percent		Numbers	Percent	p — value
Stage I:							
1	14	14	100	43	38	88	—
1.5	14	14	100	43	35	81	—
2	14	13	93	43	35	81	—
2.5	14	12	86	43	29	67	—
3	14	11	79	43	27	63	—
3.5	14	10	71	43	24	56	—
4	14	10	71	43	23	53	—
4.5	12	8	67	38	20	53	—
5	12	8	67	36	19	53	—
Stage II:							
1	15	15	100	74	54	73	0.01
1.5	15	14	93	74	45	61	0.01
2	15	13	87	74	36	49	0.006
2.5	15	11	73	74	29	39	0.02
3	15	9	60	74	25	34	—
3.5	15	9	60	74	23	31	0.04
4	15	9	60	74	21	28	0.02
4.5	11	6	55	59	13	22	0.04
5	10	5	50	51	12	24	—

munication), curves of these patients with and without adjuvant chemotherapy is shown in Fig. 3.

For patients with stage III bronchial carcinoma, the simple life table comparison reveals no difference in survival rate between patients receiving surgery and those treated with adjuvant chemotherapy (Fig. 6-left); however when the drug-treated patients were compared as leucopenic and non-leucopenic, a significant increase in survival rate was observed in the leucopenic patients (Fig. 6-right).

In these studies adjuvant chemotherapy did not result in more postoperative mortality or wound healing difficulties than is normally observed.

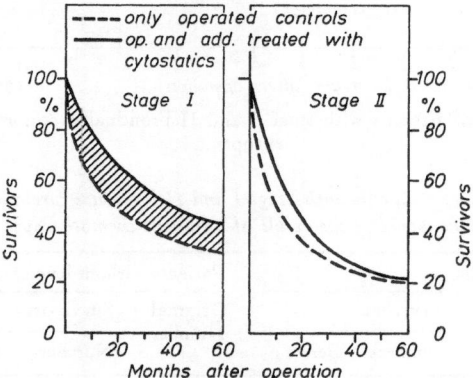

Fig. 3. Comparison of life tables of patients after radical operation (1958—1965) for bronchial carcinoma Stage I and II with and without adjuvant chemotherapy

Table III. *The number of patients receiving different numbers of courses of adjuvant chemotherapy*

Group	Tumor stage	Number of patients	Number of chemotherapeutic courses received												
			1	2	3	4	5	6	7	8	9	10	11	12	13
A lp	I	14	1	—	2	1	1	2	2	3	2	—	—	—	—
A nl	I	43	7	3	2	2	5	6	3	9	3	3	—	—	—
B lp	I	24	5	3	1	2	3	2	—	—	4	3	—	—	1
B nl	I	141	70	17	12	10	10	2	—	9	7	3	1	—	—
A	II	89	7	14	14	5	6	10	5	15	8	5	—	—	—
B	II	82	46	12	9	3	6	—	3	—	—	—	3	—	—
B lp	III	17	4	1	1	2	—	1	2	4	2	—	—	—	—
B nl	III	160	68	35	22	12	6	7	1	4	3	1	1	—	—
Total	I—III	570	208	85	63	37	37	30	16	44	29	15	5	—	1

A Group of patients according to Table I, Fig. 1. B New patients entered in study. lp, With leucopenia below 3000 per cu. mm. nl, Without leucopenia.

These studies and other similar studies (ADELBERGER and WOERN, 1964; GODÁL et al., 1962, 1964; HIGGINS, 1963; KUTSCHERA and SCHNETZER, 1965; MRAZEK, 1964; VON POULSEN, 1961; SERLIN, 1965; URABE et al., 1961; WOLBERG et al., 1965) cannot be considered conclusive because of their retrospective

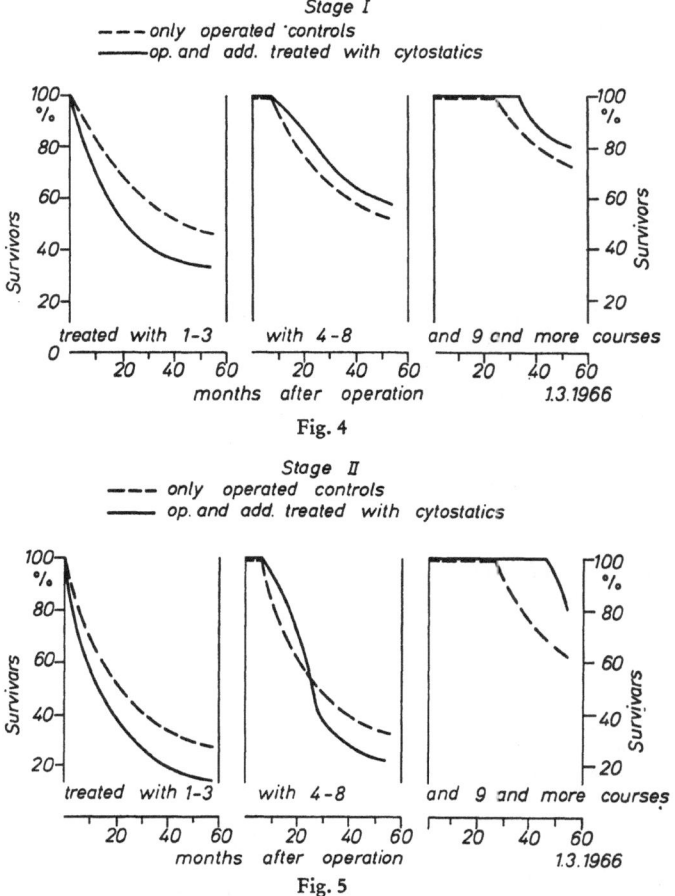

Fig. 4

Fig. 5

Fig. 4 and 5. Comparison of life tables of patients after radical operation for bronchial carcinoma stage I and II with and without adjuvant chemotherapy

nature and because of the small number of patients involved. However they are an important indication of the need for expanded and more definitive studies carried out by a larger and more authoritative group.

The differences between the two groups are less than in Fig. 1. The numbers of patients represented by different groups on the curves are given in Table III.

While compiling the data it became evident that the reliability of the protocol of treatment decreased with an increasing number of co-operating hospitals and private doctors. After classification of the patients into groups according to the actual number of courses of treatment received, the life-tables show a difference in favour of long-term adjuvant chemotherapy (Figs. 4 and 5). It should be noted that the untreated controls for each classification are the ones surviving up to or beyond the time for the minimum number of treatments for that classification. The number of patients in each classification is given in Table III.

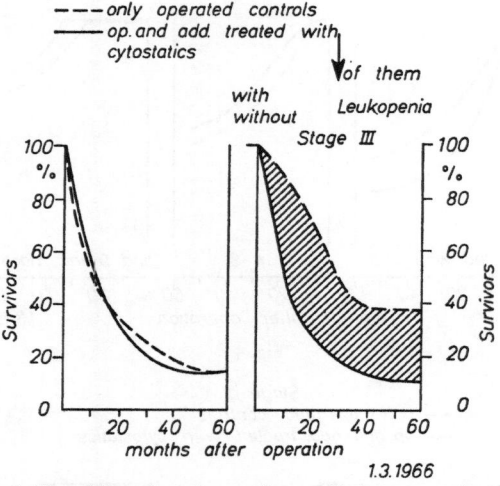

Fig. 6. Comparison of life tables of patients after radical surgery for bronchial carcinoma stage III with and without adjuvant chemotherapy and with and without leucopenia as the result of adjuvant chemotherapy

References

ADELBERGER, L., u. WOERN, H., Grundlagen und Probleme einer Rezidivprophylaxe durch Zytostatica mit besonderer Bezugnahme auf Bronchial- und Lungenkarzinome. *Mitt. Ges. zu Bekämpf. Krebskr.* 3, 612—629 (1964).

BUCHBERGER, R., u. JENNY, R. H., Ergebnisse der chirurgischen Behandlung beim Magenkarzinom. *Med. Klin.* 60, 629—633 (1965).

DENK, W., Weitere Erfahrungen mit der Rezidiv- und Metastasenprophylaxe nach Karzinomoperationen. *Klin. Med. (Wien)* 13, 426—429 (1958).

—, u. KARRER, K., Modellversuch einer Rezidivprophylaxe des Karzinoms. *Wien. klin. Wschr.* 67, 986 (1955).

— — Chemotherapie zur Rezidivprophylaxe des Karzinoms. *Wien klin. Wschr.* 68, 977—979 (1956).

DENK, W., u. KARRER, K., Chemotherapie als Versuch einer Rückfallverhütung nach Karzinomoperationen. *Krebsarzt* 14, 81—84 (1959).

— — Combined surgery and chemotherapy in the treatment of malignant tumors. *Cancer (Philad.)* 14, 1197—1204 (1961 a).

— — Chemotherapie mit Zytostatika in der Chirurgie. *Krebsforsch. u. Krebsbekämpf.* 4, 73—78 (1961 b).

—, and WURNIG, P., Über den Wert und die Risiken einer postoperativen Chemotherapie maligner Tumoren. *Arzneimittel-Forsch.* 11, 233—238 (1961).

— — — Chemotherapy as an adjuvant to the surgical treatment of cancer. *Acta. Un. int. Canc.* 20, 64—67 (1964).

FISHER, R. A., Statistical methods for research workers. Edinburgh: Oliver & Boyd (1958).

GODÁL, A., INDIN, T., KNOTZ, F., and TESAREK, T., Application of Endoxan in combination with surgical treatment in cancer of the gastrointestinal tract. *Neoplasma (Bratisl.)* 9, 537—541 (1962).

GODÁL, A., TESAREK, T., INDIN, T., and KNOTZ, F., The use of degranol in combination with surgical treatment in cancer of gastrointestinal tract *Neoplasma (Bratisl.)* 11, 89—93 (1964).

HIGGINS, G. A., The use of 5-fluorodeoxyuridine (FUDR) as a surgical adjuvant in carcinoma of the stomach and colorecum. *Arch. Surg.* 86, 926—931 (1963).

JENNY, R. H., Ergebnisse der Radicaloperationen des Bronchuskarzinoms. *Klin. Med. (Wien)* 16, 208—211 (1961).

—, and BUCHBERGER, R., Ergebnisse der chirurgischen Behandlung des Bronchuscarcinoms. *Langenbecks Arch. klin. Chir.* 299, 485—515 (1962).

KARRER, K., Probleme der Chemotherapie des Karzinoms. *Wien. klin. Wschr.* 74, 190—191 (1962).

— Zur kombinierten cytostatischen und operativen Behandlung des Karzinomas. *Arzneimittel-Forsch.* 14, 589—869, 1059—1066 (1964).

— HUMPHREYS, S. R., and GOLDIN, A., Relationship of drug toxicity to chemotherapeutic effectiveness. *Antimicr. Agents and Chemother.* 539—543 (1965).

—, u. WURNIG, P., Zur Methode der Bewertung chemotherapeutischer Rezidivprophylaxe des operierten Karzinoms. *Klin. Med. (Wien)* 17, 222—233 (1962).

KUTSCHERA, W., and SCHNETZER, J., Zytostatika nach Lungenresektion wegen Krebs. *Wien. klin. Wschr.* 77, 289—290 (1965).

MRAZEK, R. G., Chemotherapy for cancer. *Surg. Clin. N. Amer.* 44, 113—123 (1964).

POULSEN, O. VON, Prae- und postoperative cytostatische Behandlung von Lungencarcinomen mit Cyclophosphamid. *Arzneimittel.-Forsch.* 11, 238—242 (1961).

SERLIN, O., Use of thio—tepa as an adjuvant to the surgical management of carcinoma of the stomach. (V. A. Co-operative Surgied Adjuviant Study Grup.) *Cancer (Philad.)* 18, 291—297 (1965).

URABE, M., Study on chemotherapy of malignant tumors. *Stud. Mitomycin* 120, 1—13 (1961).

WOLBERG, W. H., A reappraisal of surgical adjuvant cancer chemotherapy. *Surg. Gynec. Obstet.* 120, 299—300 (1965).

WURNIG, P., Ergebnisse und Grundsätze der Rezidivprophylaxe mit Mitomen bei radikal operierten malignen Tumoren an Hand des Bronchus Karzinoms. *Wien. klin. Wschr.* 70, 63 (1958).

— SCHEUBA, J., and KARRER, K., Vorläufige Ergebnisse der chemotherapeutischen Recidivprophylaxe mit Mitomen beim operierten Bronchuscarcinom. *Acta Un. int. Cancr.* 6, 935—936 (1960).

Panel 16

Voluntary Organizations

Chairman:

J. R. HELLER (U.S.A.)

Members:

A. S. ABU-GUORA (Jordan), L. W. ADAMS (U.S.A.), K. A. GARDNER (Canada),
O. S. JACOBSEN (Norway), T. KOSZAROWSKI (Poland), K. MASUBUCHI (Japan),
A. B. DE SUSTAITA-SEEBER (Argentina)

Panel 17

Controlled Clinical Trials and their Evaluation

Chairman:

Richard Doll (U.K.)

Members:

Emil Frei, III (U.S.A.), J. Hayward (U.K.), H. Kolodziejska (Poland),
Y. Koyama (Japan), R. Nissen-Meyer (Norway), A. Rakov (U.S.S.R.),
M. Schneidermann (U.S.A.)

Introduction

Richard Doll

Medical Research Council, Statistical Research Unit, London

Whenever we treat a patient — by giving him a drug, operating on him or irradiating him — we are, whether we like it or not, performing an experiment. As scientists, our responsibility is to perform it in such a way that we are most likely to interpret the results correctly, so that the information gained may be of use to other patients in the future. As doctors, however, our primary concern must be with the good of the patient who is currently in our care. The question arises, therefore, are these two duties reconcilable, or are they mutually incompatible?

In many countries, and in many fields of medicine, the answer has come to be accepted that they can be reconciled by means of the controlled clinical trial, carried out scrupulously and under certain carefully defined conditions. And, as a result of such trials, the relative value of new treatments has been rapidly determined and old controversies have been settled — often with great saving to the patient in terms of both discomfort and expense.

In oncology, however, the use of such trials has spread only slowly and one is forced to ask whether they are equally appropriate for assessing the effects of cancer treatment, or whether there are any peculiar difficulties that make their use in this field impracticable or make modifications in their design necessary. These questions are not easy to answer — requiring, as they do, an intimate knowledge of practical therapeutics and involving basic problems of scientific method and medical ethics — and we are most grateful to the members of this panel who have undertaken the responsibility of attempting to answer them.

The Shin Tokaido* to Developing New Treatments in Medicine: Unbiasedness

Marvin A. Schneiderman

National Cancer Institute, Bethesda, Md., U.S.A.

The road you take determines where you get. Sometimes alternate ways can get you to the same place, but few are routes of choice, the king's highway. To get to answers about the efficacy of treatments in clinical medicine, and in cancer treatment in particular, my choice for the king's highway is the unbiased way. There may be some whose sense of direction is so good that they will get to the right answer no matter how they go. They don't need to use a king's highway. These remarks are not directed to them.

By unbiased I mean unprejudiced. This is not the same as "objective". Objective measurements do not assure unbiasedness. One can have objective measures which lead to biased results, and subjective measures which are unbiased. Objective measures can be gathered on a biased sample, or reported in a biased way. For example, there is hardly any measure inherently more objective than whether a patient is alive or dead. Yet, if we report survival from time of diagnosis for a treated and an untreated group of patients (who have not been assigned to "treatment", or "no treatment" by a randomization process), our results will be biased in favor of "treatment". Why? Because patients must have survived at least a little while to live long enough to be "treated". All patients who died before they could be treated must be in the nontreated group — hence the bias.

Conversely it is possible to employ subjective measures in an unbiased way. Reported pain is a subjective measure, yet it is almost the only way to assess whether a treatment reduced pain (other than, perhaps, to measure the consumption of narcotics, which is an objective expression of subjective behavior). If we made a formal random assignment of patients to "treatment" and "con-

---

* Phonetic transliteration of the Japanese for "new super-road", i.e. the royal road or king's highway.

trol" and managed the patients in such a manner that neither observer nor the patient could identify which patient was on which treatment, then the reporting of pain would lead to an unbiased assessment of the effectiveness of the treatment.

In an experimental cancer treatment our measurements are usually offered as inducements to action — to continue or discontinue the treatment. People usually have to be convinced before they take action. If the only person you need to convince is yourself, bias, or lack of it, might not even be noticed. To convince yourself that a drug is potentially useful may require that one patient do well on it — if this was your strong expectation in the first place. (Given the same expectation it is unlikely that a single patient doing badly would convince you that the drug did *not* have "potential".) To convince others is another matter, especially if their expectations are not the same as yours. Then you may have to start by first convincing them that your work and reporting have been unbiased.

The touchstone then, is unbiasedness. An affirmative answer to the question, "Was this work unbiased?" makes the rest of the argument more convincing. Unbiasedness depends on *whom* the measurements are made and *how* they are made, even more than of *what* the measurements are made. Our concern is with the "who" and "how". An approach to unbiasedness is through awareness of some of the sources of bias. Take appropriate actions to evade, avoid or reduce them and you're well on your way.

In medical research the patient is the primary source of bias. The differences in patients from one time to another and from one place to another make it difficult to compare meaningfully one investigator's results with another's — or even with his own work done at another time.

An example of this was given by GARCEAU et al. (1964). In a trial of the effectiveness of portacaval-shunt surgery for the treatment of patients with esophageal varices, the survival of treated patients was contrasted with survival of two groups of untreated patients. The first of the untreated groups was a true randomly-assigned control from the same set of patients from which the surgically-treated ones came. The second untreated group was a general collection of patients not selected for, or specifically included, in the trial. The authors called this the "unselected" group. The survival of the surgically-treated patients was far superior to the "unselected" group of patients. But so was the survival of the randomly-assigned group of untreated patients! In fact, the authors remark that "selection for the study itself ... was associated with a substantial increase in survival".

Problems of patient comparability occur at all stages in the development of a new treatment. DeVITA and his associates (DeVITA et al., 1965), trying to find the proper dose and schedule for a new anti-cancer drug, set up a sophisticated experiment having three preliminary schedule-route combinations, each given at several different doses. The plan was to find a maximum tolerated dose (in some sense a "best" dose) for each combination, and then, in a second phase of the study, use these "best" doses to then evaluate which of the three schedule-route combinations was "best" in terms of response. In the first phase, doses were found for each schedule which produced the desired level of toxicity. In the second stage doses which had been moderately toxic ("biologically active") in the first stage, now produced little or no toxicity. No decision could be made about schedule and route. Several explanations are possible: the drug had changed; the second stage patients were different; both. The author's conjecture is that sicker patients — more likely to show toxicity, had been used in the first stage of the experiment — and that the second stage patients were probably less ill. Possibly by that time the physicians had learned enough about the drug that they were more willing to risk "better" patients on it.

Examples of similar experiences could be cited almost without end — the drug effective in the hands of the originator, ineffective in the hands of someone else (minor toxicity to one investigator, major to another) — who used the same dose, schedule, route, and objective measures that the first investigators had.

Another source of patient bias is bias in patient retention. Once the patients get into the study, who is kept in? Who is reported on? One way patient-retention bias is introduced is by reporting on a portion of the patients who have been treated — rather than all the patients. A group that are often reported on separately are the "adequately-treated" patients. Talking about "adequately-treated" patients is one way of following GEORGE MOORE's (1963) instruction on, "How to Achieve Surgical Results by Really Trying". Among the techniques he noted was to "... exclude uncooperative, i. e. dead, patients from follow up ..." Defining "adequate treatment" rigidly enough can assure that all "adequately-treated" patients will live long and normal lives. Of course, no one defines it quite that rigidly — but how much less is "adequate" enough?

There are unfortunately an infinite number of definitions of "adequate treatment" — all of which lead to an upward bias in the proportion of responders, their survival, etc. Any definition of "adequate treatment" omits, from both numerator and denominator of the response fraction, only the failures or the early deaths. This means that the only unbiased "adequate treatment" includes all patients treated. If you do this all the time, all your studies will have the same base line — and will be comparable (within the limits of bias in patient selection) with everyone else's studies where all the patients are included all the time. And no one can assert that you have created a definition biased in your favor.

Bias in patient selection is not easy to overcome. One approach has been to attempt to treat and report on all patients who come to one institution or investigator in a defined, but extensive time period. Thus one sees reports that begin, "Twenty-seven consecutive patients were treated ..." This could be an unbiased procedure in the general hospital serving an isolated community — in which all cases in the community (and no others) come to that hospital. It hardly achieves unbiasedness in a referral institution or on a referral service, where cases are screened ("Can the patient travel back to us for periodic follow-up?") before admission. How many institutions treat children with acute lymphocytic leukemia similarly to the ones who, when seen at one referral institution, had a median white cell count of 9.3 thousand at start of treatment?

Since patients and diseases change with time and place, it is very useful to set up a link with other places and other times. This can usually be done by having at least two groups of patients randomly assigned — one to the new treatment (a "new" treatment includes a new dose schedule, a new route, a new dose, etc.) and one to the old treatment (or the contrasting treatment used someplace else). Results of the old treatment given to the new patients can be compared to results of the old treatment given to the old patients. If they are comparable, then one has some assurance that the patients and the disease and the ancillary services probably have not changed much in the interval. There are also strong ethical reasons for having a randomly-assigned control group who are concurrently being given the best treatment known. If we are not absolutely certain that the new treatment is better than the old, we must have a continuous comparison available to permit us to identify and drop the poorer treatment as soon as possible.

A close study of diseases sometimes reveals characteristics of the patients that are prognostic. Thus, we know that the child with acute lymphocytic leukemia will do better than the adult. The patient with the low initial white count has better survival prospects than the patient with the high count. For some diseases some investigators have gotten near creating a patient profile of important prognostic characteristics. The least this implies is that we should now stratify by major patient profiles — and attempt to compare results of treatment on comparable patients. If we do and if we assign our patients by a randomization procedure to the different treatments within strata, we may be able to make unbiased comparisons within these strata. This will help us to see interactions between patient status and treatment — and perhaps tell us when in his disease a patient should be treated by this treatment — and when he should not. A major caution is against overstratifying. This is self-defeating. Very few patients per stratum yield very few meaningful comparisons. To create too many strata is to deny similarities; it's a form of nihilism.

Summary

The key to learning and convincing from experimentation is unbiasedness: Unbiasedness in patient allocation by randomized assignment to contrasted treatments; unbiasedness in evaluation by having the trials double blind whenever possible; unbiasedness in analysis by having a randomized link to the past, and to others' work; unbiasedness in presentation of results by giving results on all patients; unbiasedness in contrasts by comparing comparable patients, gained by stratification and random assignment; unbiasedness by conducting adequately-controlled trials almost every step of the way in the development of a new treatment. The stricter the unbiasedness, the less the challenge to your work; the greater your chance of convincing others of your convincing results.

References

DeVita, V. T., Carbone, P. P., Owens jr., A. H., Gold, G. L., Krant, M. J., and Edmonson, J., Clinical trials with 1,3-Bis(2-chloroethyl)-1-nitrosourea, NSC-409962. *Cancer Res.* 25, 1876—1881 (1965).

Garceau, A. J., Donaldson jr., R. M., O'Hara, E. T., Callow, A. D., Muench, H., Chalmers, T. C., and Boston Inter-hospital Liver Group, Controlled trial of prophylactic portacaval-shunt surgery. *New Engl. J. Med.* 270. 496—500 (1964).

Moore G. E., How to achieve surgical results by really trying. *Surg. Gynec. Obstet.* 116, 497—498 (1963).

Experimental Design and Clinical Cancer Chemotherapy

Emil Frei, III

The University of Texas, M. D. Anderson Hospital and Tumor Institute, Houston, Texas, U.S.A.

There are four basic parameters for evaluating objective response to chemotherapy. These are listed on the ordinate of Fig. 1. Remission induction consists of the initial period of chemotherapy and is generally continued until maximum tumor regression has occurred. Remission duration is divided into "unmaintained remisssion" and "maintained remission". The former is the remission duration after remission induction therapy has been discontinued and the latter (maintained remission) is defined as the duration of remission when antitumor agent therapy is continued during remission. The ultimate parameter is survival and this, of course, is the major parameter for the evaluation of potentially curative therapy.

Across the top of Fig. 1 are listed three diseases: acute leukemia in children which responds excellently to chemotherapy; metastatic carcinoma of the breast which responds partially to several agents; and carcinoma of the lung which is essentially unresponsive. The degree of responsiveness of a tumor category to conventional agents plus other aspects of the natural history of the disease markedly influences the relative usefulness of the above parameters of response. For example, in acute leukemia in children a complete remission rate in excess of 80 per cent can be achieved with conventional treatment (Frei and Frei-reich, 1965). It would take a very large number of cases in a controlled study to prove that a new treatment program produced a significantly greater remission rate. Perhaps the optimal setting for evaluating a new therapeutic program in such patients is during remission (FREIREICH et al., 1963). The advantages include: 1. the number of neoplastic cells has already been reduced to low levels by remission induction therapy, 2. the patient is in much better condition generally and particularly with respect to tolerating antitumor

Parameters	Acute leukemia (Children)	Breast carcinoma (Metastatic)	Lung carcinoma
Remission Induction			
Complete	80 per cent	0—5 per cent	
Partial	Not too useful because of the very high response rate with conventional treatment *	20—30 per cent Useful	0—5 per cent Not too effective a parameter for comparative studies because of difficulties in measurement *
Remission duration			
Unmaintained	Technique for evaluating complete remission and estimating persisting neoplastic cells *	Not useful	—
Maintained	Optimal setting for evaluating new programs	Importance of continued treatment during remission emphasized	—
Survival	Relates directly to time spent in remission	Not too useful due to long survival and short responses	Most useful due to short survival and ineffectiveness of above parameters

* See text.

Fig. 1. Effectiveness of various parameters of response in three types of human tumors

(myelosuppressive) agents, 3. response is quantitative, that is duration of remission is being evaluated, rather than qualitative (remission induction yes or no) and thus is much more efficient in terms of the number of cases required to show a significant difference, and 4. the use of new therapeutic programs, even if relatively inactive, for remission maintenance does not shorten survival since active agents are not used during remission and may be subsequently more effectively employed for remission induction and maintenence. Finally this technique of evaluating agents as "remission maintainers" allows for evaluation relatively early during the course of the disease (FREIREICH et al., 1963). New agents are usually evaluated in acute leukemia for remission induction after conventional treatment is no longer effective. For many neoplastic diseases, this approach may be relatively ineffective in that the patient's poor condition precludes the administration of effective doses of antitumor agents and it is also possible that the tumor becomes intrinsically less responsive.

Unmaintained remission, survival, and the other disease catagories listed in Fig. 1 will be considered subsequently.

The comparative therapeutic trial is a powerful tool and has contributed in a major way to advancing our knowledge of cancer chemotherapy (ZUBROD, 1964). While there are aspects of the application of the comparative trial in neoplastic disease which continue to present problems, the most difficult problem in my judgement is the primary question, when is a comparative study indicated? When are controls necessary? In general, a quantitative study is indicated if it is reasonably probable that it will provide important new information. Quantitative comparative studies require a major investment in patients, time, and investigator effort. Too often such studies are undertaken, not because of a good hypothesis, but because the resources happen to be available. Some of the details relative to the decision as to whether a quantitative study is indicated are presented in Fig. 2. Let us consider a hypothetical circumstance where, in preliminary trial, an experimental chemotherapeutic program produces a 20 to 30 per cent response rate in a given tumor category. Is a placebo controlled comparative study indicated? In general, if standard treatment is at all effective, placebo controls are not justified. If standard treatment is ineffective, placebo controls are not necessary. Placebo controlled studies of selected neoplastic diseases, where the value of any treatment was questionable, have provided important information in the past, but today, with our better understanding of the natural history of most neoplastic diseases, placebo controls are rarely indicated. This does not apply to the use of placebo or untreated controls for certain studies of adjuvant chemotherapy and of remission duration.

Often in a comparative study, experimental program X (Fig. 2) is compared to standard treatment (S in Fig. 2). If the response rate to S is 10 to 40 per cent, a large number of cases will be required to demonstrate a significant difference between X and S (GEHAN, 1961). If S and X are qualitatively different drugs, what new therapeutic research leads will the study provide? These problems should be carefully considered before implementing a comparative study.

A comparative study is most strongly indicated in those circumstances where the results have a good chance of providing important new therapeutic research leads. Thus the comparison of an active analog of X (X^a) to X, where studies and experimental systems indicate important structure-activity relationships, might provide important new information. Similarly dose-response, schedule response, duration of treatment and combined treatment studies may provide important research leads and directly or indirectly lead to improved treatment (GOLDIN et al., 1956; SKIPPER et al., 1964; BRUCE et al., 1965; SELAWRY and FREI, 1964; FREI et al., 1965; FREIREICH et al., 1964; 1965 b; KARON et al., 1965).

X	= experimental program which in preliminary studies produces a 20—30 per cent response rate in a given tumor category.
?	= Is a comparative study indicated and, if so, what should X be compared to.
Placebo.	If, for remission induction, there is no effective treatment placebo controls are not necessary or justified.*
S	= Standard Treatment. If it produces a 10—40 per cent response rate in the same tumor category a large number of cases will be required to show a 10—20 per cent difference. ? biomedical significance of results.*
X^a	= analog of X. Important basis for quantitative comparison where structure activity studies suggest important therapeutic leads.
X_{1-n}	= different doses, schedules, duration of treatment of X and combinations of X with other agents. A strong experimental and clinical basis for quantitative studies with new (and conventional) agents along these lines is developing.

* See text.

Fig. 2. Comparative study: considerations in the selection of control or standard treatment

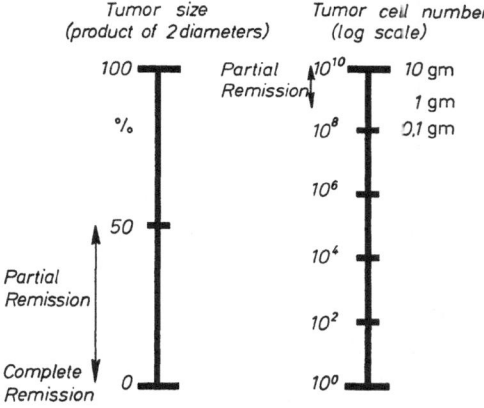

Fig. 3. Nature of remissions when measured by reduction in tumor size or reduction in proportion of surviving tumor cells

It must be emphasized that in the design of such studies it is essential to consider in detail all of the experimental data. This is particularly true with respect to the experimental biology, pharmacology, toxicology, and the cell kinetics of the host target organ and the tumor. When this is done appropriately designed quantitative clinical studies will usually provide important information with respect to our understanding of the tumor and the host and the correlation between preclinical and clinical systems even in circumstances where the results of the study are not positive in terms of demonstrating a better therapeutic program.

Selected problems relating to the above will be considered in more detail. Remission induction is usually measured by tumor regression (Fig. 3). The scale on the left in Figure 3 relates to tumor regression. A greater than 50 per cent decrease in the product of two diameters of a tumor mass is defined as a partial regression and a complete regression consists of clinical disappearance of the tumor. A 50 per cent decrease is substantial and superficially it might be interpreted as the halfway mark to our goal. Definitive studies in micro-biological systems, mammalian cells *in vitro,* and neoplastic cells *in vivo* indicate that, for chemotherapeutic agents and for x-irradiation, the *percentage of cells,* not the *absolute number of cells,* destroyed by a given treatment is constant

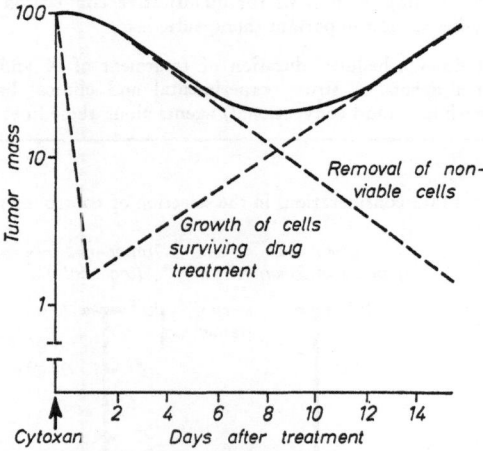

Fig. 4. Relative changes in tumor mass and number of tumor cells when experimental solid tumors are treated

(SKIPPER *et al.,* 1964). Thus twice as good as 50 per cent is 75 per cent not 100 per cent. In the light of this a better presentation of the neoplastic cell number and volume problem is presented on the right hand side of Fig. 3. Here the number of neoplastic cells are presented in log scale. On this scale a partial remission represents at best a 10 per cent inroad on the tumor rather than a 50 per cent effect. Stated another way, we would need therapy 10 times as potent as that which produceçd partial remission to approach the eradication of neoplastic cells rather than therapy which is only two or three times as potent. In view of this, partial remissions constitute relatively slight activity and one might question whether quantitative studies are indicated in a cir-cumstance where such relatively slight activity is produced in a minority of patients. A complete regression on this log scale represents at least a 10-fold reduction in neoplastic cells and in some diseases, for example acute leukemia in children, Burkitt's lymphoma, and choriocarcinoma, a much greater reduction can be achieved.

This interpretation must be somewhat qualified in the light of recent ex-perimental studies (Fig. 4). WILCOX *et al.* (1965) have evaluated the dynamics of tumor size and cell number in several experimental solid tumors. Fig. 4 is a schematic and generalized representation of their data with reference to the experimental solid tumors, sarcoma 180, and plasmacytoma. With cyclophosphamide treatment the tumor mass decreased 60 to 70 per cent for a relatively brief period of time. By volume calculation this is not impressive tumor cell destruction. However by quantitative bioassay techniques it was demonstrated that a much greater neoplastic cell destruction in fact occurred and that most of the tumor mass during the period of tumor regression and before the tumor increased exponentially was composed of dead or dying cells which are slowly resorbed. The extent to which the above is true for man is unknown. Certainly the extent and duration of remission induction therapy must be carefully reconsidered in the light of this data.

The importance of the parameter "unmaintained remission" in those diseases where a high complete remission rate can be achieved, such as acute leukemia in children and some lymphomas, should be emphasized. This parameter has been employed in experimental systems and has proven highly effective in quantitating the number of neoplastic cells persisting after a given treatment. Experimental studies by SKIPPER and his associates (1964) employing this technique have shed considerable light on problems relating to curability with chemotherapeutic agents. In diseases such as the above where intensive therapeutic programs are being employed to maximally reduce the patient's neoplastic cell burden, the duration of unmaintained remission would appear to be the most effective parameter for quantifying small "subclinical" numbers of neoplastic cells persisting after treatment. While other variables must be considered and assumptions made, it is certainly highly probable that the duration of unmaintained remission must be, at least in part, a function of the number of neoplastic cells persisting at the end of treatment. Examples of such studies are presented in Fig. 5. This is a semi-log plot of the duration of unmaintained remission after single drug treatment and after intensive combined treatment (VAMP and BIKE, FREIREICH et al., 1964; 1965 b). Not only is the median duration of remission longer following intensive treatment, but the slope of the curve and the guarantee time (time to first relapse) changes with increasingly effective therapy. Also, in any such study very long unmaintained remissions which fall outside of the straight line plot should be evaluated separately. The above factors represent important problems and opportunities in the employment and interpretation of quantitative comparative clinical trials (JOHNSON et al., 1966).

Patient survival is the ultimate parameter for evaluation of a therapeutic program. However, as a practical matter, this parameter is variously useful depending upon the therapeutic program and particularly the disease. In carcinoma of the lung where survival is short and other objective parameters, such as tumor measurement for remission induction, are difficult to apply survival is the most useful parameter. For many diseases which respond to chemotherapy it has been demonstrated that survival is directly related to the time spent in drug induced remission. In Fig. 6 the survival of patients with acute leukemia who achieve remission is compared to that of patients who have no remissions. When the time spent in remission is subtracted from the remitting

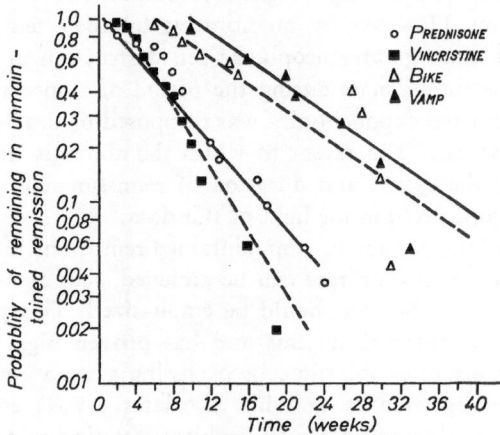

Fig. 5. Duration of unmaintained remissions with different treatments for acute lymphatic leukaemia in children

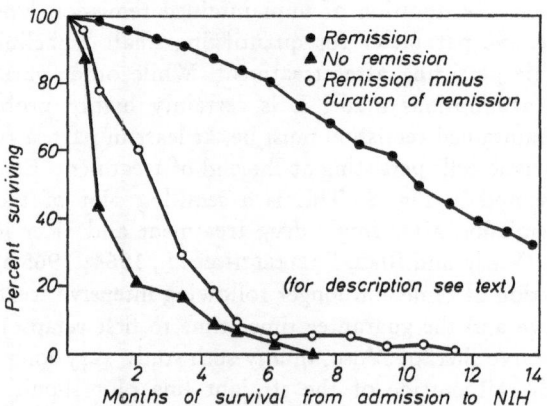

Fig. 6. Comparison of duration of survival not in remission in patients with acute leukaemia who remit and those who do not

group their survival is almost identical to that of patients who have had no remission. Thus the improved survival in children with acute leukemia is directly related to the time during which the drug controlled the disease (FREI-REICH *et al.*, 1961). This has been recently demonstrated to be true for multiple myeloma and ovarian carcinoma and should be determined for other malignancies. Again while survival is the ultimate parameter, it is, for some diseases, such as metastatic carcinoma of the breast, a difficult one to apply because of their long survival relative to the period of drug trial and drug control of the disease. Thus, it may take an extended period of time to evaluate the effect of the new therapeutic program in terms of survival, whereas the answers with respect to the other parameters will be forthcoming much sooner. To the extent that duration of tumor control by effective drug treatment correlates with survival it may be effectively employed.

References

BRUCE, W. R., VALERIOTE, F. A., and MEEKER, B. E., A comparison of the sensitivity of normal murine hematopoietic and transplanted lymphoma colony-forming cells to tritiated thymidine and vinblastine. *Proc. Amer. Ass. Cancer Res.* 6, 8 (1965).

FREI, E., III, and FREIREICH, E. J., Progress and perspectives in the chemotherapy of acute leukemia. *Adv. Chemother.* 2, 269—298 (1965).

— KARON, M., LEVIN, R. H., FREIREICH, E. J., TAYLOR, R. J., HANANIAN, J., SELAWRY, O., HOLLAND, J. F., HOOGSTRATEN, B., WOLMAN, I. J., ABIR, E., SAWITSKY, A., LEE, S., MILLS, S. D., BURGERT jr., E. O., SPURR, C. L., PATTERSON, R. B., EBAUGH, F. G., JAMES, G. W., III, and MOON, J. H., The effectiveness of combinations of antileukemic agents in inducing and maintaining remission in children with acute leukemia. *Blood* 26, 642—656 (1965).

FREIREICH, E. J., GEHAN, E., FREI, E., III, SCHROEDER, L. R., WOLMAN, I. J., ANBARI, R., BURGERT, E. O., MILLS, S. D., PINKEL, D., SELAWRY, O. S., MOON, J. H., GENDEL, B. R., SPURR, C. L., STORRS, R., HAURANI, F., HOOGSTRATEN, B., and LEE, S. (Acute Leukemia B Group), The effect of 6-mercaptopurine on the duration of steroid-induced remissions in acute leukemia: A model for evaluation of other potentially useful therapy. *Blood* 21, 699—716 (1963).

— GEHAN, E. A., SULMAN, D., BOGGS, D. R., and FREI, E., III, The effect of chemotherapy on acute leukemia in the human. *J. chron. Dis.* 14, 593—608 (1961).

— KARON, M., FLATOW, F., and FREI, E., III, Effect of intensive cyclic chemotherapy (BIKE) on remission duration in acute lymphocytic leukemia. *Proc. Amer. Ass. Cancer Res.* 6, 20 (1965).

FREIREICH, E. J., KARON, M., and FREI, E., III, Quadruple combination therapy (VAMP) for acute lymphocytic leukemia in childhood. *Proc. Amer. Ass. Cancer Res.* 5, 20 (1964).

GEHAN, F. A., The determination of the number of patients in a preliminary and a follow-up trial of a new chemotherapeutic agent. *J. chron. Dis.* 13, 346 (1961).

GOLDIN, A., VENDITTI, J. M., HUMPHREYS, S. R., and MANTEL, N., Modification of treatment schedules in the management of advanced mouse leukemia with amethopterin. *J. nat. Cancer Inst.* 17, 203—212 (1956).

JOHNSON, R. E., ZELEN, M., and FREIREICH, E. J., Evaluation of human acute leukemia data using a murine leukemia model system. *Cancer (Philad.)* 19, 481 (1966).

KARON, M., FREIREICH, E. J., and CARBONE, P., Effective combination of adult leukemia. *Proc. Amer. Ass. Cancer Res.* 6, 34 (1965).

SELAWRY, O. S., and FREI, E., III, Prolongation of remission in acute lymphocytic leukemia by alternation in dose schedule and route of administration of methotrexate. *Clin. Res.* 12, 231 (1964).

SKIPPER, H. E., SCHABEL jr., F. M., and WILCOX, W. S., Experimental evaluation of potential anticancer agents: XIII. On the criteria and kinetics associated with "curability" of experimental leukemia. *Cancer Chemother. Rep.* 35, 1—111 (1964).

WILCOX, W. S., GRISWOLD, D. P., LASTER, W. R., SCHABEL, F. M., SKIPPER, H. E., Experimental evaluation of potential anticancer agents (XVII). Kinetics of growth and regression after treatment of surgeon solid tumors.

ZUBROD, C., GORDON, Quantitative concepts in the clinical study of drugs. Advances in chemotherapy 1, 9—34 (1964).

Ethics in Clinical Trials

J. L. HAYWARD

Department of Surgery, Guy's Hospital, London

Since the turn of the century medical knowledge has progressed more rapidly than at any other period in history. Each year new treatments are introduced, some of which are but minor alterations of those in current use but many involve novel and sometimes largely untried therapies for human disease. Before this period of rapid scientific development, the few advances in therapy that became available were often minor deviations of those in current use. The assessment of their value was by clinical observation and, although the frequent worthlessness of this appreciation has since become apparent, many relics of this time can still be found in medical practice today. This was the era of the "Sayings of the great men", when because an expert said a therapy was valuable, this view was accepted and unchallenged. Thankfully this has passed; no-one believes a thing is necessarily so, because someone says it is so; proof is demanded and, because this proof relates to the treatment of human ailments, its assimilation must necessitate human experimentation. In turn this has provided its problems and in particular has meant an uneasy alliance between scientific planning and the ethical code inherent in the doctor—patient relationship.

During the past two decades it has been appreciated that for the proper elucidation of these problems use must be made of a relatively new tool, the controlled clinical trial, and because of the immediate confrontation of patient experimentation with medical ethics, many attempts have been made to provide the clinician with rules for his guidance. Many countries have elaborated codes of ethics designed to help their own investigators. In Great Britain the Medical Research Council (1964) has offered detailed rules for the guidance of doctors involved in the planning and conduct of clinical trials. More recently in 1964 the World Medical Association announced a code of ethics on Human Experimentation known as "The declaration of Helsinki". This is not the place to enumerate the various recommendations that have been made but in each case a distinction has been suggested between trials which involve treatments designed for the benefit of the patient and those involving experimental procedures which, although aimed to further medical knowledge, are not to the patients' immediate advantage. In the former case it was felt that providing a practitioner genuinely believes that a new treatment may hold advantages over, an established one he is ethically correct to compare the two by a clinical trial. Although it is suggested that he should explain the trial to his patient this may not be necessary and indeed in some cases is directly contra-indicated. The real problem arises when procedures are used which do not contribute directly to the benefit of the individual. Here permission must be sought and under circumstances where the patient will have a complete understanding of all that is involved.

Unfortunately whilst the motives that lie behind the formation of these rules are understood even their protagonists do not claim they are any more than a guidance to the doctor. No rules could be produced that would cover all circumstances and relieve the doctor of the moral obligation of considering each case on its own merits. This perhaps is the nub of clinical experimentation — that it is the investigator's own belief — or preferably that of a group of investigators — that what is being done is justified on moral grounds. The acceptance by the patient himself is not sufficient, because it is only too easy to persuade him to undergo almost any procedure the doctor suggests, due to the special relationship between them. Without the strictest personal code almost any manipulation could be carried out and would be accepted. In our own unit we have a rather homely rule which we find helps when making this decision. Would we allow members of our own family, if the occasion arose, to enter fully into the trial we were conducting and accept whatever treatment or whatever investigation was ordered by that trial? If so, then we believe it is ethical.

There are, however, other ethical considerations as well as the question of patient acceptance. The ethics of clinical investigation do not begin and end with the moral consideration of the patient's place in the controlled trial, but rather encompass the justification and design of the trial itself. If it is appropriate and ethical to test a treatment by its comparison with an established treatment then it may be inappropriate and unethical to test its clinical effect in any other way. It is, therefore, unethical to analyse the results of drug administration or operations or any new procedure by the haphazard and uncontrolled application of that procedure. Thus it is unethical — and one must admit that this frequently happens — to claim that a new drug has advantages as a result of the observation of its effects on a handful of selected patients. Moreover, if in the minds of clinicians there is doubt as to which of two treatments is the better or under which circumstance the one or the other treatment is more appropriate, then it is unethical to continue practising these treatments without attempting, providing facilities are available, to select the better by a clinical trial. It is undoubtedly wrong to continue practising a less effective therapy if, by investigation, it could be discarded. Nor does one's moral obligation end here. If one engages in a clinical trial, unless the trial is designed as appropriately as possible both from the statistical and clinical stand-point, the results may be meaningless or, worse still, even misleading. It is ethically wrong both to produce mistaken results under the guise of a scientific investigation and to subject patients to the rigour of a clinical trial when all the effort and possible discomfort will be to no avail.

Lastly, and this may be more conjectural, there are the ethical considerations inherent in the completion of a trial. If in the first place it was ethical to consider, plan and practise a clinical trial to decide which of two treatments was the more appropriate then it will be unethical to terminate the trial until a meaningful result has been obtained. By this I do not mean that one treatment need be proved statistically better or worse than the other but rather that sufficient material should have been included so that the result whether negative or positive can have some meaning. This problem obtruded in a trial on which we were recently engaged comparing adrenalectomy with hypophysectomy in the treatment of advanced cancer of the breast. At one period during the trial, hypophysectomy appeared to be drawing well ahead of adrenalectomy and although the difference was not significant we wondered if it was ethical to continue selecting the operations by random sample. The Director of our Breast Clinic, Professor HEDLEY ATKINS, consulted Sir AUSTIN BRADFORD HILL on this problem and his advice was that if it had been ethical in the first place to carry out a trial then it was unethical to terminate it until a finite conclusion had been obtained.

This is a difficult problem and much work is going on at the moment to produce so-called "Stopping Rules" to formalise the situation; in the meanwhile however, the advice must be to persist in a trial until some meaningful result has been obtained.

May I therefore, conclude by proposing certain broad ethical rules which should be considered by all those engaged in clinical experimentation.

1. It is unethical to attempt to analyse the effect of treatment by the haphazard and uncontrolled administration of that treatment.

2. It is unethical not to carry out a clinical trial when there is doubt whether a new treatment is better than an established treatment.

3. It is unethical to conduct a clinical trial unless the clinical and statistical design of the trial is appropriate.

4. It is unethical to carry out a clinical trial without due responsibility for the patients' care and, if the procedures do not contribute to the benefit of the patients, without their understanding and permission.

5. It is unethical to terminate a clinical trial unless a meaningful result has been obtained.

References

Medical Research Council. Responsibility in investigations on human subjects. In: *Report of the Medical Research Council for 1962/63* (Cmnd. 2382). London: H. M. S. O. 1964.

World Medical Association. Human experimentation, code of ethics of the World Medical Association. *Brit. med. J.* II, 177 (1964).

Experiences with Chemotherapy as an Adjunct to Surgery and Radiotherapy

Yoshiyuki Koyama

The First National Hospital of Tokyo, Japan

There are two ways to evaluate the effects of cancer chemotherapy clinically. The one is an evaluation by survival rate and the other is an evaluation by changes in objective symptoms and laboratory data brought about by anti-cancer agents. In this panel discussion, the methods and the results of the controlled clinical trials in chemotherapy adjuvant to surgery and irradiation, made by the Research Unit of the National Hospital in Japan, will be presented.

The Cancer Chemotherapy Co-operating Research Units of 17 national hospitals studied therapeutic and side effects of chemotherapeutic remedies used for cancer of the stomach, lung and cervix uteri. The first study started on 1st July, 1959, and continued to 31st October, 1961; the second was carried out from 1st November, 1961 to 31st December, 1963; and the third was from 1st January, 1964 to 30th June, 1966.

Material and Methods

Patients in each hospital participating in the program were included if diagnosed histologically as having carcinoma. New cases, that had never undergone chemotherapy, were selected. When chemotherapy was combined with an operation, curative operation was performed. Controls were included in each cancer study group, matched according to site and stage of the cancer, and the main therapeutic method used.

Patients were allocated to each treatment group at random by opening a sealed envelope. Randomization among the treatment groups was carried out separately for each hospital and for each tumor type. The chairman of the committee for planning and management of the research (which included a statistician) provided each hospital with a series of envelopes for each tumor type, on which the name of the hospital, tumor type and serial number of the patient was written, and which contained a slip indicating which therapy the patient was to receive.

The selected patients underwent the regular examinations determined by the respective study group. Such data as X-ray negatives, tissue specimens, removed lesions, etc. were stored for over five years. Patients received chemotherapy as determined by schedule; when serious side effects appeared, the therapy was discontinued.

Follow-up observations were made, as a rule at 3, 6, 9 and 12 months, respectively after the start of chemotherapy or surgery, and once every six months for five years thereafter. Evaluation on X-ray diagnosis and histological diagnosis and the final overall evaluation were rendered by the respective committees concerned in all cases. Each member of a study group, using the designated forms, sent the following reports to the chairman concerned: registration, treatment, follow-up, discontinuance and death reports, and reports of pathological and histological diagnosis and specimens.

Results of the First and Second Studies at 31st August, 1966

1. Nine National Hospitals participated in the first study of the gastric cancer group. The effects of Thio-TEPA (TSPA) and Mitomycin C (MMC) were studied in patients on whom curative resection had been performed. TSPA was given to 136 patients, MMC to 129 and 118 patients served as controls without chemotherapy. Fig. 1 shows the age distribution of the patients in the

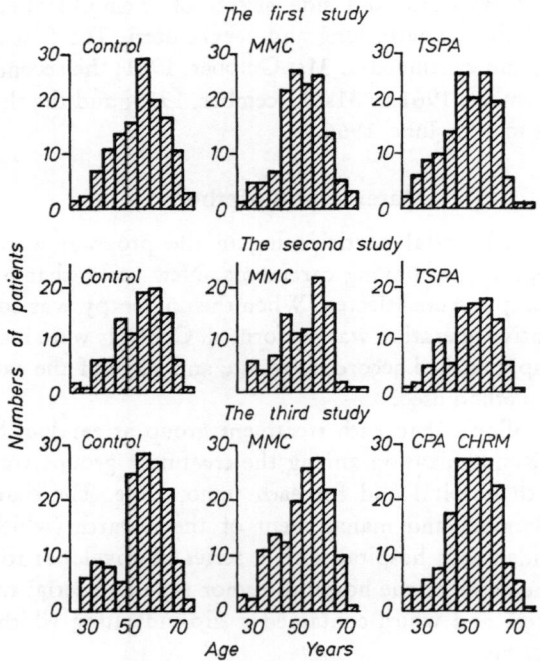

Fig. 1. Age distribution of gastric cancer patients

three treatment groups in the three studies; these were almost the same in each group. The percentages of each histological type in each study are shown in Fig. 2.

The intravenous daily dosage was 0.2 mg/kg of TSPA or 0.08 mg/kg of MMC, and the total dose was more than 50 mg of TSPA or 40 mg of MMC. During operation, 5 mg of TSPA or 4 mg of MMC was given intraperitoneally.

The procedure of the second study was the same as the first, except that the daily dose was reduced to a half and the total dose of TSPA was doubled (see Table I).

Fig. 3 shows the survival curves for the first study. The differences in survival between the control and MMC groups at one and two years are statistically significant, but no significant difference was found in survivals at five years.

These patients were divided into two groups according to histological findings: the adenocarcinoma group (ad-group) and the non-adenocarcinoma

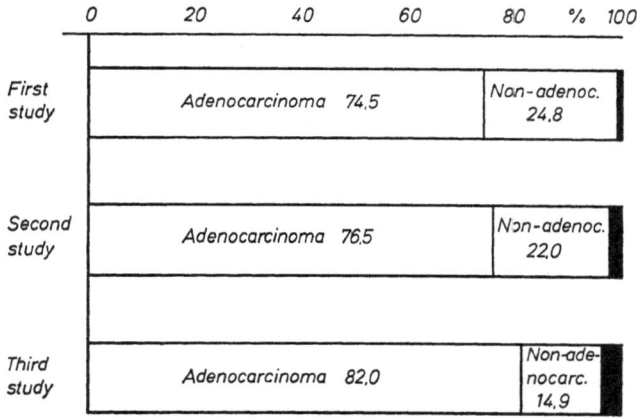

Fig. 2. Percentage of adenocarcinoma and nonadenocarcinoma in gastric cancer studies

Table I. *Method of chemotherapy in gastric carcinoma*

Study	Drug	Dosage		
		During operation	During and after operation	
			Dosage/day (i. v.)	Total dosage
First	MMC	4 mg (i. p.)	0.08 mg/kg daily	over 40 mg
	TSPA	5 mg (i. p.)	0.2 mg/kg daily	over 50 mg
	control	—	—	—
Second	MMC	4 mg (i. p.)	0.04 mg/kg daily	0.8 mg/kg
	TESPA	5 mg (i. p.)	0.1 mg/kg daily	2.0 mg/kg
	control	—	—	—
Third	MMC	4 mg (i. p.)	0.2 mg/kg twice a week	0.8 mg/kg
{	CPA	200 mg (i. p.)	2 mg/kg daily	60 mg/kg
{	CHRM	—	0.01 mg/kg daily	0.3 mg/kg
	control	—	—	—

group (non-ad-group). Two hundred and eighty six belonged to the former and 95 to the latter. Fig. 4 shows the survival curves of the "ad-group"; no significant differences were found between the treatments. In the "non-ad-group", the differences between MMC and the control treatment were statistically significant (Fig. 5).

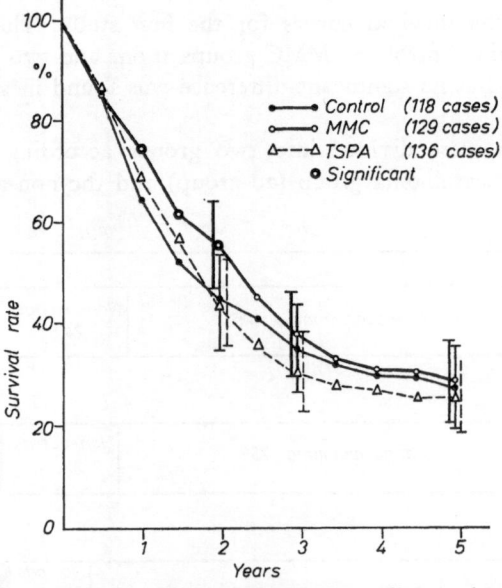

Fig. 3. Survival rates of patients with gastric carcinoma. Adjuvant chemotherapy to surgery
(the first study)

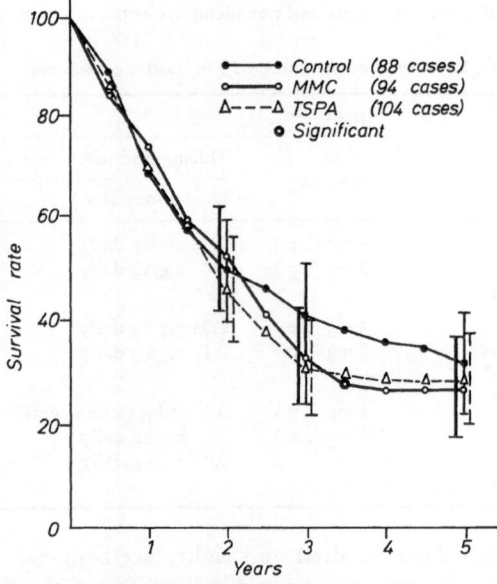

Fig. 4. Survival rates of patients with gastric carcinoma. Adjuvant chemotherapy to surgery
Adenocarcinoma group (the first study)

In the second study, three national hospitals were added and there were 277 patients in all. Fig. 6 shows the survival curves; no significant differences between the treatment groups were found.

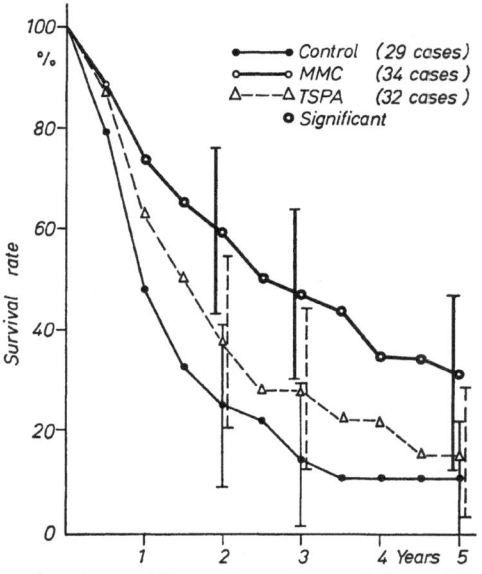

Fig. 5. Survival rates of patients with gastric carcinoma. Adjuvant chemotherapy to surgery Non-adenocarcinoma group (the first study)

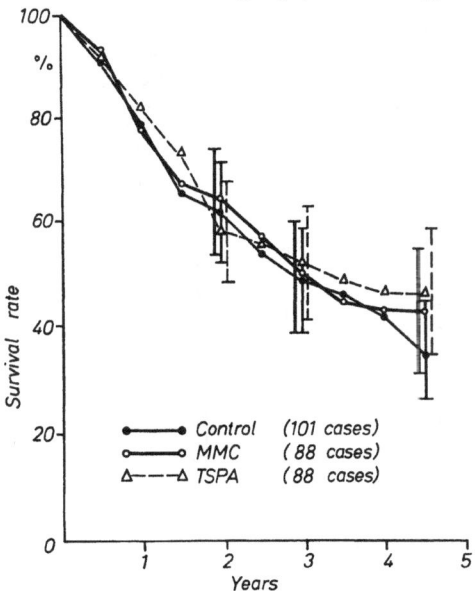

Fig. 6. Survival rates of patients with gastric carcinoma. Adjuvant chemotherapy to surgery (the second study)

Two hundred and ten patients were in the "ad-group" and 61 in the "non-ad-group". In the "ad-group" there is no significant difference between the

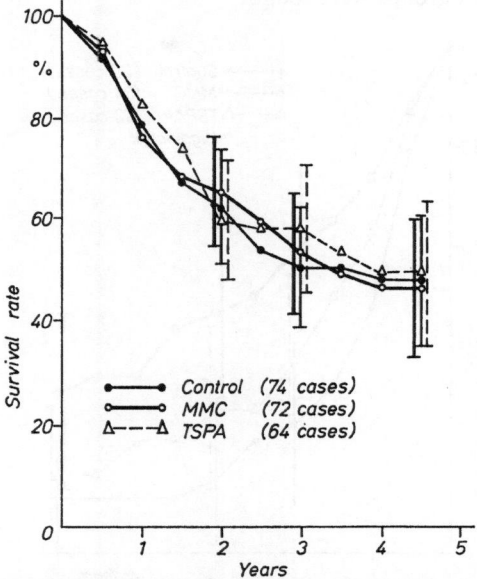

Fig. 7. Survival rates of patients with gastric carcinoma. Adjuvant chemotherapy to surgery. Adenocarcinoma group (the second study)

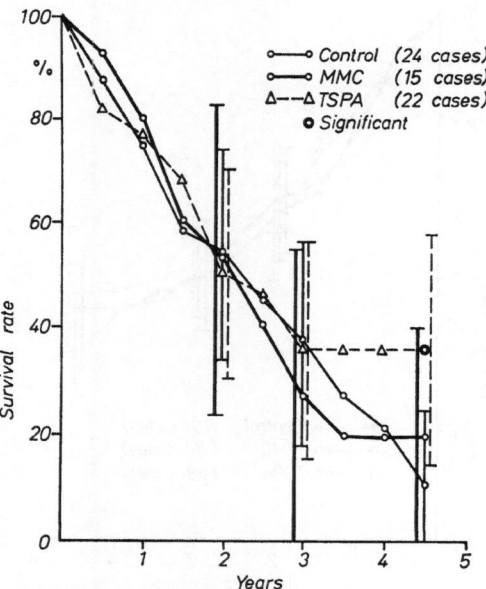

Fig. 8. Survival rates of patients with gastric carcinoma. Adjuvant chemotherapy to surgery. Non-adenocarcinoma group (the second study)

treatments (Fig. 7). Fig. 8 shows the survival curves for the "non-ad-group"; the difference between the TSPA and the control treatment is significant at $4^{1}/_{2}$ years.

The third study has been running for only two years; the results, as yet, show no appreciable differences between the treatment groups (Fig. 9).

2. The lung cancer study group consisted of nine national hospitals. Advanced cases of primary lung cancer, in which the shadow of tumors on X-ray

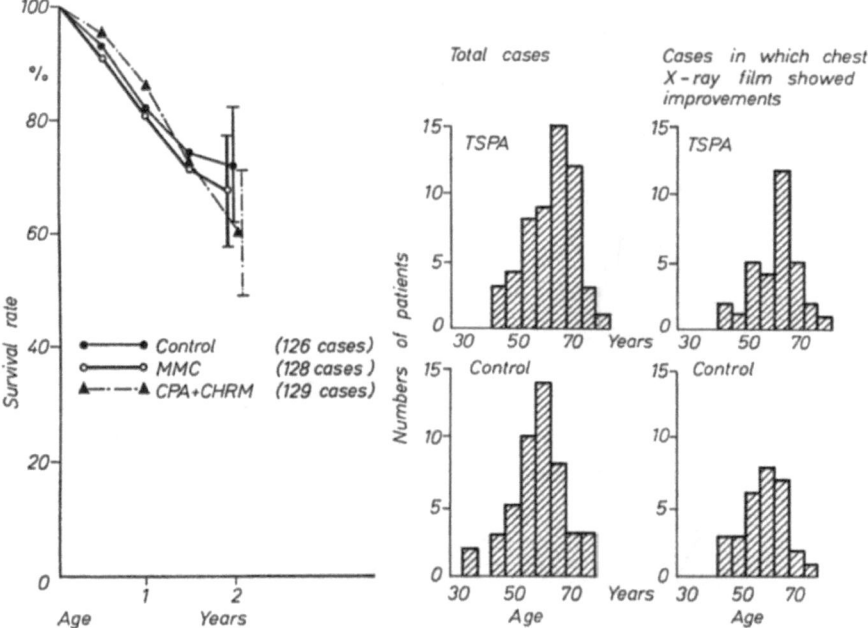

Fig. 9. Survival rates of patients with carcinoma. Adjuvant chemotherapy to surgery (the third study)

Fig. 10. Age distribution of lung cancer patients in the second and third studies

film of the chest could be estimated, were selected. The daily dose and the total dose and the route of administration are shown in Table II. In the second and third studies, 4,000 rads of irradiation with ^{60}Co was given to one lesion within three months and a daily dose of 12 mg of methylprednisolone was simultaneously administered during 30 days, totalling 400 mg. This basic treatment was combined with chemotherapy: daily dose of 0.1 mg/kg of TSPA was injected intramuscularly, totalling 3 mg/kg for one course. The age distribution of the patients is shown in Fig. 10; it was almost the same in the two treatment groups.

In the first study there were 26 patients given MMC and 23 given RC4. Fig. 11 shows the survival curves; no significant difference was found between the groups. In the second and third studies, there were 55 patients given TSPA and 48 treated as controls. No significant differences were found (Fig. 12).

Table II. *Method of chemotherapy in advanced lung cancer*

Study	Drug	Dosage	
		Daily dosage	Total dosage
First	MMC	0.04 mg/kg (i. v.)	60 mg
	RC 4	0.2 mg/kg (i. v.)	300 mg
Second and third *	TSPA control	0.1 mg/kg (i. m.) —	3 mg/kg —

* Basic treatment in the second and third studies: 4000 rads of irradiation with ^{60}Co and 12mg of methylprednisolone daily, totalling 400 mg.

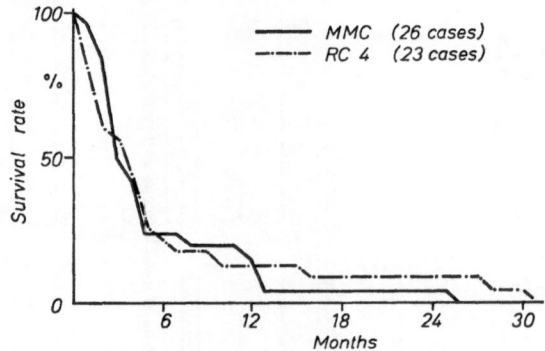

Fig. 11. Survival rates of the advanced lung cancer patients treated with RC4 and MMC

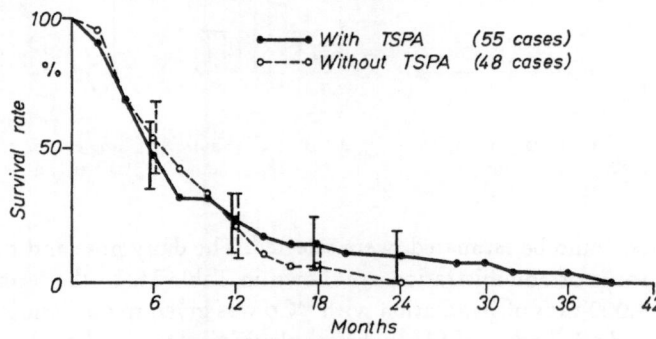

Fig. 12. Survival rates of advanced lung cancer patients treated by irradiation and methyl-prednisolone with or without TSPA

According to the evaluation of the committee on X-ray diagnosis, we had 63 patients who showed improvements on the chest X-ray film: — 29 controls and 34 on TSPA. The differences between the survival rates in these two groups at one year and one and a half years were significant (Fig. 13).

3. The cervix uteri cancer study group consisted of 13 national hospitals. Patients in the third stage from 35 to 59 years of age were irradiated with

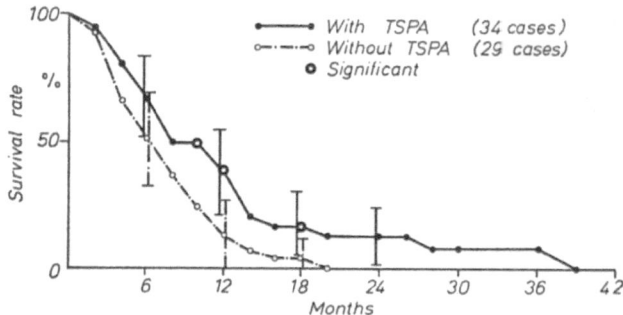

Fig. 13. Survival rates of advanced lung cancer patients treated by irradiation and methyl-prednisolone with or without TSPA (cases which showed improvements in chest X-ray film)

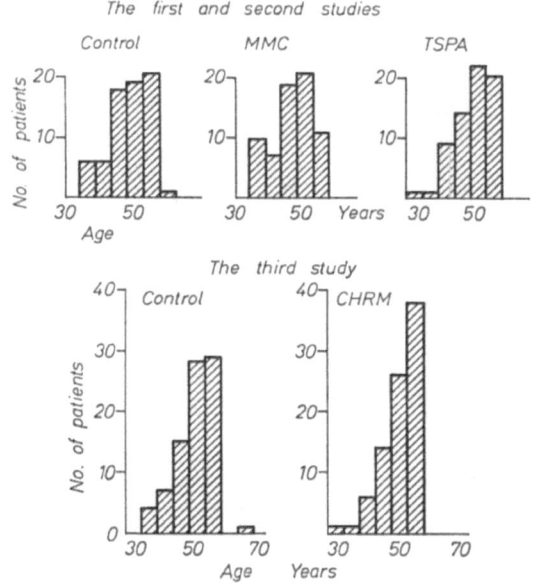

Fig. 14. Age distribution of cervix uteri cancer patients

Table III. *Method of chemotherapy in cervix uteri cancer*

Study	Drug	Dosage	
		Dosage/day	Total dosage
First and second	MMC	0.04—0.08 mg/kg i. v. every 1 to 3 days	more than 0.8 mg/kg
	TSPA	0.06—0.1 mg/kg i. v. every 1 to 3 days	more than 1 mg/kg
Third	CHRM	0.02 mg/kg i. v. every other day	0.4 mg/kg
	control	—	—

3,000 to 3,500 rads with or without chemotherapy within two months. The age
distribution of the patients is shown in Fig. 14; it was almost the same in the
three groups. In the third study 87 patients were given 0.02 mg/kg intravenously, on alternate days to a total of 0.4. The treatment schedules are shown
in Table III. In the first and second studies 68 patients were given MMC, 67

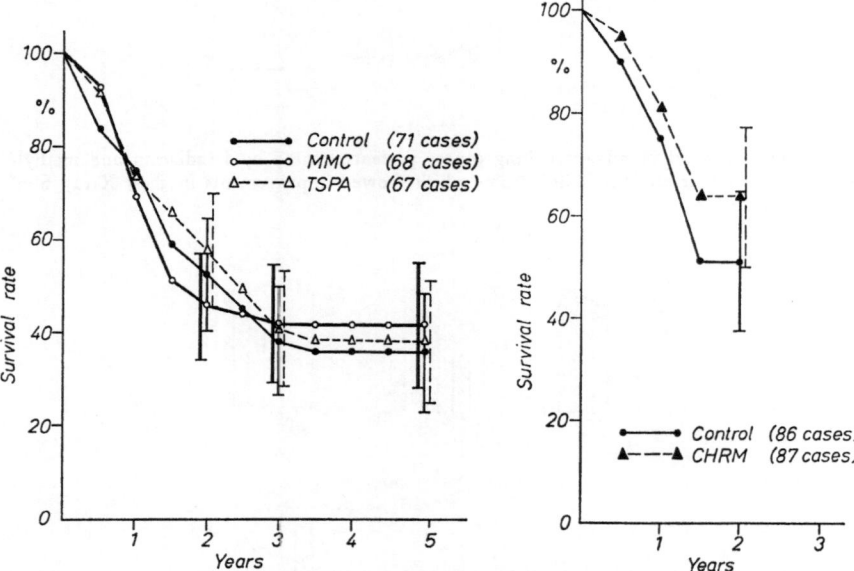

Fig. 15. Survival rates of cervix uteri cancer patients
adjuvant chemotherapy to irradiation (the first and
second studies)

Fig. 16. Survival rates of cervix uteri
cancer patients adjuvant chemotherapy
to irradiation (the third study)

Table IV. *Side effects of chemotherapy in gastric carcinoma (the first and second studies)*

Side effects	First study			Second study		
	Control (%)	TSPA (%)	MMC (%)	Control (%)	TSPA (%)	MMC (%)
Leucopenia (less than 3000)	2.9	18.3 *	24.6 **	3.8	25.8 **	24.7
(less than 1000)	0	0.8	1.5	0	1.1	1.1
Thrombocytopenia						
(less than 5×10^4)	0	2.9	4.7	0	8.7 *	12.5 **
(less than 3×10^4)	0	0	1.9	0	2.5	5.0
Disturbance of liver function	15.8	11.7	17.3	18.6	9.4	10.8
Albuminuria	1.7	7.2	8.9 *	2.0	3.3	6.7
Cases in which chemotherapy was stopped because of side effects	—	1/136	13/129 **	—	7/88	5/88

* $P < 0.05$
** $P < 0.01$

TSPA and there were 71 controls. In the third study 87 patients were given CHRM and there were 86 controls. Figs. 15 and 16 show the survival curves: there are no significant differences between the groups.

Table V. *Side effects of chemotherapy in lung cancer (the second and third studies)*

Side effects	Control (%)	TSPA (%)
Anemia		
(Hb content less than 8.0 g/dl)	0	7.7
(RBC less than 2.5×10^6)	0	7.3
Leucopenia (less than 3000)	2.3	28.9 *
(less than 1000)	0	0
Thrombocytopenia (less than 5×10^4)	5.4	12.8
(less than 3×10^4)	2.8	2.1
Hemorrhagic diathesis	4.7	2.1
Albuminuria	10.3	4.0
Weight loss (more than 1 kg)	71.5	80.5
Nausea	14.0	25.0
Vomiting	2.3	10.2

* $P < 0.01$

Table VI. *Side effects of chemotherapy in cervix uteri cancer*

Side effects	First and second studies			Third study	
	Control (%)	TSPA (%)	MMC (%)	Control (%)	CHRM (%)
Leucopenia (less than 3000)	14.1	25.7	34.3 **	7.3	15.3
(less than 1000)	0	1.5	3.0	0	0
Thrombocytopenia (less than 5×10^4)	2.8	3.0	4.5	0	3.5
(less than 3×10^4)	0	0	3.0	0	0
Hemorrhagic diathesis	0	0	6.0	0	0
Weight loss *	12.7	19.7	22.4	9.8	10.6
Vomiting	1.4	3.0	8.9	1.2	4.7
Cases in which chemotherapy was stopped because of side effects	—	2/66	6/67	—	0

* Loss of weight is more than 10 per cent of that before treatment.
** $P < 0.05$

Leucopenia, thrombocytopenia, anaemia, haemorrhagic diathesis, disturbance of liver function, albuminuria, loss of weight, nausea and vomiting were studied as side effects. Table IV shows the significant side effects in gastric cancer studies. Leucopenia of less than 3,000 was found in 18.3 per cent with TSPA and 24.6 per cent with MMC in the first study, and in 25.8 per cent with TSPA and in 24.7 per cent with MMC in the second study. Thrombocytopenia of less than

50,000 was found in 8.7 per cent with TSPA and 12.5 per cent with MMC in the second study. Albuminuria occurred in 8.9 per cent with MMC in the first study. Cases in which chemotherapy was stopped because of side effects were 13 out of 129 cases with MMC in the first study. Table V shows the side effects in the lung cancer studies. Leucopenia of less than 3,000 was found in 28.9 per cent with TSPA in the second and third studies. Other side effects were not significant. Table VI shows the side effects in the cervix uteri cancer studies. Leucopenia of less than 3,000 was found in 34.3 per cent with MMC in the first and second studies.

Conclusions

Exact clinical evaluation of cancer chemotherapeutics is very difficult. The best is a statistical estimation of the extension of survival time. Since 1st July, 1959, the Cancer Chemotherapy Co-operating Research Unit of the National Hospitals carried out studies to evaluate clinically chemotherapy. The method used and the results obtained in gastric, lung and cervix uteri cancer, especially those of chemotherapy as an adjuvant to surgery and radiotherapy, are presented.

Controlled clinical trials with randomized allocation of patients to the different treatment groups and calculation of the complete survival curves are necessary to demonstrate clearly the clinical effect of chemotherapy in cancer.

Interest of a Radiotherapist

HANNA KOLODZIEJSKA

Institute of Oncology, Krakow, Poland

Retrospective studies of clinical material played an important part in solving several crucial problems of cancer therapy such as: the correlation between end-results and stage of disease when treated, the definition of radical and palliative treatment, and the indications for surgical treatment and radiotherapy. Opinions about the curability of cancer, built up on these retrospective studies, are generally correct when the differences between the results are substantial. When, however, these differences are small, conclusions concerning the value of a given treatment are often misleading.

The present-day treatment of cancer has two distinctive characters. First, improvement of results is less significant than was expected, in spite of the development of new methods and new techniques of therapy. Secondly, the desire of doctors to increase the curability of cancer is steadily becoming more insistent. The interplay of these two factors deforms the conclusions derived from retrospective studies, and leads usually to overestimation of the benefit obtained from the treatment. The use of controlled clinical trials, excludes the factor of subjectivity and ensures more objective evaluation of relatively narrow differences in survival.

The practical value of studies based on the principles of controlled clinical trials and their effect on the progress of cancer therapy depends not only on different ethical and methodological factors but also on the proper choice of problems to be investigated, and on the proper calculation of the number of cases available for study.

From the point of view of the radiotherapist the combination of irradiation with other methods of treatment provides many controversial problems which, I think, should be studied by means of controlled trials. The use of radiotherapy combined with surgery, chemotherapy or hormonal treatment, founded more on tradition or theory than on facts, results always in prolongation of treatment and increased risk of complications. The question arises, therefore, whether these disadvantages are counterbalanced by longer or better quality survival of patients.

In the Institute of Oncology in Krakow the following problems of combined radiotherapy are under study:

1. The value of prophylactic castration in premenopausal women with breast cancer in stage III TNM, treated primarily by radiotherapy. Patients under study have been allocated to 3 groups: without castration, castration by X-rays and castration by surgery.

2. The value of pre-operative radiotherapy in women with breast cancer in "early" stage III. The group under study includes only patients classified as $T_3 N_0$ or $T_3 N_1$.

3. The value of chemotherapy (that is, nitrogranulogen) combined with irradiation in patients with lymphogranulomatoses without abdominal node involvement.

Review of these investigations after 3 years, suggests to us that they are unsatisfactory because the number of cases in each group is too small to lead to conclusive results (208, 97 and 92 patients respectively).

The total number of new cancer patients referred to our Institute annually is more than 2,000; this number, although not small, seems to be an insufficient basis for the conduct of decisive and efficient controlled trials, which should rather be organized in larger institutions or at the national level.

Experiences with Castration for Breast Cancer

R. Nissen-Meyer

Norwegian Radium Hospital, Oslo 3, Norway

At the Norwegian Radium Hospital we have used controlled clinical trials in the study of primary castration for operable breast cancer.

The questions put on trial were:

I. Does castration, performed as an adjuvant to radical mastectomy, increase the average *interval free of symptoms* in recurrence cases?

II. Is *total survival* longer with primary castration than it is if castration is postponed until recurrences are manifest?

III. May also *postmenopausal* patients benefit from a primary castration?

IV. Is *surgical removal of the ovaries* more effective than *ovarian irradiation?*

Primary castration has been frequently discussed since it was proposed by Schinzinger, nearly 80 years ago. Opinions have differed widely, from strong recommendation to total refusal, but mostly opinion was based on relatively small series without adequate control groups. During the years since we started our own investigation in 1957, several reports from other clinical trials have appeared. They show all the same trend, but we still need reliable data in order to obtain more detailed information.

Our trials were performed in a rather simple and uncomplicated way. Protocols for random allocation were prepared and kept in the Cancer Registry. All essential information about the case was plotted on special, manually operated punch-cards *before* allocation. Later, all control examinations were immediately transferred to these cards, and the progress of the study was reviewed at frequent intervals.

Only 40 per cent of our operable cases could be included in a controlled clinical trial. Random allocation was considered ethically justified only if real doubt existed whether one or other of two treatment methods was the best for the individual patient. If we were not in doubt, the patient always received the treatment considered the best for her.

According to these ethical principles we could build up two randomized statistical series:

The first study, comparing a group with *primary ovarian irradiation with a control group,* was possible only in two categories, premenopausal patients with a very good prognosis, and postmenopausal patients of both stage I and II. The reason for this was the following:

Already before we started our investigation, we believed in the effect of primary castration of premenopausal patients. Therefore we could not use such patients if their individual prognosis was not considered very good. It seemed unethical to us to place premenopausal patients with a poor prognosis in a control group without primary castration.

We did not, however, earnestly believe that primary castration could play an important role for the postmenopausal patients. On the other hand, in this age group the side-effects seemed unimportant. Therefore it was considered ethically justified to randomize all the postmenopausal patients between ovarian irradiation and control.

An important detail in this plan was the castration of all cases of the control group as soon as recurrences were diagnosed. In this way, *the time of castration was made the variable of the investigation*. The study is virtually one of so-called "prophylactic" versus "therapeutic" castration.

Premenopausal patients with a poor prognosis should, according to our view before the trial, all be given primary castration. We did not, however, know if surgical removal was better than irradiation for this purpose. We could there-fore allocate these patients at random to *one group with primary oophorectomy and one group with primary ovarian irradiation* — provided no special contra-indication was found against the surgical intervention.

Table. *Characteristics of patients with breast cancer treated by radical mastectomy, with primary castration (treatment group) or without (control group)*

	Treatment group	Control group
Number of cases	162	174
Average age	52.3 years	52.3 years
Premenopausal	45.6 %	50.0 %
Postmenopausal	54.3 %	50.0 %
Stage I	68.5 %	71.2 %
Stage II	31.5 %	23.7 %
Lateral only	46.8 %	50.5 %
Malignancy grade I + II	45.0 %	43.2 %
Malignancy grade III + IV	52.4 %	49.4 %
Not treated according to allocation	1.2 %	2.3 %

For the evaluation of primary ovarian irradiation we collected a total of 336 patients. As seen from the average age and the distribution of various prognostic factors shown in the Table, the two groups should be well com-parable.

Only 1.2 per cent of the cases in the treatment group did not receive the castration they were allocated to, and 2.3 per cent of the cases in the control group were for one reason or another castrated during the first year after mastectomy. This seems not to invalidate the significance of the trial.

The results are shown in Fig. 1. During the total observation time of 8 years a higher percentage of the castrated group was found free of disease. For the first interval of one year the difference between the two groups was significant.

Also the crude survival rates were better in the treated group during the first 7 years. For the first interval of one year the difference was highly significant.

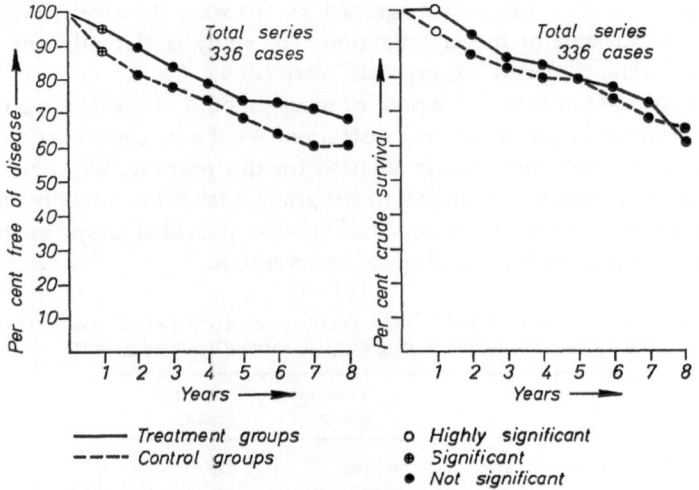

Fig. 1. Results obtained in patients with breast cancer treated by radical mastectomy with or without primary castration, at different periods after treatment

Usually, the degree of significance of a difference between two comparable groups will increase with an increasing number of cases. In this trial, the randomization was made according to the rules, and the two groups seemed well comparable. In spite of this, comparison of the total series does not provide the maximum utilization of our material of 336 cases. We remember that the series was composed of two principally different categories of patients — the premenopausal women with a good prognosis and the postmenopausal women. Let us now try to split up the total series in this way.

We then find (Fig. 2) that in the subseries with postmenopausal women the difference between the groups is clearly marked already during the first few years after treatment. Although the number of cases, 175, is only half the number in the total series, the difference is highly significant, both in terms of years free of disease and crude survival.

In the other subseries, the 161 premenopausal women with good prognosis, the disease is progressing very slowly. It therefore necessarily takes many years before a possible effect in the treatment group may be demonstrated.

Already in 1960 it was clear that the castrated group of the postmenopausal women did significantly better than the control group. We therefore had to stop collection of new cases for this part of the study, and after 1960 ovarian irradiation was given to all new postmenopausal patients up to the age of 70 years. In the other part of the study collection of new cases continued to the end of 1963, and we still wait for more significant results to come.

In Fig. 3 the postmenopausal subseries is further sub-divided into stage I and stage II cases. Even with the small number of cases in each group, statistical

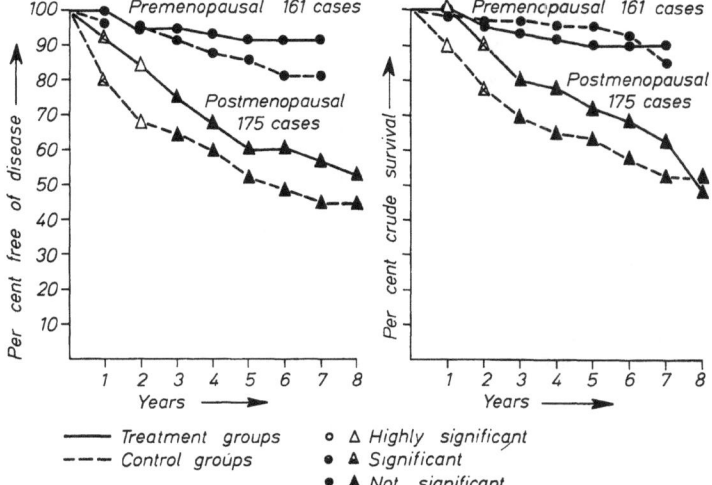

Fig. 2. Results obtained in patients with breast cancer treated by radical mastectomy with or without primary castration, subdivided according to menopausal state at time of treatment

significance is still obtained. This demonstrates the advantages of evaluating series with a homogeneous composition.

In Fig. 4 are shown the results of the comparison between oophorectomy and ovarian irradiation in the series of premenopausal patients with a poor prognosis. Formally we may only state that in this trial, with this limited number of patients, we were not able to demonstrate any significant difference. The fact that in this series the ovarian irradiation group did somewhat better than the oophorectomy group, we may believe is due to chance alone. On the other hand, the trial has reduced the possibility that oophorectomy might be much better than ovarian irradiation for this special purpose.

The practical results which have come out of these trials are: it has been shown that in patients who were not cured by mastectomy, primary ovarian irradiation increased the interval free of symptoms with an average of about 1 1/2 years. The total survival time was also increased. The difference was found highly significant for the postmenopausal patients up to the age of 70 years. A formal statistical significance cannot for the present time be claimed for the premenopausal patients, but it may still appear when we have a longer observation time in this part of the trial.

Surgical removal of the ovaries was not found superior to ovarian irradiation as a method of primary castration.

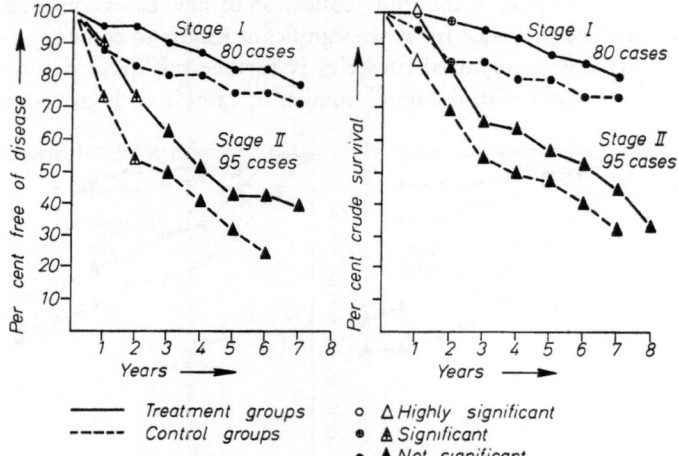

Fig. 3. Results obtained in patients with breast cancer treated by radical mastectomy with or without primary castration, postmenopausal women at time of treatment subdivided by stage of disease

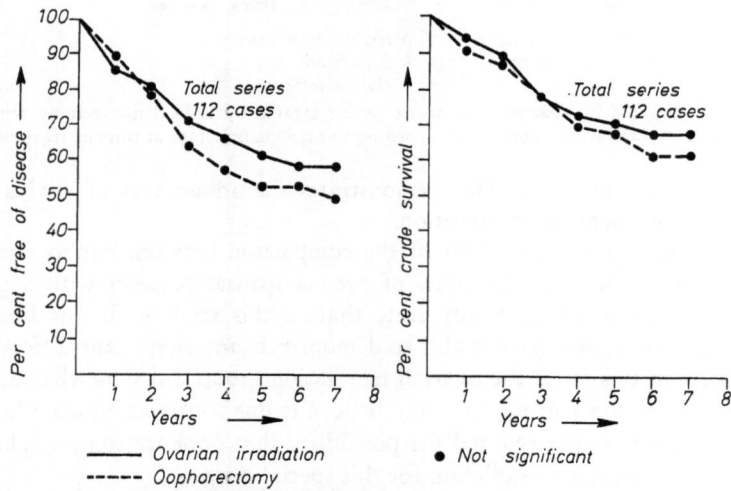

Fig. 4. Results obtained in patients with breast cancer treated by radical mastectomy combined with ovarian irradiation or oophorectomy

The methodological points I want to underline are the following:

1. Calculation of the complete survival curves may be necessary to demonstrate the effect of a treatment. — Calculation of only the 5-year survival rates is often insufficient.

2. The effect of the treatment may reach its maximum at different time periods in the different categories of patients. It may therefore be necessary to split up a randomized series into subseries of more homogeneous prognosis, even if the original allocation has resulted in apparently comparable groups.

3. Such splitting up of large, mixed series may be undertaken also *after* the randomization, for example, at the time of evaluation of the results. *But,* and this is very important, there must be no doubt about the criteria upon which such a division of the series is based. Classification according to such criteria should have been clearly stated for each individual patient *before* the allocation.

4. Continuous follow-up may soon demonstrate significant results in certain categories of patients. Allocation of cases to these categories should then be stopped, and new patients should be given the treatment found to be the best for them. The trial should be continued only in categories of patients for whom no definite results have yet been found.

I may perhaps add that during the study period we treated a total number of 1129 cases in stages I and II. Of these 60 per cent had a primary castration. An extensive analysis has shown that the results obtained in the groups *not* included in the controlled clinical trial were in complete accordance with the results I have just shown for the groups that were included. Detailed results are given elsewhere (NISSEN-MEYER, 1965).

References

NISSEN-MEYER, R., Castration as part of the primary treatment for operable female breast cancer. A statistical evaluation of clinical results. *Acta radiol. (Stockh.),* Suppl. 249 (1965).

Discussion opened by A. I. Rakov

I should like to make some comments concerning Dr. HAYWARD's presentation.

The first point is: whether a clinical trial is applicable to cancer patients? In principle, my answer is positive, but in each case it should be justified by the interests of the patient.

I am ready to agree with all five points presented by Dr. HAYWARD as unethical approaches to a clinical trial, except perhaps for the last. I have a doubt whether it is ethical to continue any clinical trial if it is obvious that the immediate result of the treatment given is bad. The example mentioned by Dr. HAYWARD with hypophysectomy and adrenalectomy in the treatment of breast cancer is not quite convincing.

Certainly, it is extremely difficult in each specific case to decide whether a clinical trial is ethical or unethical. In general, we use the same homely rule that Dr. HAYWARD suggested. If a new method can be applied to a relative of the doctor who provides the treatment, it is suitable to try it. I was the witness of such an episode that took place in one surgical clinic. A young doctor came to the chief and asked his permission to perform a very complicated operation. The chief answered him: "If you believe you have enough experience in surgery, please find your relative who needs such an intervention and then operate on him." It is a wise rule to remember when we organize a clinical trial, that treatment is for patients, not patients for treatment.

I have also some comments on Professor KOLODZIEJSKA's presentation.

The main purpose of a clinical trial is to find the best method of treatment. In order to have comparable data we should use unique designations of the extent of disease, i. e. an international clinical language. The TNM system, elaborated by the U. I. C. C. Clinical Classification Committee, provides such a language for almost all sites of tumors. The TNM system is a very good basis for a clinical trial.

The second point is to accumulate enough material for evaluation of the method of treatment. It is difficult to do so in one oncological clinic. Therefore the necessity arises to arrange some clinical trials on the national level. Perhaps, for some sites of tumors, where cancer is not so frequent, it is desirable to organize special international groups, as is done for the study of melanotic tumors. Yesterday afternoon we had a meeting of that group. Agreement was reached to organize a clinical trial concerning the expediency of prophylactic groin dissection for melanoma of the lower extremities. Proceeding in such a way we can reach our common purpose more quickly.

Conclusion

During discussion many important practical questions were raised, particularly in regard to legal restrictions and the codification of medical ethics. In reply to some of these questions, the Chairman summed up the position of the members of the panel as follows.

A controlled trial did not necessarily imply a comparison with a placebo. From the point of view of pure science it might be of considerable interest to know whether the treatment had any biological effect at all, but in a clinical trial one was usually concerned to know whether the new treatment was better than an old one. In most trials the control treatment was, therefore, the previously accepted best treatment for the special group of patients under consideration — irrespective of whether that treatment was operative, radiotherapeutic or medical.

A controlled trial was required — and was justifiable — only when there was genuine doubt about the relative value of different methods of treatment. Doubt was nearly always present when a new treatment was introduced, because one had to take into consideration not only immediate effects, but also the long-term effects of the treatment on both survival and the quality of life. In exceptional circumstances, if no doubt existed — as would be the case if 3 or 4 adults with acute leukaemia were apparently cured — further "controlled" trials would be unethical. Apart from when new treatments are introduced, genuine doubt still exists about the relative merits of many classical forms of treatment and controlled trials are urgently needed to establish the facts. But they should not be undertaken by doctors who feel convinced, either intellectually or emotionally, that one or other treatment is certainly superior.

The exact conditions under which a particular trial can be carried out, can be decided only by the doctor concerned with their treatment. If wise, however, he will always consult with his colleagues. Lawyers cannot relieve the individual doctor of his own ethical responsibilities. Attempts to codify the conditions under which trials may be conducted are valuable so long as they lay down only broad general principles, but individual circumstances vary greatly and exceptions must always be allowed for.

A regulation that doctors must always tell patients that they are to be included in a controlled trial is inimical to the best practice of medicine. Is it reasonable, for example, to ask a surgeon to say to his patient "I don't know whether it is better to remove your ovaries at the time I operate on your breast or not, but I want to find out and I propose, with your agreement, to decide what to do by the toss of a coin"? In our opinion it is not. That is not to say that the surgeon cannot do the trial, but that he should shoulder the burden of the decision himself and not attempt to salve his conscience by throwing it on the patient. That the patient's consent should always be required before subjecting him to any risk that is not a part of his treatment is not disputed; but that is no justification for demanding that he should also have to give his consent for taking part in a trial, the object of which is to find out how to improve the treatment of the condition from which he is suffering.

The interests of the patient are best protected by the collective concern of the medical profession in maintaining its own ethics and not by legislation; by the application of Professor RAKOV's and Dr. HAYWARD's homely rules and by insisting that new trials are begun only after the doctors immediately concerned have consulted with their colleagues.

Panel 18

Prognostic Criteria in Relation to Treatment

Chairman:

S. J. CUTLER (U.S.A)

Members:

J. W. BERG (U.S.A.), T. KAJITANI (Japan), A. I. RAKOV (U.S.S.R.)

Panel 19

Experimental Animals in Cancer Research

Chairman:

O. MÜHLBOCK (Netherlands)

Members:

W. HESTON (U.S.A.), T. NOMURA (Japan), C. CHANY (France),
M. POLLARD (U.S.A.), C. J. DAWE (U.S.A.)

Panel 20

Advances in the Management of Leukaemias and Lymphomas

Chairman:

J. H. Burchenal (U.S.A.)

Members:

A. Aguirre (Mexico), D. P. Burkitt (U.K.), P. Clifford (Kenya), P. B. Desai (India), E. C. Easson (U.K.), E. Frei (U.S.A.), S. Hibino (Japan), G. Martz (Switzerland), V. Ngu (Nigeria), J. Ramos (Brazil), D. H. Wright (Uganda)

This panel discussion dealt with the newer developments in the treatment of leukemias and lymphomas with particular attention to the possibilities of cure as well as to the palliative management. Since the current status and new developments in the management of Burkitt's tumor were the subject of a conference organized by the U.I.C.C. in Kampala, Uganda in January 1966, and since there had been new developments of interest in this tumor since this time, a significant portion of the discussion was reserved for summary of this conference which was presented by Ngu and discussed in considerable detail by Burkitt, Clifford and Wright. It was considered that the studies on Burkitt's tumor had broad implications for the whole problem of the management of the leukemias and lymphomas.

The reasons for this concentration on Burkitt's tumor are first, that it is a serious problem in tropical Africa comprising about 50 per cent of all tumors in children in these areas. Second, its epidemiology suggests an arthropod vector. Third, it is apparently curable by chemotherapy alone in a significant percentage of African patients even when far advanced. Fourth, since Burkitt's tumor has also been found in Europe and the Americas, it would be extremely important to ascertain whether this same disease in other areas of the world responds similarly to the same types of chemotherapy. If differences were found in the response to chemotherapy, this would suggest that environmental or hereditary factors play a rôle in the response to chemotherapy.

The paper by Ngu summarizing the Kampala Conference on the Treatment of Burkitt's tumor follows:

The Burkitt Tumour

V. ANOMAH NGU

Department of Surgery, University of Ibadan, Nigeria

I. Introduction

It is right and proper that I should begin by paying tribute to Mr. DENIS BURKITT for his many and important contributions to the so-called African Lymphoma which now bears his name. His tumour safaris have helped to define a clinical entity which only a few will deny (DORFMAN, 1965; O'CONOR *et al.*, 1965) is unique in the realm of childhood tumours (BURKITT, 1958). Its restricted geographical distribution (BURKITT, 1962) (Fig. 1) in parts of Africa, coupled with BURKITT's other epidemiological studies (BURKITT, 1966 a) first called attention to the possibility that a human cancer might be caused by a virus and

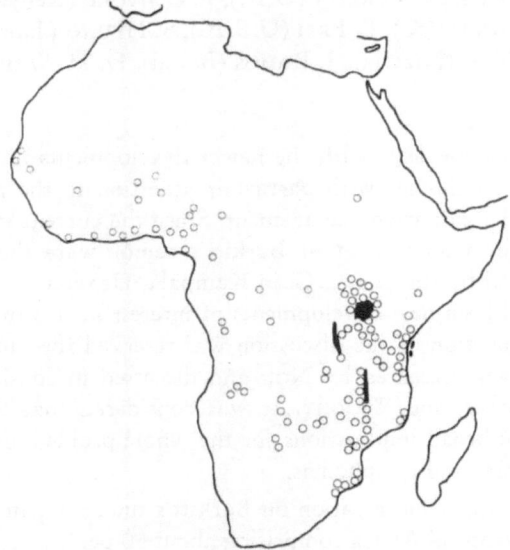

Fig. 1. Map of Africa showing Burkitt tumour incidence

spread by an insect (HADDOW, 1963). His treatment of this tumour has revealed the existence of immunological factors and recent reappraisals of the chemotherapy of other lymphomas is based on the hope that similar factors to those seen in the Burkitt lymphoma may also be uncovered. We admire DENIS BURKITT's achievements for themselves and for the difficult circumstances under which he worked in Africa!

In tribute to his work in Africa, I was asked to summarize some data presented at a recent Conference on the Chemotherapy of the Burkitt Tumour held at Kampala, Uganda, under the auspices of U. I. C. C. in order to present, for those not familiar with this tumour, a brief but complete picture of the disease. I accepted this honoured but difficult task on the assurance that Dr. BURCHENAL and Mr. BURKITT who were co-Chairmen of the Kampala Conference, and Mr. P. CLIFFORD and Dr. E. FREI will supplement my presentation.

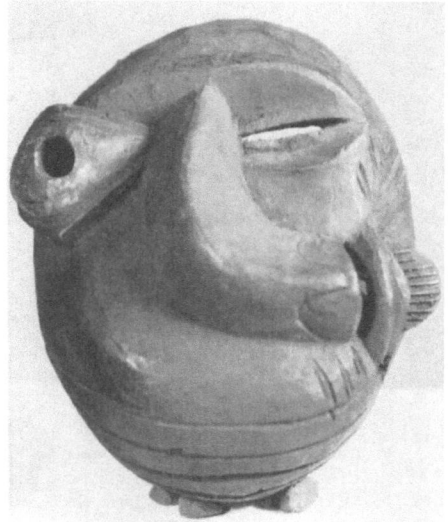

Fig. 2. Old mask from Lagos — showing Burkitt tumour

The Burkitt lymphoma is not, of course, a new disease. Records at the old Mengo Hospital at Kampala (unpublished) show that this tumour was seen there in the early part of this century. The old mask (Fig. 2) from our museum in Lagos is claimed by some to represent a case of Burkitt tumour. With a greater awareness of this tumour and improvements in medical facilities, its incidence will probably increase in those underdeveloped parts of the world where the climatic conditions are similar to those in Africa.

II. Pathology

O'CONOR and DAVIES (1960) first classified the Burkitt tumour as a poorly differentiated lymphocytic lymphoma and noted the presence of foamy histiocytes scattered among the lymphoid cells giving the so-called "starry sky" pattern. This pattern is seen in other lymphomas including the cat lymphoma (SQUIRE, 1966) (Fig. 3). Imprint preparations show the lymphoid cells to be 20—30 μ in diameter with round, oval or deeply cleft nuclei with prominent nucleoli. The thin basophilic cytoplasm contains a variable number of vacuoles. PULVERTAFT (1966) and OSUNKOYA (1966a) by phase contrast cytology have shown that these vacuoles contain lipoid granules and are characteristic of this tumour (Fig. 4).

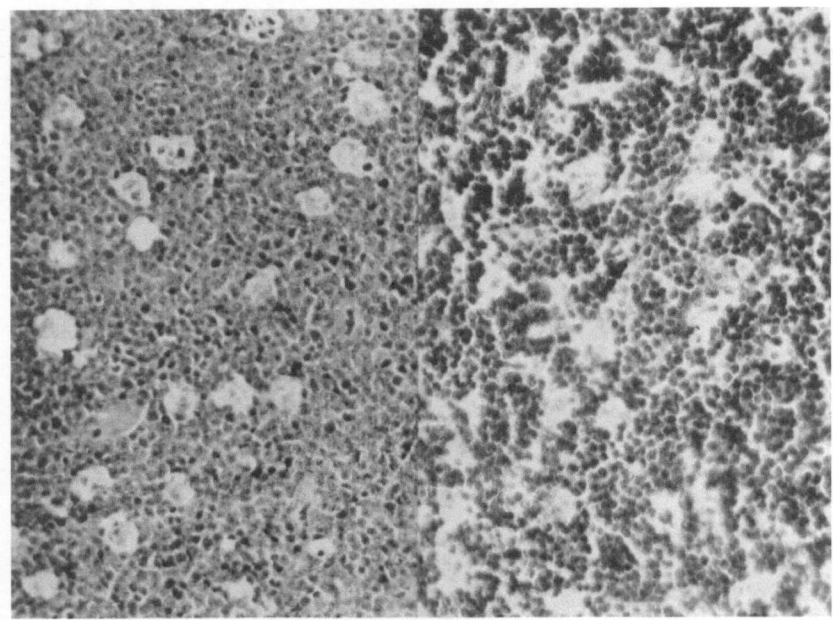

Fig. 3. Starry sky pattern in Burkitt tumour and cat lymphoma

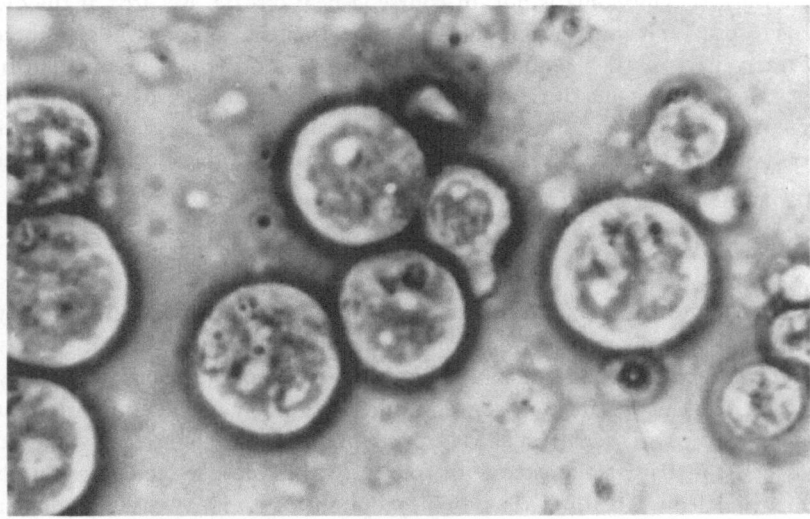

Fig. 4. Phase contrast photograph of Burkitt cells showing lipoid granules

III. Epidemiology

1. Incidence

The Burkitt lymphoma is the most common childhood tumour in tropical Africa south of the Sahara comprising more than half of all childhood malignancies (DAVIES and DAVIES, 1960; O'CONOR and DAVIES, 1960; EDINGTON and McLEAN, 1964). It has been reported from New Guinea (TEN SELDAM et al., 1966), Brazil (LUISI et al., 1965), and Colombia (BELTRAM et al., 1966) in reasonable numbers. It is however rare or only occasionally seen in South

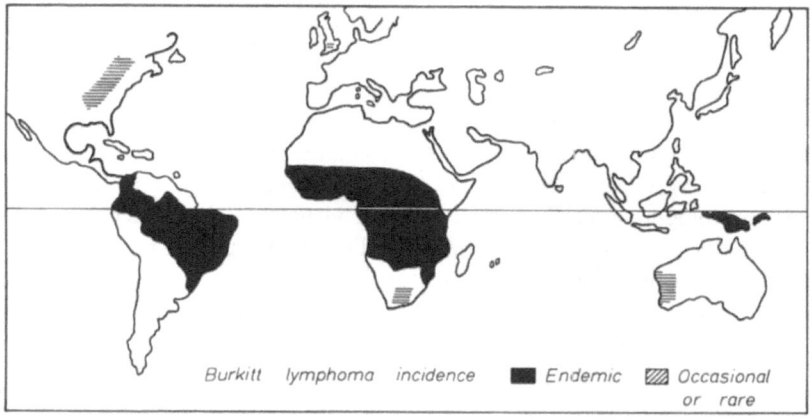

Fig. 5. Map of World showing areas with high and low incidence of Burkitt tumour

Africa (GLUCKMAN, 1963; SCHMAMAN et al., 1965), parts of Australia (TEN SELDAM et al., 1966), England (WRIGHT, 1964) and North America (DORFMAN, 1965; O'CONOR et al., 1965) (Fig. 5). The reasons for these differences in incidence are not clear, but they may be related to differences in the incidence of the vector, or to differences in host susceptibility. Detailed epidemiological studies in both high and low incidence areas may help to resolve these various differences.

2. Age Incidence

In a series of 545 cases recorded by BURKITT (1966c) in Uganda, only one was seen below the age of 2 years of age, and only 9 below 3. Over 60 per cent occurred between 4—8 years inclusive and only 10 per cent occurred above 15. A detailed study further showed that the average age was related to the intensity of the tumour distribution. In south west Uganda where the tumour was rare, the average age was twice that recorded in north east Uganda where it was most common. Adult emigrants from non-endemic into endemic areas were as liable to the disease as local children. In Western Nigeria, our experience is almost identical and the few patients coming from Northern Nigeria, which borders on the Sahara desert, and where tumour incidence is low are much older than those from Western Nigeria with a high tumour incidence. The geographic distribution and the age incidence of this tumour have immunological implications which support the theory that a virus may be responsible for it.

3. Viruses

As far as possible aetiological viruses are concerned, three groups have so far been isolated from the tumour. The first, the herpes-like viruses were seen by Epstein et al. (1964), Stewart et al. (1965) and O'Conor and Rabson (1965), not only from Ugandan and Nigerian patients but from indigenous North American cases. Bell and his colleagues (1966) have isolated reovirus type 3 on 10 occasions from 7 patients. He has also shown by immunological methods that 73 per cent of Burkitt lymphoma patients as compared with 18 per cent of controls carried antibodies to reovirus 3 (Bell, 1966). Stanley et al., (1966) reported that this virus had been found to infect mosquitoes and to produce runting in mice. Splenic cells from such runted mice produced lymphomas in isologous mice. The third group of viruses are the unidentified agents isolated from 6 cases of this tumour by Dalldorf and Bergamini (1964). There ist therefore no lack of evidence for the presence of viruses in the Burkitt tumour but it is as yet undecided whether they are merely passengers or have any aetiological significance.

IV. Clinical Features

This tumour has the same easily recognizable features from different countries (Fig. 6).

Distribution of Lesions

Facial lesions have varied in the different series. In our own, they form 52 per cent of cases. Below the age of 8, 2 out of 3 patients had facial lesions but above 8 only one out of 3 had such lesions. With a few exceptions practically all organs especially the intra-abdominal organs of the body can be involved. Long and pelvic bones are frequently involved although leukaemic transformation is rarely seen (Clift et al., 1963). The central nervous system is usually involved by extension of primary facial or paravertebral tumour. A frank meningitic form of the disease is now well recognized and may occur in the absence of systematic disease in the follow-up period. Only the lung and peripheral lymph nodes appear to be relatively immune to this tumour and are seldom affected.

The familiar presentation of the tumour with facial lesions or abdominal masses (Fig. 7) may be absent and may thus delay diagnosis or lead to errors. In endemic areas, this tumour frequently enters into the differential diagnoses of unusual disease syndromes in children and young adults. For example, pyrexia and pancytopenia of undetermined origin, a gouty type arthritis with high uric acid, unexplained cardiac arrythmia, were all shown to be due to Burkitt lymphoma. Similarly, a flaccid paraplegia of rapid onset or breast tumours in girls have been due to this tumour. A high index of suspicion is thus essential to the correct diagnosis in such cases.

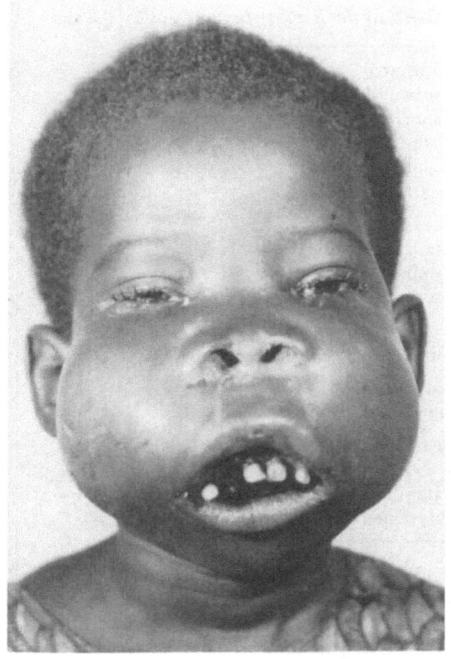 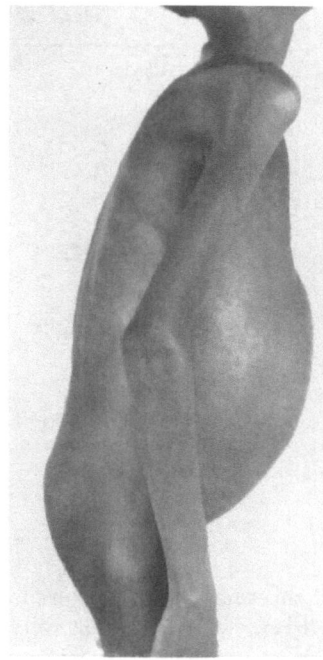

Fig. 6   Fig. 7

Fig. 6. Burkitt tumour from Nigeria and New Guinea. (By courtesy of editors of "Cancer" and R. E. J. TEN SELDAM et al.)

Fig. 7. Burkitt tumour of the abdomen

An unusual feature of the Burkitt tumour is its very rapid growth rate especially in the younger child, mimicking an acute infection. The natural course of the disease may thus be as short as 8 weeks! In the older child, it however runs a slower course requiring 3—8 months or more for a fatal termination.

Associated with the rapid growth is a corresponding rapid tumour necrosis as shown by the very high uric acid levels, some of which may be 5—7 times the normal values (CLIFFORD, 1966; NGU, unpublished). The uricaemia appears to be related to the size or number of tumour masses present.

V. Chemotherapy

Table I shows the categories of drugs that have been used or tried in the treatment of this lymphoma. Of these, only cytoxan, methotrexate and nitrogen mustard by the intra-arterial route have given consistent and worthwhile results (BURKITT, 1966 b; NGU, 1966 a; CLIFFORD, 1966). An intriguing aspect

Table I. *Drugs used or tried in the Burkitt tumour*

Alkylating:	Nitrogen mustard Cyclophosphamide (Endoxan, Cytoxan) L-Sarcolysin (Melphalan) O-Sarcolysin (O-merphalan) Chlorambucil (Leukeran) Mannitol — Myleran Epodyl
Antimetabolites:	Methotrexate Pyrimethamine (Daraprim) 6-Mercaptopurine
Antibiotics:	Actinomycin D Mytomycin C
Alkaloids:	Vincaleukoblastin (VLB) Vincristine (Leurocristine VCR)
Miscellaneous:	Steroids (Prednisolone) Colcimid Terephthalanilide (Wander drug) Methylhydrazine (Ro4 — 6467)

of this tumour is the prompt and rapid tumour regression that is achieved with cytoxan when it is sensitive. BURKITT (1958) has suggested that this prompt response, in doubtful cases, may serve as a useful diagnostic test.

Other drugs such as melphalan, orthomerphalan, chlorambucil (CLIFFORD, 1966) and vincristine have also given good but short-lived tumour responses. Steroids and velban, so useful in other lymphomas, have proved disappointing in the few cases that have been studied.

Results of Treatment

Table II presents the results of treatment reported at the Kampala Conference using mainly cytoxan and methotrexate (BURKITT, 1966 b; NGU, 1966 a; CLIFFORD, 1966). Twenty-five of them or 14 per cent were well, without evidence of disease, and were not receiving maintenance therapy. Three of these had gone for between 6 months and 1 year, 6 for 1 and 2 years, 6 for 2 and 3 years, 7 for 3—4 years and 3 over 4 years. Most of them may be described as "cured". A large number of patients were lost to follow up and it is highly probable that some of these may still be alive. Indeed, since the Kampala Conference, we conducted a moderate search for such patients at Ibadan and were rewarded with 6 more patients who had been lost and considered dead. They are all symptom free and on no drugs between 2 and over 4 years after treatment. Of our total 11 patients now in long term remissions, 4 have survived over 4 years, 2 over 3 years and 5 over 2 years. A more determined search and a better follow up of patients will undoubtedly improve the results reported and place them amongst the best so far achieved in the treatment of lymphomas.

Table II. *Results of treatment of Burkitt tumour*

Author and treatment centre	No. of cases treated	Percentage of cases with total regression	No. of cases in long term remission "cures"
D. Burkitt, Kampala	88	40 %	14
V. Ngu, Ibadan	54	24 %	5
P. Clifford, Nairobi	39	21 %	6
Total	181	—	25 (or 14 %)

Problems of Treatment

There are still many problems that beset our treatment programmes.

As immunological factors seem to play a part in our results (Ngu, 1965; Burkitt, 1966 d), it is essential that we do nothing that might damage them. Inadequate treatment will however fail to control the tumour. Burkitt (1966 d) has achieved his good results by giving 30—40 mg/kg body weight of cytoxan as a single injection which is repeated after about 10—14 days if necessary. Marrow toxicity is absent or minimal by this schedule. With an eye on the varying size of tumour masses, we do not give a fixed dose but choose one or vary the number of days it is given to ensure total regression with minimal marrow toxicity. We certainly do not deliberately push treatment to severe marrow toxicity in order to ensure adequate treatment. With the rapid tumour regression that occurs we cannot, however, exclude the possibility that our results may be partly due to achieving a total tumour cell kill (Skipper, 1966).

Resistance in this tumour may arise at the initial treatment or during a recurrence. Resistance at the initial treatment is frequently seen although not exclusively in patients with very large tumour masses or in those who have severe local infection. Considering its pale, relatively avascular appearance, it is probable that failure of adequate amounts of drug to reach the center of large tumours may contribute to their apparent resistance. Clifford (1966) has achieved complete regression in some cases following partial excision of large tumour masses which were at first unresponsive. Limited surgical excisions at *special sites* may thus facilitate complete regression.

Small ineffective doses may be carried to eventual marrow toxicity and at the same time lead to resistance of the tumour at the initial treatment. Moderate doses for short periods are preferable to small doses over a long period. Those on prolonged maintenance therapy generally prove resistant when they recur. We therefore discontinue treatment as soon as it is clear that regression is complete and treat recurrences as they appear.

C. N. S. disease continues to prove difficult. We have, however, observed significant falls in tumour cell counts in the C. S. F. following systemic cytoxan, as well as intrathecal methotrexate. A few paraplegics with cord compression have made acceptable recovery after long periods and it is probable that many more may recover if they can be kept alive long enough.

As stated earlier, uricaemia may constitute a real hazard of treatment. Allopurinol, a xanthine oxidase inhibitor, has proved useful in the few cases tried (NGU, unpublished).

It is evident that there is no room whatsoever for complacency. The search must continue for new and better drugs. At the Kampala Conference GOLDIN (1966) reported that most compounds which had shown activity against the Burkitt tumour were picked up when screened against Leukaemia L 1210 in the mouse and Walker Carcinoma 256 in the rat. These systems may therefore be useful in selecting new agents for trial against the Burkitt lymphoma. Tissue culture methods, using various cell lines, were reported by OSUNKOYA (1966 b) and BURCHENAL et al. (1966) as potential methods for evaluating new drugs but it is still too early to attempt any clinical correlation.

VI. Recent Developments

Immunolgy

In addition to the reported regression that is sometimes seen after inadequate treatment (BURKITT, 1966 b; NGU 1965), temporary tumour remissions lasting 2—3 weeks have been observed after the intravenous infusion of 100—150 ml of plasma from Burkitt tumour patients in complete remission (NGU, 1966 b; BURKITT, 1966 d) (Figs. 8A and B).

KLEIN et al. (1966) using indirect membrane immunofluorescence techniques showed that sera from patients and indigenous adults from East Africa were positive when tested against live Burkitt cells whereas sera of Swedish controls were generally negative. OSUNKOYA (in press, 1966) at Ibadan using Burkitt cell lines (OB3) studied the sera of various groups of patients. Table III presents his results which are in general, similar to those of KLEIN et al. He has also observed that serum from indigenous adults increased the tendency to autolysis of Burkitt cells. These cells survived much longer in medium containing serum from the donor of the tumour cells (OSUNKOYA, 1966 a).

Protein Studies

Preliminary studies of immunoglobulins in Burkitt tumour and various groups of children have shown very low IgM values only in the Burkitt patient. Such low values were not observed in either normal or sick children (NGU et al.,

1966 a) or in patients with other lymphomas (NGU *et al.*, 1966 b). A correlation of the immunoglobulin values and their growth effects on tissue culture of Burkitt tumour cells showed that in Burkitt patients and sick children, increasing values of IgM produced increasing growth suppression (NGU *et al.*, 1966 a). In preliminary studies of the C. S. F., Udeozo (unpublished) observed that the

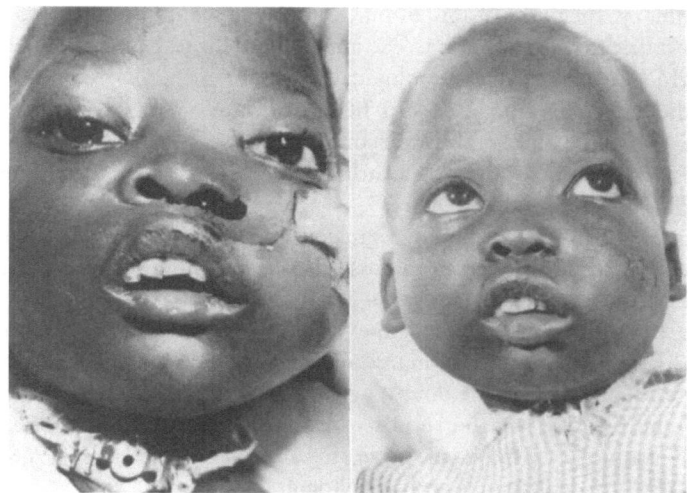

Fig. 8 A   Fig. 8 B

Fig. 8 A. Burkitt tumour before the infusion of "immune" plasma

Fig. 8 B. Burkitt tumour 10 days after the infusion of "immune" plasma

Table III. *Membrane immunofluorescence reaction on OB 3 cells cultured in sera from various individuals*

Groups of individuals	Age (yrs.)	Number tested	Number of positive sera	% positive sera
Nigerian blood donors	18—50	107	44	41
Parents of Burkitt tumour patients	Not known	14	9	64
Burkitt tumour patients	4—20	37	21	57
Sick Nigerian children with miscellaneous complaints	3—12	21	4	19
Malignant lymphoma patients (Nigerians)	20—50	14	6	43
New York blood donors. Negroes	25—51	39	9	22
New York blood donors. Caucasians	20—59	44	8	18
American Peace Corps volunteers. Newly arrived in Nigeria	22—27	15	1	7
American Peace Corps volunteers. 2 years resident in Nigeria	23—27	21	7	33

presence of IgM was associated with that of Burkitt cells and high IgG values. The significance of these various protein studies remains to be determined but it is clear that they offer yet another fruitful line of research into this fascinating tumour.

Summary and Conclusions

In summary, the present state of our knowledge would permit us to say that

1. The Burkitt lymphoma has certain unique clinical and epidemiological features which *suggest* a viral aetiological agent.

2. Although viruses have indeed been associated with this tumour, their significance remains to be established conclusively.

3. Treatment of this tumour has achieved 14 per cent of long term remissions which may be considered "cures".

4. Finally some of the tumour regressions and various immunological and protein studies strongly suggest the possibility that immunological factors may contribute to the good result achieved.

In the short time available, it is inevitable that I should have touched only briefly on some, and omitted many important, aspects of this fascinating tumour. Yet there can be little doubt, even from this brief sketch, of the importance and the promise for the future which the Burkitt tumour holds for the lymphoma problem. It may yet serve, in BURCHENAL's words (1966), as "a stalking horse" for leukaemias and lymphomas.

References

BELL, T. M., Review of the evidence for a viral aetiology for Burkitt's lymphoma. In: J. H. BURCHENAL and D. BURKITT (eds.), *Treatment of Burkitt's tumour.* Berlin, Heidelberg, New York: Springer 1966.
— MASSIE, A., ROSS, M. G. R., SIMPSON, D. I. H., and GRIFFIN, E., Further isolation of reovirus type 3 from cases of Burkitt's lymphoma. *Brit. med. J.* I, 1514—1517 (1966).
BELTRAM, G., BAEZ, A., and CORREA, P., Burkitt's lymphoma in Colombia. *Amer. J. Med,* 40, 211—216 (1966).
BURCHENAL, J. H., Geographic chemotherapy — Burkitt tumour as a stalking horse for leukaemia. Presidential address to the American Association for Cancer Research, Denver, May 1966. *Cancer Res.* 26, 2393—2405 (1966).
— WIGGINS, R. M., and GUTHRIE, E. D., Cell culture as a technique for evaluating potential chemotherapeutic agents for Burkitt's tumour. In: J. H. BURCHENAL and D.

BURKITT *(eds.), Treatment of Burkitt's tumour,* Berlin—Heidelberg—New York: 1966.
BURKITT, D., A sarcoma involving the jaws in African children. *Brit. J. Surg.* 46, 218—223 (1958).
— Determining the climatic limitations of a children's cancer common in Africa. *Brit. med. J.* II, 1019—1023 (1962).
— Recent developments in geographical distribution. In: J. H. BURCHENAL and D. BURKITT (eds.) *Treatment of Burkitt's tumour.* Berlin—Heidelberg—New York: Springer 1966 a.
— Chemotherapy of jaw tumours. In: J. H. BURCHENAL and D. BURKITT (eds.), *Treatment of Burkitt's tumour.* Berlin—Heidelberg—New York: Springer 1966 b.
— Some clinical features. In: J. H. BURCHENAL and D. BURKITT (eds.), *Treatment of Burkitt's tumour* (in press). Berlin—Heidelberg—New York: Springer 1966 c.
— Clinical evidence suggesting the development of an immunological response against

the African lymphoma. In: J. H. BUR-CHENAL and D. BURKITT (eds.), *Treatment of Burkitt's tumour*. Berlin—Heidelberg—New York: Springer 1966 d.

CLIFFORD, P., Further studies in the treatment of the Burkitt's lymphoma. *E. Afr. med. J.* 43, 179—199 (1966).

CLIFT, R. A., WRIGHT, D. H., and CLIFFORD, P., Leukemia in Burkitt's lymphoma. *Blood* 22, 243—250 (1963).

DALLDORF, G., and BERGAMINI, F., Unidentified filtrable agents isolated from African children with malignant lymphoma. *Proc. nat. Acad. Sci. (Wash.)* 51, 263—265 (1964).

DAVIES, A. G. H., and DAVIES, J. N. P., Tumours of the jaw in Uganda Africans. *Acta Un. int. Cancr.* 16, 320 (1960).

DORFMAN, R. F., Childhood lymphosarcoma in St. Louis, Missouri, clinically and histologically resembling Burkitt tumor. *Cancer (Philad.)* 18, 418—430 (1965).

EDINGTON, G. M., and McLEAN, C. M. U., Incidence of the Burkitt tumour in Ibadan, Western Nigeria. *Brit. med. J.* I, 264—266 (1964).

EPSTEIN, M. A., ACHONG, B. G., and BARR, Y. M., Virus particles in cultured lymphoblasts from Burkitt's lymphoma. *Lancet* 1964 II, 702—703.

GLUCKMAN, J. F., Multifocal lymphoma in South Africa. Its first observations in South African and white children. *S. Afr. Cancer Bull.* 7, 7—12 (1963).

GOLDIN, A., Potential techniques for developing new chemotherapeutic agents for use in Burkitt's tumour. In: J. H. BURCHENAL and D. BURKITT (eds.), *Treatment of Burkitt's tumour*. Berlin—Heidelberg—New York: Springer 1966.

HADDOW, A. J., An improved map for the study of Burkitt's lymphoma syndrome in Africa. *E. Afr. med. J.* 40, 9, 429 (1963).

KLEIN, G., CLIFFORD, P., KLEIN, E., and STJERNSWARD, J., Search for tumour specific immune reactions in Burkitt lymphoma patients by the membrane immunofluorescence reaction. In: J. H. BUR-CHENAL and D. BURKITT (eds.), *Treatment of Burkitt's tumour* (in press). Berlin—Heidelberg—New York: Springer 1966.

LUISI, A., PADUA BERTELLI, A. DE, MACHADO, J. C., and ACHE DE FREITAS, J. P., "Linfoma Africano" em Criancas Brasileiras. *Rev. bras. Chirurg.* 49, 280—295 (1965).

NGU, V. A., The African lymphoma (Burkitt tumour): survival exceeding two years. *Brit. J. Cancer* 19, 101—107 (1965).

— Clinical experience in the therapy of Burkitt's tumour. In: J. H. BURCHENAL and D. BURKITT (eds), *Treatment of Burkitt's tumour* (in press). Berlin—Heidelberg—New York: Springer 1966 a.

— Clinical evidence of host defences in Burkitt tumour. In: J. H. BURCHENAL and D. BURKITT (eds.), *Treatment of Burkitt's tumour* (in press). Berlin—Heidelberg—New York: Springer 1966 b.

— McFARLANE, H., OSUNKOYA, B. O., and UDEOZO, I. O. K., Immunoglobulins in Burkitt's lymphoma. *Lancet* II, 414—416 (1966 a).

— UDEOZO, I. O. K., McFARLANE, H., and OSUNKOYA, B. O., Unpublished 1966 b.

O'CONOR, G. T., and DAVIES, J. N. P., Malignant tumours in African children with special reference to malignant lymphoma. *J. Paediat.* 56, 526—535 (1960).

—, and RABSON, A. S., Herpes-like particles in an American lymphoma (Preliminary note), *J. nat. Cancer Inst.* 35, 899 (1965).

— Rappaport, H., and SMITH, E. B., Childhood lymphoma resembling Burkitt's tumor in the United States. *Cancer (Philad.)* 18, 411—417 (1965).

OSUNKOYA, B. O., Various aspects of the Burkitt tumour cell in tissue culture. In: J. H. BURCHENAL and D. BURKITT (eds.), *Treatment of Burkitt's tumour* (in press). Berlin—Heidelberg—New York: Springer 1966 a.

— The effect of some anticancer agents and steroid hormones on Burkitt cells *in vitro*. In: J. H. BURCHENAL and D. BURKITT (eds.), *Treatment of Burkitt's tumour* (in press). Berlin—Heidelberg—New York: Springer 1966 b.

PULVERTAFT, R. J. V., The use of tissue culture in the diagnosis of Burkitt tumours. In: J. H. BURCHENAL and D. BURKITT (eds.) *Treatment of Burkitt's tumour* (in press). Berlin—Heidelberg—New York 1966 a.

SCHMAMAN, A., GAMPEL, B., and LIMTZ, C. H., The Burkitt lymphoma syndrome in Johannesburg. *S. Afr. med J.* 39, 741 (1965).

SKIPPER, H. E., Some types of quantitative and kinetic information worth seeking and considering in the design of therapeutic trials. In: J. H. BURCHENAL and D. BUR-

KITT (eds.), *Treatment of Burkitt's tumour* 1966 a.

SQUIRE, R. A., Feline lymphoma: A comparison with the Burkitt tumour of children. *Cancer (Philad.)* 19, 447—453 (1966).

STANLEY, N. F., WALTER, M. N. I., LEAK, P. J., and KEAST, D., The association of murine lymphoma with Reovirus type 3 infection. *Proc. Soc. exp. Biol. (N. Y.)* 121, 90—96 (1966).

STEWART, S. E., LOVELACE, E., WHANG, J., and NGU, V. A., Burkitt tumour: tissue culture, cytogenetic and virus studies. *J. nat. Cancer Inst.* 34, 319—327 (1965).

TEN SELDAM, R. E. J., COOKE, R., and ATKINSON, L., Childhood lymphoma in the territories of Papua and New Guinea. *Cancer (Philad.)* 19, 437—446 (1966).

WRIGHT, D. H., *A. R. Brit. Emp. Cancer Campgn.* 42, 535 (1964).

Discussion

In his comments on NGU's summary of the Conference, BURKITT emphasized that the ideal chemotherapy was the least possible amount of drug which would produce a complete regression of all tumours. He presented data on patients who had had what would ordinarily be considered inadequate therapy and had still responded with long-term remissions. He stated that he had never seen a treated patient relapse who had remained in remission without maintenance therapy without any evidence of disease for over a year.

WRIGHT described the diagnosis of the disease. Characteristically it involves the jaws, abdominal viscera, and abdominal nodes sparing the peripheral nodes. He noted the presence of large foamy histiocytes between the lymphoid cells giving the so-called "starry sky" pattern to the tumour. He stressed the importance of cytologic imprint preparations from the tumour stained with May-Grunwald-Geimsa or Wright's stain. He described the cells of Burkitt's tumour on such imprint preparations as lymphoid cells 20—30 μ in diameter, which vary in size but not in apparent maturity. Their nuclei are round, oval or deeply cleft and have a stippled chromatin pattern. Nucleoli number 2 to 5 but are not conspicuous in deeply stained preparations. The cytoplasm forms a well defined rim around the nucleus. It is intensely basophilic, apart from a pale-staining area adjacent to the nuclear indentation. Cytoplasmic vacuoles are always present in at least some of the cells but their number varies widely. Detached fragments of vacuolated cytoplasm can usually be seen between the lymphoid cells. In Africa generalized marrow involvement is rare, although this may not be true in the United States, and a leukemic blood picture is extremely rare.

CLIFFORD showed cases with far advanced Burkitt's tumour which had responded well to chemotherapy and it was his opinion that the size of the tumour at the beginning of treatment was less important than its sensitivity to chemotherapy and the defenses of the host against the tumour. He felt that Cytoxan and Orthomerphalan were the drugs of choice and that of the two he prefered Orthomerphalan in doses of 1.0—1.2 mg/kg intravenously, repeated once after 10 days to 2 weeks. In collaboration with the KLEINS, he is studying the effects of inoculations of BCG and of irradiated autologous tumour tissue on host defenses and long-term survival following chemotherapy in patients whose tumour is in regression.

DESAI in discussing lymphoma and Burkitt's tumour in India noted that 23 per cent of all the lymphomas in his series arose in extranodal sites. Although the extranodal lymphomas in India predominantly appear in the head and neck areas (75 per cent), they have also been found to appear in the gastro-intestinal tract, the skeleton and the soft tissues. The overall control and prognosis of these extranodal lymphomas was distinctly better considering the fact that about 30 per cent of these patients had survived for more than 5 years. In his series there were about 30 lymphomas occurring in the jaw and paranasal sinuses of which he believed that 11 or 12 could justifiably be called Burkitt's tumour. Two of these came for treatment from Africa, 3 from Pakistan, and 7 from India.

AGUIRRE reporting from Mexico on 50 cases of lymphosarcoma, found 46 per cent in the intestine, and 16 per cent with primary localization in the face area, some involving the facial bones and others only soft tissue. Of 28 cases of reticulum cell sarcoma, 19 had begun in soft tissues including the head, abdominal wall or extremities. Eight of the cases were seen during the first year of life. In an analysis of 44 cases of lymphosarcoma and reticulum cell sarcoma, he found that most of the cases lived in towns located in tropical, and a few in sub-equatorial, climate with low altitude and heavy rainfall. Eleven of the towns were so small as not even to be located on maps. He felt that this finding might be significant since his hospital is in Mexico City at a high altitude, yet most of the cases of lymphosarcoma have appeared to come from lower altitudes. He expressed the opinion that the lymphomas of Mexico might be somewhere between the lymphomas of Africa and those of the United States with less tendency to involve the bone marrow and the blood than in the United States. It had been hoped that Professor Ramos of São Paulo would be able to report on his experience in treating Burkitt's tumour in Brazil, but unfortunately he was unable to be present.

MARTZ discussed the uses of the Ibenzmethycin (Natulan) in the treatment of Hodgkin's disease and the lymphomas. He mentioned that several of these derivatives have been studied in mice and two or three in patients and this was the best clinically. It can be given by mouth and will produce remissions not only in patients previously untreated but also in those whose disease has become resistant to the alkylating agents and to the vinca alkaloids. He also mentioned that this drug is very effective in lowering the immune response and that as such there was the thought that it might be valuable in certain autoimmune diseases and also in organ transplantation. The fact that high carcinogenicity has been noted with this drug in animals however, suggests that it should not be used except in patients with lymphomas, leukemias or widespread cancer with limited life expectancy. Natulan represents another useful drug in the armamentarium of the clinician engaged in treating the lymphomas.

HIBINO discussed the use of Mitomycin C in the treatment of chronic granulocytic leukemia. This drug affords a practical method of management of this disease but seems to have very little advantage over Myleran. Although early work had suggested less acute blast crises in those patients treated with Mitomycin C, more recent studies show that they do occur about as frequently as with Myleran.

HIBINO also discussed the registry of long term survivors of acute leukemia which is being set up in Japan.

FREI discussed the concept of total cell kill in the leukemias. He reviewed the work of SKIPPER and his group showing that a given dose of a compound would kill a fixed percentage of the leukemic cell population regardless of whether the population was 10 million or 10,000. The percentage of the leukemic cell population destroyed by a single LD_{10} dose of compound varied from compound to compound with some drugs giving 99 per cent whereas others might give 99.999 per cent cell kill. The objective is to discover a drug and a schedule which would increase this percentage cell kill to a point where there is less than one single cell surviving. Dr. FREI carried this concept over to the patient with acute leukemia and showed that after the induction of a complete remission, the duration of unmaintained remission to relapse might be taken as an indicator of the percentage of total cell kill. Certain drugs such as Prednisone and Vincristine, while inducing excellent remissions, had apparently not killed off an adequate percentage of the cells and thus the remission was very short when treatment was stopped. On the other hand, if courses of intensive treatment such as those employed in the VAMP or BIKE programs were given, the unmaintained remissions appeared to be much longer. Indeed, of the 23 patients in these two programs there were three who survived over 3 years in unmaintained remission and two of these are still continuing, whereas one has relapsed with a typical Burkitt-like ovarian involvement. He also showed the advantages to be gained by different schedules of a single drug such as Methotrexate, where a dose of 30 mg/M² twice weekly appears to be markedly superior to the daily oral administration of the drug. It would seem that in the treatment of acute leukemia, rapid induction of remission by Prednisone and Vincristine followed by intermittent methotrexate alone or in combination with various other active agents is the best therapeutic regimen.

One of the more interesting and important developments in the treatment of the lymphomas was discussed in detail by EASSON. He presented the concept that Stage I and II lymphomas are curable. He defined a cure as occurring when in time, probably a decade or so after treatment, there remains a group of disease-free survivors whose progressive death rate from all causes is similar to that of a normal population of the same sex and age constitution. He felt that this was the most practical and realistic interpretation of the word cure and that it certainly is the most acceptable definition from the patient's point of view. This concept of curability is based on the assumption that Hodgkin's disease and some of the other lymphomas originate as a unicentric tumour. Since these tumours are usually very sensitive to radiation therapy, localized disease could be completely obliterated by treating agressively with massive doses of radiation therapy. By adding to this the assumption that Hodgkin's disease not only originates unicentrically but also spreads at first to contiguous areas, investigators arrived at a plan of irradiating not only the involved nodes but also the contiguous uninvolved node bearing areas. This type of aggressive therapy has been pioneered by EASSON, PETERS and KAPLAN. EASSON showed that in more than 1,000 cases of Hodgkin's disease treated from 1934 through 1959 at the Christie Hospital in Manchester, England, of more than 300 with clinically localized disease, 50 per cent survived 5 years and about 40 per cent could be expected to survive 15 years. He presented evidence to show that the survival of patients with localized Hodgkin's disease after 10 years was similar to the expected survival curves in an age adjusted population from that same area of England. With localized lymphosarcoma and reticulum cell sarcoma, after 5 years there appeared to be similar evidence of cure. He felt that 3,000 to 3,250 rads in a period of three weeks using a Cobalt source constituted adequate therapy. KAPLAN in previous discussions had suggested a dose of 3,500 to 4,000 rads over 4 weeks using a 6 MEV Linear Accelerator.

EASSON stressed the fact that the pessimism concerning Hodgkin's disease and lymphosarcoma must be challenged, since Stage I and II disease is definitely curable in a high percentage of patients. He felt that it was extremely important to institute a vigorous program of re-education of the medical population to the concept that Hodgkin's disease, in the early stages, is a definitely curable disease.

Panel 21

Management of Patients with Advanced Cancer

Chairman:

DAVID A. KARNOFSKY (U.S.A)

Members:

A. HOCHMAN (Israel), A. C. JUNQUEIRA (Brazil), D. J. JUSSAWALLA (India),
M. PAREDES (Mexico), H. J. TAGNON (Belgium)

Introduction

With Comments on the Management of Advanced Cancer in the United States

DAVID A. KARNOFSKY

*Division of Chemotherapy Research, Sloan-Kettering Institute and Department
of Medicine, Memorial and James Ewing Hospitals, New York, N.Y.*

Cancer is a worldwide problem, and it is appropriate to discuss it as such at an international meeting. At present, despite the advances in diagnosis and treatment, the majority of patients with cancer are not cured. The progression of the disease causes disability, pain, cachexia, dysfunction of various organ systems and death.

Participants in this symposium have been asked to tell the story of advanced cancer treatment in their area of the world, as it is, without attempting to justify or rationalize the situation. Progress can be made if the truth is known. We hope that their candor and objectivity will be respected. It is the purpose of the International Union Against Cancer to improve the lot of the cancer patient, not only by research, but by optimal applications of the effective means we have available, and not only for the wealthy, the informed and the members of highly developed modern societies, but for all the people of the world.

Under conditions where anti-cancer therapy and supportive measures are used intensively, the survival time data on patients with non-resectable or disseminated cancer from clinical onset are shown in Table I. These data were obtained from the files of the Division of Chemotherapy Research of the Sloan-Kettering Institute and from the Department of Medicine, Memorial Hospital. Depending on the type of cancer, 50 per cent of the patients who ultimately die of their cancer survive beyond 7 to 71 months from clinical onset, and 10 per

Table I. *Survival time of patients with non-resectable and disseminated neoplastic disease from clinical onset to death (treated 1956—1962)*

Type of neoplastic disease	No. of patients	percent survival (months after clinical onset)	
		50	10
Acute leukemia, adults	160	7	23
Acute leukemia, children	205	14	32
Carcinoma of lung	159	10	23
Carcinoma of stomach	85	15	39
Reticulum cell sarcoma	66	16	66
Multiple myeloma	21	17	106
Carcinoma of testes	67	18	53
Carcinoma of ovary	108	21	71
Carcinoma of uterus	43	22	81
Carcinoma of bowel	240	25	62
Carcinoma of kidney	60	26	74
Soft part sarcomas	80	28	145
Melanoma	107	32	83
Chronic myelocytic leukemia	27	34	83
Hodgkin's disease	109	42	119
Carcinoma of breast	509	47	128
Lymphosarcoma	25	71	131
Chronic lymphocytic leukemia	34	62	144

cent beyond 2 years to 12 years. As a general figure, 50 per cent of patients who die of progressive cancer survive for 2 to 3 years and beyond and 10 per cent for 5 to 8 years and longer after the clinical onset. Active treatment may not be needed during the major period of the illness; and the disabling medical problems proliferate in the last few months of life.

The management of advanced cancer is only temporarily effective, in the vast majority of patients, in relieving pain, correcting organ dysfunction, and prolonging life. The availability and application of treatment for the individual patient vary in different countries, and in different social strata within each country. Some preliminary estimates of the effort involved in the United States in the management of patients with advanced cancer are presented in this report. Therapeutic methods may be classified as *specific*, in that they are intended to control the growth of the cancer, and *supportive*, in that they are designed to sustain the patient or alleviate complications, without acting on the cancer. It is sometimes difficult to separate these objectives.

Surgery (Table II) is used to relieve intestinal or ureteral obstruction, to resect fungating masses, to remove tumors pressing on vital structures, and to correct incidental complications. Radiotherapy is widely used in order to control local disease and to relieve symptoms (Table II). It is estimated that there is about 1 radiotherapy unit of 250 KV or higher voltage per 50,000

Table II. *Specific local therapy*

Surgical

　Relief of obstruction

　　Intestinal
　　Tracheal
　　Urinary tract
　　Cord compression

　Removal of fungating masses

　　Extremity
　　Breast

　Treatment of incidental complications

　　Abscess
　　Intestinal perforation
　　Bleeding
　　Pinning of pathological fractures

Radiotherapy

　　To inhibit the growth of local and non-resectable metastases.
　　To relieve pain; to relieve obstruction produced by cancer.

Table III. *Chemotherapy*

May eliminate the disease
　Choriocarcinoma in females

May prolong life
　Acute leukemia　　　　　Carcinoma of prostate
　Lymphomas

May produce predictable palliation
　Lymphomas　　　　　　Carcinoma of ovary
　Chronic leukemias　　　Carcinoma of testes
　Multiple myeloma　　　　Carcinoma of breast
　　　　　　　　　　　　Carcinoma of uterus

May occasionally produce measurable benefit
　Soft-part tumors　　　　Carcinoma of stomach
　Melanoma　　　　　　　Carcinoma of large bowel
　　　　　　　　　　　　Carcinoma of lung
　　　　　　　　　　　　Carcinoma of pancreas
　　　　　　　　　　　　Carcinoma of kidney

people in the United States, and about 70 per cent of the X-ray treatments are given with the limited objective of palliation.

Chemotherapy is assuming a larger role in the management of advanced cancer. While its value is limited, it has been widely accepted as worthy of trial in many situations (Table III). An estimate of the number of patients receiving chemotherapy for cancer each year in the United States and the cost of the drugs is shown in Table IV. Approximately 150,000 patients received

Table IV. *Estimated cost of anti-cancer drugs in the United States in 1965, excluding steroid hormones, and estiminated number of patients treated per year*

	Approx. value to producer	No. of patients who receive treatment
Alkylating agents	$ 2,225,000	97,000
Nitrogen mustard, Chlorambucil Melphalan, Cyclophosphamide, Thio-TEPA, Busulfan		
Antimetabolites	850,000	36,000
Methotrexate 6-Mercaptopurine 5-Fluorouracil		
Antibiotics	75,000	2,500
Actinomycin D		
Plant alkaloids	500,000	9,000
Vinca alkaloids		
	$ 3,650,000	144,500

anti-cancer drugs during 1965, or about 35—50 per cent of those patients who die of their disease. This estimate is subject to considerable error since in some cases, such as chronic myelocytic leukemia, the patient may be maintained on chemotherapy for 2—4 years. The total value of these anticancer drugs in the United States, at the manufacturer's cost, is about $ 3,650,000 per year, and this does not include the steroid hormones.

The supportive measures that may be helpful to the patient with advanced cancer are almost unlimited (Table V). They include the use of blood and platelet transfusions and antibiotics, the availability of biochemical, radiographic and microbiologic laboratories for diagnostic studies, the advice of consultants in the various medical specialities, such as internal medicine, physiology, hematology, cardiology, psychiatry, etc., and the trained teams of physicians who can apply measures to relieve pain, to correct life-threatening complications and to sustain life.

It is estimated that about 300,000 persons die of cancer in the United States each year, and the usual period of hospitalization, during which a well-trained staff and elaborate diagnostic and therapeutic facilities are needed, may average 2–3 months per patient (Table VI). This means that an estimated 100,000 hospital beds per year as well as a proportional level of out-patient, home care and nursing home services, are in use in the United States for the care of advanced cancer. Some patients are cared for in small community hospitals, some in general, governmental, military or university hospitals, and others in specialized research institutions where new forms of treatment are being evaluated. One can estimate that the yearly cost of the care of patients with progressive cancer is about $ 1.5 to $ 2.0 billion dollars.

In highly developed countries cancer has become a major medical problem, second only to cardiovascular disease. In the United States the public has high

Table V. *Supportive measures*	Table VI. *Facilities needed*
Blood transfusions	Hospitals
Platelet transfusions	Trained physicians
Nutritional support	Nursing staff, hospital and visiting
Antibiotics	X-ray therapy facilities
Psychiatric assistance	Surgical teams
Special measures for complications of	Chemotherapists
respiratory tract, liver,	Research units
central nervous system, etc.	Terminal care facilities
	Medical specialties

expectations of good medical care, and doctors, hospitals, and the government are making every effort to comply with the demand. The cost of medical care is of lessening concern, since funds to care for the sick are increasingly provided by insurance, local, State and Federal sources. The factors which are leading to improved patient care are:

1. an increase in hospital facilities and medical and para-medical personnel
2. availability of governmental and private insurance funds to provide the cost of the care, and
3. an inculcation in the public of the philosophy that everyone, irrespective of means, is entitled to the security of high-level, continuing, and readily available medical care from conception to death.

This panel proposes to examine, in various parts of the world, the attitudes of patients and their families at various social levels, and of physicians, hospitals and governments, as related to the management of advanced cancer. It plans to review the medical facilities and trained personnel available in relation to the total number of patients requiring care. The panel hopes to indicate the requirements for the proper care of advanced cancer patients throughout the world, and to discuss how well these needs are being met. Relevant to these conclusions is the stage of development of each country, its medical and financial resources, and the priorities of other pressing medical and public health problems.

Management of Advanced Cancer in Belgium

HENRI J. TAGNON

*Service de Médecine et d'Investigation Clinique, Institut Jules Bordet,
Centre des Tumeurs de l'Université Libre de Bruxelles, Brussels, Belgium*

In Belgium, approximately 20 per cent of all patients with the diagnosis of cancer are treated in the official Government supported and university affiliated Cancer Centers. The remainder are treated in general hospitals, including the university hospitals, or privately in their homes. Although all Cancer Centers are fully equipped for the administration of roentgenotherapy, they differ organizationally as far as medical and surgical participation in patient care are concerned. For instance the Cancer Center in Brussels has fully organized departments of medicine and surgery besides the department of roentgeno-therapy. On the other hand, certain other centers consist exclusively of a department of roentgenotherapy and rely on the general hospital for necessary medical and surgical assistance.

The relatively small proportion of cases of cancer treated in the Cancer Centers is not necessarily to be deplored and can be explained by two main reasons: first, the Centers act as pilot institutions, where new treatments originating inside or outside the country are tested before they are applied to the general medical population. Too many patients would impose a heavy routine burden on the staff. Secondly, the surgical departments in general hospitals often specialize in certain types of cancer: for instance the University Hospital in Brussels specializes in cancer of the digestive tract and as a result few stomach and colon cancers are treated at the Brussels Cancer Center.

The following statistical data obtained at the Brussels Center, therefore, do not necessarily reflect the general situation in the country, but they present the situation as it occurs in a Cancer Center.

Table VII is a comparison of the incidence of different types of cancer in the Brussels Cancer Center and in the general population in Belgium.

Table VII. *Distribution of cancer patients*

	Brussels Cancer Center (per cent)	Belgium (per cent)
Skin cancer	23.5	13.2
Cervix	13	10
Breast	19.4	13.2
Digestive	1.8	24
Respiratory	9.6	10
Sarcomas	11.1	5.1
Leukemia	11.1	5.1
Lymphomas	11.1	5.1

Table VIII shows the operable, Stages I and II, cases of cancer and the inoperable, Stages III and IV, cases of cancer as seen at the Cancer Institute.

Table VIII. *Stage of disease when first seen at Brussels Cancer Center*

	Per cent
Stage I and II, operable	49.1
Stage III, inoperable	23.2
Stage IV, usually inoperable (lung, esophagus, bladder, nervous system, sarcomas, leukemia, lymphoma)	17.2
Not treated	10.5

Table IX. *The results of treatment on the total patient population of the Brussels center*

	Curable cases Stage I and II (per cent)	Advanced cases Stage III and IV (per cent)	All cases (per cent)
1. Five year survival with no evidence of disease	49.2	15.7	39.4
2. Died of other diseases	9.5	7.6	11.1
3. Temporarily asymptomatic	27.9	19	17.1
1 year survival with no evidence of disease	37.3	46.1	39.1
2 year survival with no evidence of disease	32.8	31.4	33
3 year survival with no evidence of disease	16.5	13.2	16.1
4 year survival with no evidence of disease	9.7	6.3	8.6
5 year survival with no evidence of disease	3.7	3	3.2
4. Living at five years with evidence of cancer	2	2.2	2.1
5. Temporary improvement	1.8	12.3	7.8
6. No improvement	7.3	41.8	21.6
7. Deaths during treatment	1.6	1.1	1
8. Lost to follow up	0.8	0.3	0.6

These data indicate that approximately 50 per cent of our patients are potentially curable when seen at the Brussels Center, and 50 per cent are in the advanced stage where cures are uncommon and improbable.

Table IX presents the results of treatment in the whole patient population of the Brussels Center.

Similar statistics are available from our Institute for the different types of cancer and have been published by SIMON and LAGNEAU [*Bull. Cancer* 48, 585 (1961)].

From these data, limited conclusions can be derived. These data confirm well-known statistics and are compatible with the position of Belgium as a Western European country having a population characterized by a long life expectancy and high incidence of diseases associated with old age. Cancer mortality occupies the second rank as a cause of death in Belgium. Fifty per cent of the patients when first seen at the Institute are advanced, of whom 15 per cent survive five years with no evidence of disease. The number of surviving patients in this group drops sharply after 2 years.

These data indicate the present limits of the conventional forms of treatment of cancer. They indicate that, even in this group, conventional treatment may be of palliative value but that the real solution of the problem depends wholly on the results of basic and clinical research.

Management of Advanced Cancer in Israel

ABRAHAM HOCHMAN

Head, Department of Oncology, Hadassah Medical Organization, Jerusalem, Israel

As a first step, let us look more deeply into the meaning of the term "Advanced Cancer". Advanced cancer includes all malignancies that are not amenable to cure by surgery or radiotherapy. These agents are effective only locally, therefore their scope of action is limited to localized disease. Their area of application is strictly demarcated by certain anatomical limitations and biological rules, and cancers which at the time of treatment have spread over and beyond these anatomical and biological boundaries are beyond control by surgery or radiation. Some of these difficulties have been overcome by improvements in surgery and radiation therapy; yet while local results are better, the total cure rate has not been markedly altered.

There is a turning point in the life history of any malignancy when it changes from a localized lesion to a generalized disease. The greater the malignancy of the tumor, the earlier the turning point occurs. Some tumors, because of their high malignancy, are never detected in their localized form; and these highly malignant tumors constitute the majority of all cancer cases.

One wonders whether any organized detection program can overcome the tendency of some tumors to spread early and thereby increase the proportion of curable cases. If we exclude skin cancer, it is assumed that about 80 per cent

of all cancers come under medical care and treatment when already in the
incurable or advanced stage. Advanced cancer progresses to the stage of terminal illness, a situation not difficult to define. At this point means to restrain
the progression of the disease are not available and the patient is thereafter
managed by nursing care. To state categorically that the patient is to be
abandoned to nursing care only, without specific therapy, is a difficult decision
to make. When surgery was the only method of treatment, this nursing stage
set in early. The advent of radiotherapy relegated terminal nursing care to a
more distant future. Hormone therapy and chemotherapy have pushed back
this stage even further and have allowed us to bring palliation and help to
the formerly hopeless patient. If we may speak of progress made in the treatment of cancer patients it is just this aspect of the treatment of advanced cancer
which is of the greatest importance to the clinician. Surgery, radiotherapy,
chemotherapy and hormone therapy can achieve palliation and alleviate suffering for days or weeks in the life of the cancer patient. It is true that when we
exclude patients in whom the disease has produced a life-threatening com-
plication, such as a mediastinal tumor or an obstructing lesion of the bowel,
which is relieved by therapy, the overall prolongation of life with palliative
therapy in negligible. The length of survival is not the most relevant yardstick
in evaluating the achievements of modern cancer therapy.

After the curable stage is passed, the cancer runs a course of its own from
which it can only be slightly diverted or suppressed by the available forms of
treatment. The fate of an incurable breast cancer patient depends on the extent
and rate of spread to viscera, on whose physiological integrity life is dependent.
Those cases where signal therapeutic success has reversed a mortal situation and
saved the patient's life, for the time being, do not weigh heavily in statistical
analysis of survival time for a given type of cancer. At present the only
relevant point in the discussion of treatment of advanced cancer, the only
practical goal to be aimed at, is maximum palliation and maximum physical
fitness. Prolongation of life *per se* is not the goal of therapy, unless the patient
is restored to sufficiently good health to lead a useful life.

This practical goal is attainable; but its achievement requires the services
of a team of specialists familiar with all the facets of the surgical, radiological
and chemotherapeutical treatment of cancer. We often notice a specialist in one
therapeutic field deprecating the efforts of a specialist in another field; thus a
surgical colleague may discourage a patient with advanced cancer from seeking
another form of treatment. This negative attitude may stem from a lack of
knowledge of chemotherapy and radiotherapy, but it is often accompanied by
a philosophy of defeatism and resignation; the expressed principle being: Let
him end his life peacefully, the sooner the better; any treatment will only add
needless pain.

To some extent this attitude toward disease is a function of the cultural
and religious background of the physician and the patient, and the psycho-social

attitude of the community. Jewish patients and their families do not accept and will vigorously oppose defeatism and resignation. Life for them has a value *per se*, a kind of transcendental value. Life in itself is a mission which the human being has a duty to take to full course, irrespective of suffering. Prolongation of life is a sacred duty in itself, both for the patient and the family. Respect for human life and human dignity is of the highest order in the Jewish religion. Whenever someone saves the life of a human being — it is said — it is as if he has created the Universe from its beginnings. Naturally Jewish patients want their doctor to be a fighter, and they will not accept the hopelessness of a death warrant. They will look for someone who has the knowledge, the ambition and the subtlety to aid the patient. Therefore, in Israel we are faced with a situation where we treat patients who might be abandoned elsewhere. We admit patients to our ward who elsewhere might be diagnosed as hopeless and beyond benefit from cancer therapy. It is surprising how some individuals can still be salvaged even in this far-advanced condition, and two examples are described.

Case 1. The patient, a lecturer in economics, aged 42, had a surgical resection in August, 1962 for an astrocytoma of the left frontal lobe. He felt well postoperatively and returned to work. Six months later he developed Jacksonian seizures, with right hemiparesis and aphasia, and in February 1963, another craniotomy was performed. The tumor in the left frontal lobe was incompletely excised; and he received Co^{60} 6,000 rads to the left frontal area. In August, 1963 he had repeated episodes of unconsciousness, right motor weakness, and he received another 3,000 rads. He remained well for over a year, continued to lecture and published a book on financial and economic problems. His condition remained stationary until November, 1965 when he became bedridden because of right hemiplegia, left motor weakness and aphasia. A therapeutic decision was difficult since his brain had already been exposed to 9,000 rads in two series of treatment, as well as two craniotomies. Surprisingly, these extreme procedures did not affect the patient's intellectual performance. On the family's insistence, and even the patient's prayers, further treatment was undertaken. He received injections of vincristine, and small daily doses of radiation therapy at the rate of 500 rads per week for six weeks. The motor deficit improved, asphasia disappeared and the patient plans to resume his academic work.

Case 2. The patient, aged 40, had a radical mastectomy for a Stage II infiltrating duct carcinoma in December, 1962. By October, 1963 extensive bone metastases appeared and were treated by radiation castration and testosterone. The patient was relieved of pain and led an active life as a housewife, mother and teacher. In December, 1964 there was a sudden change for the worse; the liver increased rapidly in size, with a high alkaline phosphatase and the patient developed anorexia and somnolence. Hypophysectomy by $Yttrium^{90}$ implant was discussed but rejected because of her poor condition. Prednisone was ineffective, and the patient then received cyclophosphamide. The liver returned to almost normal size, she showed remarkable clinical improvement and was able to leave the hospital and return to work. She was maintained on cyclo-phosphamide for almost one year, when in November, 1965 hepatomegaly recurred with weakness, loss of appetite and low-grade fever. The patient received a course of thioTEPA and considerable improvement occurred, but less than that after cyclophosphamide. This treatment produced a leukopenia and it was discontinued. A pituitary Yttrium^{90} implant was discussed a second time and performed, but there was no improvement. The liver again increased considerably in size with a mixed obstructive and hepatocellular jaundice and a trial of 5-fluorouracil produced a partial response and the patient was able to leave the hospital.

These two cases illustrate to what length we will go in treating the advanced and practically hopeless stages of cancer. This is done because of the particular mental attitude of the Jewish patient towards sickness, and of his and his family's insistence on fighting for the life of the patient even if the margin of success seems narrow. No wonder then, that a patient if abandoned, will turn to seek the help of charlatans. It is surprising that when an aggressive thera-peutic policy for very advanced cases is pursued, there is a considerable salvage among apparently hopeless cases.

Israel has a population of about 2,250,000. There are two cancer registries, one for mortality and one for incidence. The cancer mortality in the country during the past few years was about 100 cases per 100,000, and the cancer in-cidence was about 200 per 100,000. If we deduct incidence of skin cancer — about 35 per 100,000, other types of cancer have an incidence of 165 cases per 100,000 of which roughly 65 per cent cannot be cured. The figures probably should be 10—15 per cent higher or closer to 75 per cent. The mortality statistics are based on death certificates, which are not highly reliable. We may estimate the prevalence of advanced cases at 6,000—8,000 in the whole country.

This is a high figure and if we adopt an aggressive policy in the treatment of advanced cancer patients, adequate facilities must be available. This means hospital beds, proper radiation equipment, proper facilities for chemotherapy and, of course, research facilities. Without the latter, it is not possible to operate a good clinic for advanced cancer patients. It will not attract the skilled scien-tists who are willing to dedicate themselves to this, mostly frustrating, effort to salvage the lives of hopeless patients if, by working in the meagre and sad present, their work does not show promise of leading to a brighter future.

In a recent publication of the W.H.O. Expert Committee on Cancer Treat-ment, it is estimated that some 130,000 nursing days will be required per 1,000,000 persons, effectively to apply the various measures presently available. This amounts to 350 beds per 100,000 population, and may well be a con-servative estimate. About half the beds would be surgical, and the other half for chemotherapy, hormone therapy and radiotherapy. The report further recommends the establishment of a network of specialized cancer treatment centers of different levels staffed by qualified personnel and furnished with appropriate diagnostic and therapeutic equipment; the organizational details would vary from country to country, with appropriate attention to local conditions.

The trend in Israel for many years has been to organize cancer treatment by pattern similar to that recommended by the World Health Organization; and that of major cancer centers in England, Scandinavia and the USA. In the near future cancer centers will be established in the major cities in Israel. The Center in the Hadassah University Hospital in Jerusalem will be enlarged, its bed capacity increased, the facilities for out-patient care in the form of comprehensive day care and home care programs will be widened and facilities for clinical research extended. Clinical research will be an important effort, since a proper effort has not been made to utilize our clinical material for cancer research.

The University Hospital Department of Oncology in Jerusalem functions as a center for diagnosis, treatment and follow-up of cancer patients and for undergraduate instruction in Oncology in the Medical School, and the training of specialists in radiotherapy and chemotherapy.

The relative incidence of cancer in the population of Israel reflects some particular features characteristic of this group (Table X). The incidence of prostatic carcinoma is about 10 per 100,000 — a third of the incidence in other countries. Carcinoma of the penis is non-existent, although it constitutes about five per cent of the total cancer incidence in some population groups in the United States and is much higher in Eastern and Southern Asia. Skin cancer has about the same incidence as in other countries, despite the high intensity of sunlight. Bronchus carcinoma in males is lower than in England and the United States and is about 21 per 100,000, whereas the incidence of stomach cancer is similar to that of the western countries. The female group is characterized by a low incidence of cervical carcinoma, 5 per 100,000, and a rather high breast carcinoma incidence — 46 per 100,000.

We selected some types of cancer which are either more or less common in Israel than in other countries, and would like to discuss other possible differences, such as the relative proportion in advanced stages and the success of treatment.

Cancer of the cervix has a low incidence among Jews, being about a tenth of the incidence in Western countries. However, when diagnosed, the disease is usually in an advanced stage: 66 per cent of the patients are in Stage II and Stage III, and only 12 per cent are in Stage I. Our 5 year survival rates are remarkably good; in Stage II — 55 per cent, in Stage III — 25 per cent. In carcinoma of the cervix radium was applied to the cervical tumor, and external radiation to the parametrium.

Cancer of the ovary appears mostly in the incurable stage, with about 70 per cent in the advanced stages with local extension or widespread disease. Treatment was, in general, surgery and postoperative radiation or, in advanced

17*

Table X. *Israel cancer registry annual incidence — rate per 100,000 persons*

Site	Males	Females
All sites	200.5	220.1
Lip	3.8	1.0
Oral, salivary, nasopharynx	2.3	1.0
Esophagus	3.0	2.0
Stomach	22.5	14.1
Colon	8.9	10.8
Rectum	6.1	6.7
Gall-bladder, extrahepatic ducts	2.5	6.9
Liver primary	1.7	—
Liver, secondary or unspecified	2.0	2.3
Pancreas	7.1	4.9
Larynx	6.6	—
Bronchus, lung	21.2	6.5
Breast	1.2	46.8
Prostate	10.2	—
Testis	1.4	—
Cervix uteri	—	5.5
Corpus uteri	—	9.0
Uterus, unspecified	—	1.2
Ovary	—	10.9
Other female genital organs	—	1.5
Kidney	5.3	3.5
Bladder	9.8	2.2
Melanoma of skin	2.2	2.9
Skin	33.6	30.2
Eye	1.1	1.0
Brain, other parts of CNS	9.8	9.1
Thyroid	1.8	4.1
Bone	1.2	—
Connective tissue	2.5	2.4
Lymphosarcoma	8.3	5.5
Hodgkin's disease	2.7	2.1
Multiple myeloma	1.8	1.8
Leukemia	8.4	6.6

cases, chemotherapy combined with radiation when possible. Fifty per cent of all cases die within the first year. Only about 15 per cent remain alive after 5 years (Fig. 1).

Advanced or recurrent cancer of the breast in most frequently seen on our wards. It is also the type of carcinoma which, even in the advanced stages, is still amenable to palliation for long periods of time. Radiation, surgery, chemotherapy, endocrine therapy — each of them alone or in combination can lead to improvement. We studied the end results of treatment in a group of 338 patients suffering from recurrent disease or inoperable carcinoma of the breast. Apparently the most critical period is the first two years after diagnosis. At the end of the first year 90 patients (33 per cent) and at the end of second year another 70 patients (25 per cent) (out of 268 patients) showed objective signs of recurrence, and after 5 years only 11 per cent were alive without symptoms of renewed activity of the disease. In a few exceptional cases metastases appeared after 10 and in one case after 25 years (Fig. 2).

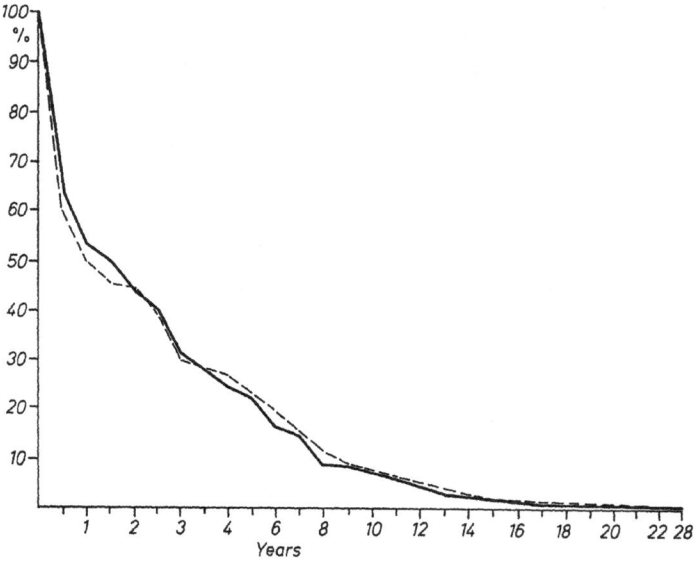

Fig. 1. Survival in 135 cases of ovarian carcinoma. The solid line shows survival in all 135 patients, the broken line shows survival in 70 patients with complete follow-up. [From IVAN RATZKOWSKI and HOCHMAN, *Cancer (Philad.)* 16, 1578 (1963)]

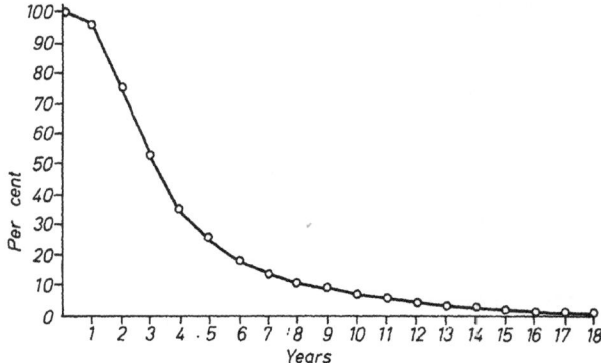

Fig. 2. Percentage survival of 338 breast cancer patients with recurrent disease. [From IVAN RATZKOWSKI and HOCHMAN, *Cancer (Philad.)* 14, 300 (1961)]

The duration of the so-called free period did not influence the survival after manifestation of occurrence, proving that the host factors which contributed during the free cancer period in inhibiting the cancer manifestations, ceased to exercise their influence on the tumor at the time of recurrence. The type of first recurrence had a certain influence on survival. We could establish that locally recurrent disease has a more benign course and therefore the mean survival of these patients was considerably higher than that for the other patterns of recurrence.

Practically every patient who showed signs of recurrence or had inoperable disease when first seen, received some attempt at altering the hormonal environ-

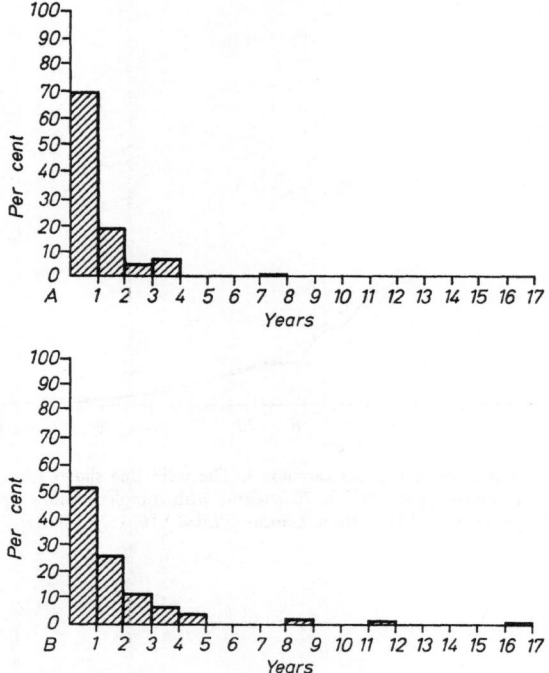

Fig. 3. Percentage of deaths per year for 336 patients after the appearance of recurrence. A, Percentage of deaths among 66 who did not have hormonal therapy. B, Percentage of deaths among 270 patients who had hormonal therapy. (Of the 338 patients studied, in 2 it could not be ascertained whether or not there had been hormonal therapy.) [From Ivan Ratzkowski and Hochman, *Cancer (Philad.)* 14, 300 (1961)]

ment of the cancer by castration, addition of androgens, estrogens and adrenal steroids, by irradiation of the pituitary or by adrenalectomy. Many patients, in addition, received local irradiation. Seventy per cent of patients derived benefit from these various treatments, either objective or subjective, or both.

About 50 per cent of patients on hormonal treatment died during the first year after recurrence but, in contrast, about 70 per cent of those who did not receive hormonal treatment died during the same period. Three per cent treated by hormones survived for more than five years, whereas one per cent of the other group stayed alive for more than five years (Fig. 3).

The question of prolongation of life by hormonal treatment has been studied, and in our series hormonally-treated patients had a mean survival time of 20.2 months after recurrence, whereas those not receiving hormones had a mean survival time of 14 months.

Malignant lymphomas are considered to be more frequent in people of Jewish extraction. This is not confirmed in the statistical figures in Israel. Malignant lymphomas in males were 11/100,000 and in females 7.6/100,000; figures close to those observed in Western countries. These patients received radiotherapy for Stages I and II, and chemotherapy for Stage III. In Stage II almost a third of the patients survived for five years and about six per cent for ten years. Women lived longer than men in similar stages of the disease.

In reviewing the survival figures of patients with advanced cancer, one cannot escape the conclusion that though the disease ultimately is fatal, death is not necessarily imminent, and prolongation of life is possible in many instances, particularly in certain types of cancer. However, prolongation of life *per se* cannot be the aim of treatment, if it means prolonging the patient's suffering. It is of value only when accompanied by a restoration of the patient's well-being and improved physical performance. This is attainable with the present methods of treatment. Many patients can benefit from treatment, their suffering can be alleviated, and their useful life prolonged. Not only should more knowledge concerning the importance of early diagnosis be taught and spread, but also knowledge concerning progress that has been made in the management of advanced cancer. The handling of the advanced cancer patient is a medical speciality when skill is acquired by special training.

In summary it can be stated that under optimal conditions, expert knowledge, a well-trained staff, adequate technical equipment and outpatient hospital facilities, much can be done for the advanced cancer patient to alleviate his suffering and to prolong his useful life.

Management of Advanced Cancer in Brazil

ANTONIO CARLOS JUNQUEIRA

Chief, Service of Clinical Research on Radio- and Chemotherapy, Central Institute of Cancer, S͂ao Paulo, Brazil

Cancer, together with cardiovascular diseases, is responsible for the greatest percentage of deaths in the developed countries. In South America, approximately 60 per cent of patients with cancer are in an advanced stage when first seen, and the management of advanced cancer is thus a major problem.

This report is composed of three parts: (A) a picture of the general situation in the treatment of advanced cancer in South America; (B) a review of some important facts directly related to the management of the advanced cancer patient; and (C) suggestions which may be helpful in improving the present situation.

Unfortunately, the almost complete lack of statistics and official data creates great difficulties in determining the real situation. We will present data based on personal communications from a survey among physicians in several countries and from our own observations. Most of the figures will be estimates, although real data could be obtained from some cancer institutes; these, however, show the local situation only, and are usually the best in the country.

A. General Situation of South America

The reasons for the present condition in South America, and the scarcity of statistical data are mainly:

1. Little interest on the part of governments and health authorities to face the problem of treating patients and obtaining statistical data on incidence, mortality, and epidemiology of cancer. This is, in part, explained by the pressing necessity to deal also with other important sanitary problems among which are mainly infectious and nutritional diseases.

2. The very low index of literacy and, also, the almost absolute lack of knowledge related to cancer among the rural population. Their ignorance is astounding. The disease is left to progress to a late stage, with the development of great masses, because they do not know the danger they are facing. The patient only seeks treatment when the disease is advanced and there is pain or other forms of discomfort. The patient's family does not believe in the possibility of cure — there is a general belief that cancer is always fatal and cannot be cured — and does not insist that the patient follow therapeutic recommendation. When improvement is not rapid, it is common to abandon the treatment and turn to charlatans.

3. Differences in economic and social conditions and medical facilities between urban and rural areas. The cities have better facilities and town people are also more inclined to look for medical attention.

4. Lack of professional cancer education. Clinicians and surgeons attending the patients in the country and small towns do not have the knowledge to carry out the necessary diagnostic and treatment procedures. The physicians frequently continue caring for the patients for economic reasons, but this happens also in the big cities.

5. Deficiency of tumor registries. Only three or four South American countries have general tumor registries. Regional ones are found in some cities of Brazil. Almost all of them were created in recent years and are still inadequate. The few cancer institutes have their own registries, but their figures are not

useful for this report since they reflect the situation in the city where they are located and where the best facilities are available. Statistical data based on these registries are useful for other purposes, but do not give a true picture of the situation in South America.

6. Cancer is not a compulsorily reportable disease. Many advanced cases die at home, without the benefit of proper attention. These deaths are never recorded and thus cannot contribute to a better understanding of the cancer situation in each nation.

7. Death certificates are frequently incomplete. Several items are not recorded, and in patients who die of complications of cancer, these complications are registered as the cause of death.

8. Extensive areas and long distances make access to the cancer clinics difficult. This is a major reason why the patient may not go for treatment initially, or remains at home after the first treatment or abandons long-term therapy.

9. Follow-up data are very deficient. Long distances and poor communications are responsible for this. A characteristic attitude of general surgeons is to lose interest in the cancer patient after surgery, and the patient's ignorance of his own situation also contributes to inadequate follow-up.

10. The most important factor responsible, in great part, for all the above mentioned, is the very low economic level in South America. On the one hand are the people with a small income, insufficient to pay for the medical services, hospitalization, travel, drugs, etc. On the other, the government does not allocate sufficient funds to attack all aspects of the cancer problem.

All these facts contribute to make even more complex and difficult the cancer situation in South America.

B. Some Facts Related to the Management of Advanced Cancer

1. Incidence of the major forms of advanced cancer.

In the absence of official statistical data we have to rely on information based on personal communications, or from published reports on cancer. The most frequent forms of cancer in South America are those arising in breast, cervix, uterus, stomach, lung, skin and the lymphomas. With the exception of skin cancer, which has a high percentage of cure, the others provide most of the patients with advanced cancer. Table XI shows the incidence of major forms of cancer treated at the Cancer Institute of São Paulo, from 1953 to 1965 (*Ann. Rep.*, 1965). It also shows that a highly active unit of an institution expresses an erroneous picture of the incidence of the various forms of cancer. The Head and Neck Department, an active and efficient one, is responsible for a great number of cases treated at the Hospital.

Table XII shows the great proportion of patients who, when first seen, were already too advanced for radical treatment. Considering the facts above mentioned, and the difficulty in obtaining an early diagnosis in some cases, about 60—70 per cent of the patients are in advanced stages when first seen. In Uruguay for instance, 87 per cent of lung cancer, 75 per cent of lymphomas, 53 per cent of cervix cancers and 40 per cent of breast cancers are advanced when first seen (KASDORF, personal communication).

The high incidence of advanced cancer, when the patient is first seen, occurs all over South America (ESTEVEZ; GAYTAN YANGUAS; MIRRA; PAULSON BEJAR; UDIHARA; VAUTHIER DE SOUZA — all personal communications). When we

Table XI. Incidence of do the major forms of cancer in patients registered at the Instituto Central Câncer, São Paulo, Brazil, 1953—1965

	Number	Per cent
Skin	4,859	23.8
Cervix	3,012	14.8
Breast	2,315	11.3
Stomach	1,045	5.1
Lip	1,004	4.9
Lymphomas	761	3.7
Tongue	745	3.6
Naso-pharynx	557	2.7
Larynx	457	2.2
Esophagus	437	2.1
Lung	428	2.1
Others	4,738	23.7
	20,358	100.0

Table XII. Proportion of untreated advanced cases among the major forms of cancer (Instituto Central do Câncer, São Paulo, Brazil)

Year	Number of Patients	Stage III	IV	Per cent	
1961	267	131	26	58	Cervix
1962	278	128	34	58	Cervix
1961	201	73	31	51	Breast
1962	238	80	50	54	Breast
Advanced					
1961	184	126		68	Mouth
1962	174	107		61	Mouth
1961	81	47		58	Stomach
1962	111	62		56	Stomach

deal with cancer, we are, in effect, concerned with advanced cancer. The situation is a little better in the Cancer Institutes because of the better facilities and greater educational and economic status among its patients.

2. Survival time of patients who died of specific forms of cancer.

The lack of statistical data also affects a consideration of this item. As a rule, the patient with advanced cancer is kept at home. The hospital beds are used mainly for the early stages and even these patients must wait, sometimes for months, for hospital admission. It is common for an early case to lose a possibility of cure because those better placed on the admission list are treated first. A great number of patients are lost to follow-up after the first treatment. The great distances and difficulties of communication are the main reasons for the poor follow-up. It is almost impossible to establish an accurate estimation for survival rates, and we have had to rely on personal communications. In Montevideo's Institute of Radiology the average survival time, after treatment, for lung cancer was 5 months and for lymphomas 14 months (KASDORF, personal communication). In a recent survey of 48 private patients with advanced ovarian cancer who received adequate treatment, we found only 10 or 20.8 per cent survived one year from the beginning of treatment (JUNQUEIRA, 1966).

3. Facilities available and the per cent of the population with cancer which benefit from these facilities.

In the discussion of this item we have to consider two situations.

a) The major cities usually have cancer institutes or cancer clinics in the general hospitals. These cancer institutes, as a rule, have the conventional facilities for treating cancer. They do not have, with very rare exceptions, facilities for research, but are able to offer adequate treatment to a *limited* number of patients. The surgeons are capable and experienced; radiotherapy departments are equipped with standard machines and radium. There is no super-

Table XIII. New patients registered during 1965 (Instituto Central do Câncer, São Paulo, Brazil)

		Per cent
1. From Bolivia	2	
2. From other states in Brazil	452	14.9
3. From the state of São Paulo	1,264	41.9
4. From the capital (São Paulo)	1,298	43.0
Total	3,016	
Patients treated	1,603	53.0

voltage apparatus, although telecobalt units are available in several places. In Brazil, there are approximately 20 units, of which 10 are in São Paulo. Chemotherapy is done by surgeons and clinicians who do their best with the drugs available. The major difficulty is the lack of hospital beds in specialized centers. These few centers have to deal with an excessive number of patients. As a consequence, patients are kept waiting and treatment, as a rule, is not optimal. As an example, Table XIII shows the number of patients registered at the Cancer Institute of São Paulo in 1965. Only 53 per cent were treated; the others either did not have cancer, had disease which was considered too advanced for treatment, or were not treated for other reasons. Table XIII also shows that only 43 per cent of the patients were from the city of São Paulo and that 14.9 per cent came from other states.

Even the best hospitals may not have research facilities, essential radiotherapy units, chemotherapeutic agents, domiciliary service, terminal care beds, follow-up programs, etc.

These centers can treat, we believe, around 10 to 40 per cent of the cancer patients who apply, and as the early cases are to be preferred, the advanced ones receive practically no specific treatment.

b) The country and the great majority of cities do not have cancer institutes or tumor clinics. Patients are managed by general surgeons and clinicians, not by specialists. When possible, these patients are referred to the cancer centers, but the advanced cases rarely receive adequate assistance.

As an estimate, we could say that in the whole of South America, not more than 10 per cent of the advanced cancer patients have the benefit of adequate facilities for management of their situation.

4. The attitude of hospitals, governments, physicians and patients towards the efforts to sustain life in advanced stages of the disease.

We can say that, as a rule, there is a growing interest in the cancer problem everywhere. The government and health authorities have, in South America, several other medical problems as important as cancer; these are mainly parasitic, infectious, and nutritional diseases. The financial support must be distributed to care for a number of pressing medical problems, and for this reason cancer patients cannot receive a bigger contribution. Nevertheless, lately the general attitude, at least in Brazil, has changed for the better, and more understanding is found regarding the cancer problem. It seems that soon this may be translated into more generous economic support.

The physicians, through a better understanding of the complexity of the problem, are more cooperative in referring patients to specialized institutions, where they are managed by a team of experts. This is happening in the big cities and also in some rural areas, but in other areas, the problem remains the same. Everybody treats cancer as best he can, a consequence of economic, social and educational conditions.

The general opinion is in favor of making efforts to sustain life when there is the possibility of prolonging useful life.

The family of the poor and indigent patient, as a rule, looks at his death with equanimity. In the rich families, however, it is common to ask the physician to do everything possible to sustain the patient, and the request to "try anything", is heard with great frequency.

An important aspect related to the cancer problem, which should be considered is that of charlatanism. Charlatanism is found in all countries, but South America, where the social, economic and educational conditions are favorable and medical facilities for the advanced cancer patient are few, is one of the best places for it to grow and spread. The use of concoctions, plant extracts, magic formulae and "special" treatments is widespread with all its disadvantages.

5. Requirements for the optimal medical care for advanced cancer patients in comparison to what is actually available.

Surgery, in advanced patients, is used only as a palliative, to relieve obstruction, resect infected and fungating masses, perform tracheostomy, etc. This kind of surgery can be done everywhere by any surgeon.

Radiotherapy is very useful in controlling some forms of local disease and to relieve symptoms. Radium is not used as a palliative. As a rule, there is also no necessity to use super-voltage radiation in palliation. The isotopes, for example Au^{198} for the control of pleural or peritoneal effusions, can be replaced by chemotherapy. Thus, as long as there are sufficient 250 KV units, practically everything there is to be done by radiotherapy, for the advanced patient, can be done. But, unfortunately, the machines are very expensive and need staff, technicians and adequate installation to be properly used. As a rule, radiotherapy services are found only in hospitals or in large cities, and as advanced cancer patients usually have to be in hospital beds, the number of beds is also a limiting factor.

Chemotherapy, lately, is assuming a much larger and important role in cancer palliation. It is used, not only on those forms of cancer where it has already proved its value, but also on others, and, in some places, on almost all cases of advanced cancer. As there is no limitation to its use, any physician can prescribe a drug and the majority of cases can be treated at home. It has been substituted, almost entirely, for other forms of specific treatment.

Unfortunately, the limitations characteristic of the presently known drugs, the high prices, and difficulty in obtaining some of them, the stage of the disease and the lack of knowledge and experience of the physicians not familiar with their use, produce very poor results as a rule. Nevertheless, properly administered chemotherapy could be very useful in the rural areas and small cities. The more elaborate technics, as perfusion, infusion, and experimental chemotherapy should be conducted only in specialized centers.

Supportive measures include practically all fields of medicine; some of them, as blood transfusion, antibiotics, drugs to relieve pain and laboratory tests can be provided almost everywhere. Others are to be found only in large centers, as are consultants in the various specialties, trained nursing staff for hospitals and home care, etc.

At present, we believe that not more than 10 per cent of the advanced cases receive proper assistance. These patients usually belong to rich families, pay for all that is necessary, and are treated in the best institutions with the assistance of private doctors.

6. Clinical situations, where the use of the presently available treatments may yield important results in terms of increased survival time, patient comfort, and social effectiveness.

The more frequent advanced tumors in South America are, as mentioned before, those arising in the breast, cervix, lung, stomach, and the lymphomas. The lymphomas properly treated by radiotherapy and chemotherapy, even in the late stages, can have an increased survival time, sometimes with the disappearance of symptoms and masses, and restoration to a useful life.

Breast cancer also can be benefitted by the control of symptoms mainly in those cases with bone metastases. These cases, properly treated, can have good palliation for months and years.

The same applies, in a smaller degree, to cervix carcinoma. Radiation and chemotherapy by arterial infusion can reduce large masses and relieve symptoms.

For gastric and lung cancer, specific treatment is less efficient but, in some cases, offers benefits.

The supportive measures are useful for all cases.

Other forms of cancer, less frequent in South America, which can be helped by specific treatment, are the chronic and acute leukemias, multiple myeloma, choriocarcinoma, ovarian carcinoma, seminoma and prostatic carcinoma.

7. Distinction between clinical research in order to evaluate new forms of treatment and the practical application of elaborate but inconsistently effective ones.

New forms of therapy, mainly in the fields of chemotherapy and immunology, can be tried in some selected institutions where the facilities and personnel are available. They are contra-indicated in other places. Doctors should be instructed about the dangers and disadvantages of trying new procedures in sporadic cases, or in places or institutions without the necessary facilities.

C. Suggestions to Improve the Situation

There is no doubt that the main reason for the deficiencies in the management of advanced cancer in South America is its low economic status. Almost all the problems could be solved, in due time, if there were enough financial support, but unfortunately, at the moment, this is not possible.

However, in a Panel of this importance, we should not only present and discuss the difficulties and negative aspects of the subject, but also try, with a practical and optimistic mind, to take the necessary steps to correct what is possible with the resources available and to improve the situation.

Considering that one of the purposes of UICC is to improve the treatment and control of cancer, this Panel represents a good occasion to make some suggestions which could be useful in this regard.

1. Professional education — The lack of knowledge about cancer, among the physicians, could be corrected, in part, if the schools of medicine introduced oncology as a discipline in their curriculum. Only some of the more recently created schools have presented the subject.

Visiting teams of experts could also be very useful. They would spend one or two months in a country giving lectures and demonstrations on the several aspects of cancer.

Journals and papers more concerned with the clinical and therapeutical aspects of cancer should be increased. The majority of the presently available journals are dedicated, mostly, to research and cannot attract interest in South America, where clinical investigation is almost nonexistent.

2. Public education — An elementary knowledge about cancer, its danger signals, the possibility of cure, and the importance of an early diagnosis would improve the situation. This could be done through well-planned public campaigns in newspaper articles, etc.

3. Organization of tumor clinics in general hospitals of small towns. Even without the necessary equipment, these clinics should be very useful for diagnosis and for maintaining follow-up records on local patients who have been treated at the cancer institutes.

4. Tumor registries — Great emphasis should be put on the creation of general and local registries, and those existing should be improved. For large countries, like Brazil and Argentina, with a great diversity of social, geographic and economic conditions, regional registries are more feasible.

5. Every effort should be made to obtain follow-up records. In the country and small towns non-medical groups, such as the police departments, voluntary organizations, etc. could be useful in obtaining information on patients.

6. Charlatanism should be fought at all costs. The already existing laws should be enforced, and, if necessary, new ones introduced. Physicians should avoid all the unproven methods of treatment, and legitimate research should be conducted in cancer institutes. Terminal cases should not be abandoned to charlatans, and the people should be instructed about the disadvantages of charlatanism.

7. Compulsory registration of cancer should be adopted universally, and doctors should be instructed about its importance.

8. Knowledge about the conventional use of chemotherapy should be increased in the country and small towns. It is a useful weapon, when properly employed, in the management of advanced cancer and can be of great assistance in the outlying areas.

If the above suggestions were implemented, it would represent a great help in the management of cancer, and, as a consequence, of advanced cases, at relatively little expense.

Acknowledgements: The information gathered from the answers to a questionnaire sent to well-known cancerologists in South America was of great assistance in the preparation of this report. We want to express our gratitude for their generous cooperation to Drs. HELMUT KASDORF, ROBERTO ESTEVEZ, MARIO GAITAN YANGUAS, GUILLERMO PAULSON BEJAR, ROBERTO VAUTHIER DE SOUZA, MASSAKI UDIHARA, and ANTONIO PEDRO MIRRA.

References

Annu. Rep. — Associação Paulista de Combate co Cancer — São Paulo, Brazil 1965.

JUNQUEIRA, A. C. C., Report to be presented at the UICC Symposium on Ovarian Cancer to be held at Houston (USA), October 12—15, 1966.

Management of Advanced Cancer in Mexico and Central America

MARIO PAREDES and RODOLFO MORAN

Departments of Medicine and Preventive Medicine, University of Guadalajara School of Medicine and the Cancer Clinic, City Hospital of Guadalajara, Guadalajara, Mexico.

Our area of the world, with a total population of over 56 million inhabitants, comprises 7 quite different republics of Latin America with many common economic, educational, sanitary and health problems (Fig. 4). Some thought ought to be given to these problems properly to place in perspective the situation of our advanced cancer cases.

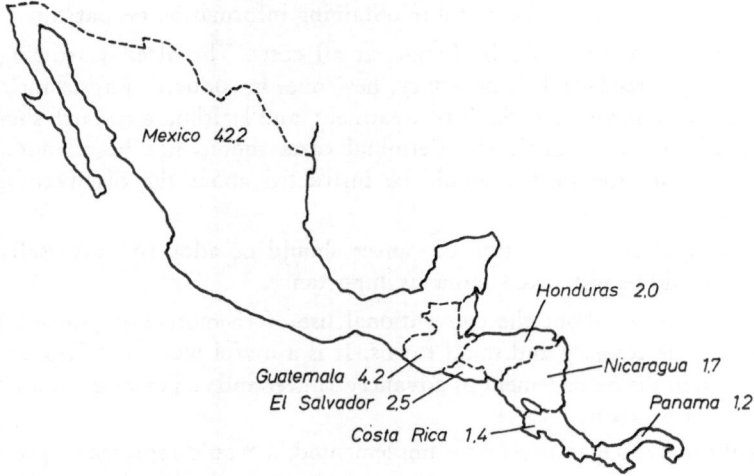

Fig. 4. Population (millions) in Mexico and Central America. (From Compendio Mundial, 1966. Selecciones del Reader's Digest pp. 96—100, 103—106, 107—121, 133—136, Mexico)

Income distribution in Mexico and Central America is badly balanced in favor of the privileged classes. Total production is low, housing is deplorably bad and health facilities are not adequate. Malnutrition and diarrheal disease are leading causes of death. Infantile mortality is alarmingly high; thus, one in ten babies dies before it is a year old. For every child that dies of malnutrition in the United States, more than 300 die of the same deficiency in some of our countries (EISENHOWER, 1963). Only about 12 per cent of the population in Mexico is 50 years of age or older.

The income of workers is incredibly low, ranging from 150 to 410 dollars a year in the best areas of Mexico and Central America. Only as few as 3.5 per cent of the families in some of the states of Mexico earn more than 250 dollars a month per family (Ingresos..., 1965); thus, it is estimated that up to 60 per cent of our people are medically indigent. Education is a rare privilege. Illiteracy is as high as 70 per cent in Guatemala. Only 16 per cent of children in Nicaragua attend public or private schools. Taxes bear heavily on the poor and tangible reform movements are developing much too slowly; nevertheless, things seem to be moving in the right direction in some of our countries. Costa Rica, for instance, points with pride to the fact that it has more teachers than soldiers. Her people have a literacy rate of 80 per cent. Mexico's progress in the last 30 years stands in sharp contrast to the slowness with which other Latin American peoples have moved (EISENHOWER, 1963). There are reasons to hope for a better future.

Table XIV. *Cancer mortality (1960—1962)*

Country	Rank	Country	Rank
Panama	3rd	El Salvador	8th
Costa Rica	5th	Nicaragua	11th
Honduras	6th	Guatemala	18th
Mexico	6th		

This is the area of Latin America where we attempted to estimate the true magnitude of the cancer problem. It must be said at the outset that we have not succeeded. Official statistics when available are grossly inaccurate. The incidence of cancer, or for that matter of advanced cancer, in Mexico and Central America is not known. Cancer is not a reportable disease. Hospital records are incomplete in most instances. Private doctors who keep files on their patients are the exception. Sporadic studies give an approximate idea of the incidence of specific types of cancer (MARTÍNEZ *et al.*, 1964; GARCÍA and GARZA, 1964). In Mexico for instance, Arizaga (personal communication) found an incidence of 0.66 per cent of positive vaginal cytologies in 1500 asymptomatic women 30 years of age or older and there are some 6 million Mexican women in this age group. Similar results have been reported from Honduras (CARDONA DE HERRERA, 1965) and Panama (MONDRAGON, and FIGUEROA, 1965). It is only through mortality statistics that we learn a bit more about the cancer problem. Thus, cancer is the third cause of death in Panama, the sixth cause of death in Mexico, and the eigteenth cause of death in Guatemala (O.M.S., 1964). (Tables XIV and XV.) Admittedly, death statistics are not wholly representative, but at least they reflect the fact that malnutrition and communicable diseases are a much more common problem in our countries. However, cancer is becoming a more important cause of death, at least in Mexico. Isolated reports show that whereas about 8 per cent of all autopsies showed cancer in 1939, this figure had increased to 26 per cent in 1959 and this increase was due in large part to the reduction of infectious and parasitic diseases (STEINER, 1960). Our data on the incidence of the major forms of advanced cancer are based principally on autopsy studies done by STEINER (1960) and by PEREZ-TAMAYO (personal communication) in two of our largest university hospitals and on our own recent analysis of over 3000 medical histories of patients with specific forms of cancer

Table XV. *Mortality in Guatemala (1962)*

Rank	Disease	Per 100,000
1.	Senility, unknown and ill-defined causes	257.3
2.	Gastroenteritis	223.5
3.	Diseases of early childhood	186.4
4.	Influenza	145.8
5.	Pneumonia	140.3
6.	Malaria	108.1
7.	Other infectious and parasitic diseases	99.3
8.	Whooping cough	91.5
9.	Measles	53.5
10.	Anemia	39.2
11.	Dysentery	35.8
12.	Liver cirrhosis	35.8
13.	Cardiovascular diseases	34.7
14.	Motor vehicle accidents	32.4
15.	Tuberculosis	31.4
16.	Bronchitis	29.0
17.	Avitaminosis	26.7
18.	Cancer	25.9

Table XVI. *Incidence of specific types of cancer (per cent)*

Type	STEINER	PEREZ-TAMAYO	PAREDES-MORAN
Cervix	28.3	20.1	31.3
Lymphoma and Leukemia	10.3	—	6.8
Breast	7.0	6.0	8.3
Stomach	7.0	7.0	4.8
Head and Neck	6.6	4.9	5.7
Lung	3.7	7.1	4.3
Liver and Bile Ducts	3.3	3.9	2.4
Ovary	3.3	—	0.9
CNS Tumors	2.9	5.8	0.4
Testis	2.6	—	0.6

seen in our cancer clinic, one of the five free cancer clinics in Mexico (Table XVI). The little information we could obtain from other similar hospitals of Mexico and Central America seems to coincide with our data. Thus, about 3 out of 4 patients presenting to our clinics for the first time have nonresectable disease. Our patients usually wait an average of two years after first symptoms appear before they are started on specific therapy (MACÍAS and MORÁN, 1965).

Lack of medical education on cancer among doctors and laymen is an important contributory factor.

Cancer of the cervix is of course, a major killer; it is four times as frequent as cancer of the breast. Early pregnancy and multiparity of our women as well as inadequate postpartum care and meager facilities for cancer prevention are among the factors resposible for this high incidence. Other neoplasias attacking young people are also common; leukemias and lymphomas, as well as breast carcinomas, are high in the list. Myeloid leukemia would seem to be much more frequent than the lymphocytic type. Head and neck — including larynx and thyroid — and stomach cancer are commonest in the male population. Lung cancer is also common and, in this type of cancer, our autopsies do not show an important difference between sexes. Thus, a ratio of 1.7:1 and 1.5:1 between males and females respectively was obtained in our two pathological studies. STEINER and others (BUECHLEY et al., 1957) have encountered similar data in the Mexican population of California. Ovarian and testicular carcinomas were common in STEINER's series but not in ours. Likewise our study showed that large bowel cancer is the tenth most common but STEINER did not find a single instance of cancer of the colon in his series. No attempt will be made to explain these differences.

Survival figures of our advanced cancer patients are nearly always meaningless in Mexico and Central America. Most free cancer centers have large numbers of patients abandoning treatment either before, or soon after, primary treatment is started. In our clinic, for instance, during the period from 1957 through 1961, 89 per cent of our cervix carcinomas were lost to observation; more than two thirds of these cases did receive primary treatment. We have had better luck in the ensuing years but we still have a desertion rate of well over 50 per cent. Our survival statistics are then thoroughly based upon the small percentage of cases that do not escape observation. What happens to the rest of the patients is anyone's guess.

Reasons for abandoning treatment include the fact that free treatment centers do dot offer optimal facilities at present available to the large mass of people constituting our medically indigent population. Many of these patients manage to save enough money to pay for initial private medical attention and are only referred to the clinics with disseminated disease for complementary radio- or chemotherapy. Diagnostic workups are limited to the essentials and treatments are given almost selectively to cases who benefit most from standard methods of therapy; breast, cervix and lymphoma cases excluded, a large majority of advanced cases are given only the most needed and urgent palliation. They are seldom admitted to hospitals and are usually sent home to die. This attitude is conditioned by a budget that allows us a maximum of about 20 dollars per case, one extra dollar per day for cases needing hospitalization. Similar conditions prevail in most of our free treatment cancer centers throughout Northern Latin America.

Better facilities are to be found in general and cancer hospitals under the program of our National Social Security Institutions. Roughly about one fourth of Mexico's total population, representing most of her middle class, enjoy its advantages. Cancer survival and incidence figures from these hospitals are seemingly unavailable. We have reasons to suspect that they too have a high desertion rate. Other countries with similar programs of socialized medicine, like Guatemala, El Salvador and Panama, do not have statistical studies available either.

The general attitude of our peoples towards official institutions, medical or otherwise, is one of distrust. Many of them belong to what LEWIS (1965) has called the culture of poverty. These people have "a sense of resignation and fatalism based upon the realities of their difficult life situation. They only know or care about their problems, about their local conditions, about their own way of life. They are only partially integrated into national institutions and are marginal people even when they live in the heart of a great city. They are like foreigners in their own country, convinced that existing institutions do not serve their interests or their needs". In a recent survey done by us in 100 families they frequently stated they are suspicious of hospitals where "one goes only to die". Advanced cancer cases and their families do not protest too strongly for being refused adequate medical attention in official institutions. Many look upon lethal disease as a blessing to end their constant struggle for survival. Although the ideal of family solidarity is rarely achieved, it prevails as a foundation for caring for the ill at home. Affection, compassion, limited medical assistance (ZUCKERMANN, personal communication) and a fairly good share of herb concoctions and sortileges of all types are the principal pillars to sustain life to the very end.

We have heretofore intended to portray a realistic view of our cancer problem. Specific recommendations to improve the level of medical care for our advanced cancer cases would require a much deeper knowledge of our economic and human potentials. Massive financial and technical assistance properly channeled through better integrated and more extensive programs of socialized medicine could result in overall improvement of medical attention but parallel efforts for sympathetic understanding of our peoples' makeup would have to be made to help repair the damage done by poverty to the poor. Scientific educational programs for doctors and laymen alike and improvement in the material conditions of living should be decisive to help us shatter our bonds of ignorance, injustice and poverty.

Summary

Attempts were made to estimate the extent of the cancer problem and the management of advanced cancer in Mexico and Central America. Neither incidence figures nor accurate survival data could be obtained. Mortality statistics would seem to indicate that infectious and nutritional diseases overshadow the cancer problem. A general outlook was given on the problems affecting this area of the world and their relationship to the management of advanced cancer.

Although expenditures by our governments for public health in general and for national cancer campaigns in particular are pitifully small, they may be generous in the context of our poverty. Improvement of our present cultural, economic and sanitary conditions has to be accomplished before cancer cases can enjoy their share of modern medical attention in our countries.

References

BUECHLEY, R., DUNN jr., J. E., LINDEN, G., and BRESLOW,, L. Excess lung cancer mortality rates among Mexican women in California. *Cancer (Philad.)* 10, 63—66 (1957).

CARDONA DE HERRERA, H., Detección de Cancer Cervico-Uterino en Honduras. *Pren. méd. mex.* 128, Marzo-Abril (1965).

EISENHOWER M. S., *The wine is bitter,* p. 14, 20—29. Garden, City, New York: Doubleday & Co., Inc. 1963.

GARCÍA, G., y GARZA, T., La epidemiología del cancer cervico-uterino en Mexico. *Rev. Inst. nac. Cancer (Méx.),* "Symposium de Cancer del Utero." 16, 372—386 (1964).

Ingresos y Egresos de la Población de Mexico. Secretaría de Industria y Comercio 1965.

LEWIS, O., Antropologia de la Pobreza, p. 16—32. Fondo de Cultura Económica. Mexico-Buenos Aires. 5A. Edicion 1965.

MACÍAS, E., and MORÁN, R., Estudio Epidemiológico de las Neoplasias Malignas en Guadalajara. *Bol. méd. Hosp. Mex.-Amer.* 1 (1965).

MARTÍNEZ, G. R., ALVAREZ, A. R., GALLEGOS, V. G., RAQUEL, O. B., and VALENZUELA, D. P., Resultados preliminares de la Campaña del Instituto Mexicano del Seguro Social para el Descubrimiento del Cancer Cervico-Uterino. *Rev. Inst. nac. Cancer (Méx.)* "Symposium de Cancer del Utero" 16, 470—474 (1964).

MONDRAGON, H., and FIGUEROA, J. M., Informe citopatológico del servicio de laboratorio del hospital Gorgas, Zona del Canal, Panama. *Pren. méd. mex.* 128, Marzo-Abril (1965).

O. M. S. "Las Condiciones de Salud en Las Americas" 1961—1962. Publicaciones Científicas No. 104 (1964).

STEINER, E. P., Cancer en Autopsias Hechas en la Ciudad de Guadalajara. *Actualid. méd.* 1, 88—96 (1960).

Management of Advanced Cancer, the Indian Problem

DALI J. JUSSAWALLA

Indian Cancer Society, Parel-Bombay 12, India

Dr. PAREDES' presentation demonstrates the socio-economic climate that exists in the poorer countries of the world today. Most of the problems are likely to be similar in diverse underdeveloped areas the world over, with individual variations depending on habits, customs and nutritional status of the population, as modified by climatic and economic conditions. The burden of caring for vast numbers of patients with advanced disease is even more pronounced in a country like India, because of the crushing impost of a population of half a billion hungry souls.

If we were to analyze the medical and health problems of non-industrialized countries merely by statistical computation, it would make dismal reading. Even if realistic statistical information was obtainable in such countries, it could at best give a static view of the situation. Only by assessing the trend of the changing scene, and the tempo of over-all socio-economic development over a period of time, can future possibilities be gauged with any degree of accuracy.

To deduce from Tables of Disease Incidence that only a handful of public health problems merit exclusive attention, would seem to us to indicate a somewhat monocular outlook. But such indeed was the official view-point in India until 1950, perhaps justifiably so because infant mortality, pneumonia, malaria, tuberculosis and infectious diseases claimed dubious distinction in ranking, in public health analyses. But during the past 15 years a fair amount of control has been achieved over these diseases, and with this changing scene chronic diseases have now begun to show a relative increase in incidence. In no underdeveloped country, however, can cancer claim to deserve high priority in the over-all public health program.

In India, since the past decade, it is being increasingly recognized by the Central Department of Public Health, that cancer as a disease entity needs to be treated at a specialized institutional level. The Indian Cancer Society has played a significant part in creating this opinion. In the past 25 years, five cancer hospitals have been established from private and public sources, and cancer departments have also been created at a few medical centers. But this is a mere drop in the ocean of demand for such facilities.

As the majority of our people live in villages, management of advanced cancer depends on the facilities available locally in the rural areas of our country. Relief from pain can probably be obtained by most of the advanced cancer patients, but only a minority can expect surgical help, in the thousands of towns and villages scattered in all directions across the country (Table XVII).

Table XVII

Distribution of population in towns:		Distribution of population in villages:	
Population	Number	Population	Number
Over 100,000	73	Over 10,000	721
Over 50,000—100,000	110	Over 5,000—10,000	1,916
Over 5,000— 50,000	2,223	Over 500— 5,000	555,858
Less than 5,000	661		
Total number of towns	3,067	Total number of villages	557,989

This gives a ratio of 1 town to 180 villages.

Prolongation of life in advanced cancer often necessitates surgical inter-
ference to curb hemorrhage, relieve obstruction or control fungation. This
entails minor surgery well within the capacity of a small-town surgeon, even
though laboratory and radiological investigations are not always available in
our villages and small towns. But lack of available hospital beds is the main
reason why advanced cancer patients do not get the surgical attention they need.
In India there is a great need to attend to the medico-social welfare of such
patients and their families.

This matter is occupying the attention of the Indian Cancer Society which is
planning through its branches to organize minimal-care units to look after such
patients with advanced disease.

To understand the magnitude of our problem one should realize that India
occupies 2.4 per cent of the total land area of the world, but strives to support
nearly 15 per cent of the total world population, 60 per cent of whom are non-
earning. Only 12 per cent of the total working group are covered by Health
Insurance Schemes. To care for the health of this colossal mass of humanity,
only 130,000 doctors will be available by 1970 giving a ratio of 1 doctor per
4,000 of population as compared to 1 in 1,000 in the United Kingdom. At the
same time 90,000 trained nurses (an increase from 15,000 in 1950) and 300,000
hospital beds will become available. Medical colleges have been established in
112 centers. (There were only 61 in 1961 and 25 in 1947.)

By 1965 the death rate had been reduced to under 20 per thousand and
expectation of life at birth had gone up to 50 years. The birth-rate is expected
to be reduced to 25 per 1,000 within the next 5 years and could well mark the
beginning of the slow rise to long cherished self-sufficiency.

On analysing 650,000 deaths that occurred in the city of Bombay between
1941 and 1943, Pai has shown that cancer and heart disease have increased in
frequency 3 and 4 times, respectively within 2 decades. By 1963 cancer had
achieved the 8th rank as a cause of death, the commonest causes being due to
respiratory and infectious diseases. It is interesting to note that in the age-group
of 45 and above, cancer was the *THIRD* commonest cause of death, after heart
diseases and tuberculosis.

The age structure of the population according to the 1961 Census of India
was:

Age	per cent
0— 4 years	13.5
5—14 years	24.8
15—54 years	53.4
55—75 years	8.3

In India cancer occurs most commonly in men in the region of the head and
neck. Approximately 30 per cent of male cancer occurs in this region. In women
the commonest sites are the cervix (21 per cent) and breast (17 per cent). The

incidence rate of oesophageal cancer is 8 per cent both sexes. These figures are quoted from the Bombay Cancer Registry.

From the Health Survey Report published by the Central Ministry of Health, excellent results seem to have been achieved since 1950 by the National Malaria Eradication Programme. This disease has for many centuries past dominated the scene as the most important public health problem, but it has been nearly wiped out today. Similarly, tuberculosis is being better controlled with mass BCG vaccination programs and easy availability of efficacious drugs. Infectious diseases are being increasingly curbed with improvement in hygiene and by the rising indigenous manufacture of antibiotics.

To analyse the health situation further, it has been estimated that out of a population of 500 million, 10 million could fall ill on any one day, of whom 40,000 would definitely need hospital admission.

The Cancer Society's Bombay Registry computed a crude cancer incidence rate of 685 per million of population of Greater Bombay. But if age-correction is carried out by applying SEGI's standard population, the rate goes up to 1366. This rate is higher than the age-adjusted rate computed for Poland.

On the basis of age specific rates computed for Bombay, one can estimate that about 411,000 persons are likely to develop cancer in India every year. About 70 per cent of these patients, i. e. 287,700, would already have had advanced disease by the time they reach a medical centre; so obviously the vast majority cannot expect to be cured. (We assume that any cancer which has spread beyond its primary site of origin should be considered as advanced.) About 211,800 persons are estimated to die of the disease in India every year.

It is difficult correctly to assess the optimal facilities available in India today for the treatment of advanced cancer, but we can safely assume that such facilities are totally inadequate. A remarkable change seems to have occurred within 10 years in the outlook of the indigent patient with regard to acceptance of hospital treatment. Institutional admission is now sought early, in contrast to the previous antagonistic attitude towards hospitals. There is also an increasing tendency on the part of Government and other official agencies to help sustain the life of patients suffering from even advanced diseases such as cancer. In the economic depression prevalent today this attitude may seem unrealistic. Religious philosophy, strong family ties and traditional respect for all forms of life, have helped to create this contrary outlook, of fatalism on the one hand, and the urge to prolong life (even of the hopelessly ill) on the other.

There is a tendency today to create special cancer departments in general hospitals but it will take a long time before sufficient numbers of such units can be established. So far cancer is treated throughout India in the general hospitals, by medical and surgical specialists. This situation results in a patient receiving treatment at various levels of efficiency, depending on the medical training, philosophical outlook and psychological bias of the specialist responsible.

Optimal medical care for advanced cancer patients entails an integrated service capable of utilising the skill of a number of scientific disciplines, such as surgery (including its many sub-divisions), radiology, radiotherapy, nuclear medicine, pathology, biochemistry and chemotherapy. Generally speaking the district hospitals and medical centers even in the larger towns, have but a few such men on their staff. So the majority of district centers send their patients whenever possible, to the major city hospitals for treatment. Thus 7,000 cancer patients (mostly referred) are seen at the Tata Memorial Hospital in Bombay every year; and other hospitals in the city account for 5,000 more. Of these 12,000 approximately 70 per cent are found to be suffering from advanced cancer.

Until now, radiotherapy had necessitated the use of X-ray generators, the maintenance of which still leaves much to be desired in India. It is most frustrating to find that nearly 60 per cent of the few radiotherapy units available in the country are constantly out of order, because of inadequate maintenance facilities or non-availability of spare parts. The Indian Atomic Energy Establishment started functioning in the early fifties, and this fact may eventually lead to a change in the current scene, as far as radiotherapy is concerned. May I venture to suggest that instead of acquiring deep X-ray generators, under-developed countries should obtain Tele-caesium units. This isotope has a long half-life, and the apparatus needs only a minimal amount of maintenance. The cost factor also is reasonably low. A pilot plant has been completely designed and manufactured by the Atomic Energy Establishment at Bombay, and is now under test. The caesium source could also be charged to a high level of activity in the reactor built with Canadian collaboration at the same center, because of the high neutron flux already achieved. Such facilities for radiotherapy cannot as yet be made available in the small-towns and villages, because of a lack of other ancillary medical facilities.

Excellent nuclear medicine workshops are conducted twice a year by the Atomic Energy Establishment, which has also assumed the responsibility for advising on the set-up of radiotherapy units to hospital administrators throughout the country.

To facilitate public health measures, rural India has been grouped into 5,000 blocks, each unit having a family planning and primary health centre. A general hospital serves a number of such blocks. Radiotherapy units when made available, can serve as a king-pins around which could be organised a cancer department in a number of such hospitals.

Each Indian State is traditionally divided into numerous districts for administrative purposes, and a general hospital usually has served as the district medical center. These District Hospitals are in the charge of Civil Surgeons who as a rule are usually qualified specialists, capable of treating a variety of cancers. A general hospital may drain a varying number of districts, but unfortunately few of them have any facilities for undertaking radiotherapy.

Statistical information is only available from those district hospitals where the administrative personnel are interested in collecting such information, which is unusual.

Numerous Christian Missionary Hospitals are dotted all over the country. A few have grown into large medical centers having adequate facilities for the treatment of a variety of diseases including cancer. A number of such mission hospitals have achieved the distinction of evolving into medical colleges, staffed by highly qualified specialists trained in various disciplines of medicine and surgery. A few of these medical centers also attract highly qualified European and American missionary doctors and specialists.

Even though the majority of cancer patients are still seen in India in the late stages of the disease there is a demand to have some form of medical aid available if only to ease the few remaining years or months of life. Without the facilities special cancer units could offer, such help cannot be given adequately. The chronic shortage of hospital beds does not encourage the admission of advanced cancer patients even in the large urban medical centers, for what at best would be palliative procedures. A Cancer Department would make it easier to provide for the treatment of advanced cases, whenever indicated.

It is understandable that this austere scene does not encourage any other reaction amongst the poorer masses of the population but one of despair. The amount of suffering that can be silently borne by the Indian peasant is truly remarkable, and blind acceptance of what is termed fate is directly responsible for the philosophy to face every trying situation with resignation, and even to meet death with equanimity. Unlike the Western countries, there is no vociferous public demand yet heard for providing adequate medical facilities for patients with advanced cancer.

The situation is probably somewhat different in the larger towns, where education in the facts about cancer, undertaken by the local branch of the Cancer Society, encourages the public to ask for even palliative aid, in increasing numbers. In fact today, the general outlook towards the treatment of a patient with advanced cancer varies greatly in urban and rural India.

Conclusions and Comments

The treatment of advanced cancer is woefully inadequate in India as in every other underdeveloped country with an agricultural economy.

An unbalanced view can easily be obtained from a brief visit to the principal urban population centers, as isolated examples of efficient hospital groups would usually be found today in underdeveloped nations making serious efforts to improve their medico-socio-economic status.

Thus the Tata Cancer Centre at Bombay has 12 therapy units including 3 Tele-Cobalt units. It boasts of a specialized staff well trained in various branches of medicine and surgery. It has a chemotherapy clinical unit conducted by the Cancer Society and a fundamental research division which has a staff of 400 scientists.

There is a very sophisticated nuclear medicine facility, and a host of other departments maintained by the Cancer Society, including a social service research unit, a rehabilitation center, a publication office for "The Indian Journal of Cancer" and a Registry to survey the cancer problem in Greater Bombay.

A few of the smaller developing countries may have better opportunities to improve their lot in a hurry, because of the lesser burden of looking after a smaller population. A much bigger effort is indicated in India if currently accepted standards of medical care are to be achieved in the foreseeable future, because of the enormous burden of supporting half a billion people. Unless international agencies, private foundations and the governments of the richer highly industrialized nations step in to establish pilot projects to serve as guiding lights, progress will be painfully slow. The situation is made worse by the current restrictions, due to economic crisis, on the import of modern drugs and medical and scientific apparatus not yet available locally. General hospitals will continue to shun the care of advanced cancer patients until cancer departments are included as a part of their organizational set-up.

Conclusions and Panel Recommendation

This panel has undertaken a difficult and unpleasantly probing assignment, and it deserves our gratitude for its willingness to examine the problem of advanced cancer in various parts of the world in a fair, honest, and realistic manner. We are concerned about patients with cancer not susceptible to a curative procedure; while the more highly developed countries have active programs, meager facilities, patient ignorance and medical neglect are common in large areas of the world. It is noted that cancer is an individual and lonely disease; society is not threatened by cancer as by a contagious or transmissible disease, and consequently urgent public health measures are not instituted to help stamp out the disease and to isolate the affected individuals. The victims do not tend to band together, society does not react vigorously in meeting the individual problems, and the care of these patients is ultimately dependent on the conscience and not the evident self-interest of society. The care of patients with cancer is expensive. The result of intensive medical effort is not often rewarding in terms of long-term survival and increased patient productivity. Yet it is essential that the physician and society struggle to improve the lot of the cancer patient, and not subordinate his needs to what appear to be the more pressing social and health problems. The panel has unanimously approved the following recommendations to the governing body of the International Union

Against Cancer, as the international body dedicated to the struggle against cancer.

The Panel on the Management of Advanced Cancer, held on October 25, 1966 in Tokyo, Japan wishes to bring the following statement and recommendation to the attention of the governing body of the International Union Against Cancer.

"The care of the advanced cancer patient is a matter of concern to the U.I.C.C. Advanced cancer presents many complex economic, psychological, social and medical problems involving patient attitudes, hospital facilities, physician motivation and responsibility and governmental support. It is apparent that, whereas the Western World, including the USA, Europe and the USSR, and Japan in the East, is making strenuous efforts to provide adequate care for advanced cancer patients, such programs are practically non-existent in many other areas of the world. An explanation for these negligible facilities is the existence of more pressing medical and public health problems within these underdeveloped countries. It is the function of the U.I.C.C, nevertheless, to lead the fight against cancer wherever in the world it is found.

"The panel recommends that the U.I.C.C. establish a committee with representation from developed and underdeveloped countries to survey the resources available and the needs of patients in various countries throughout the world, to be conducted in cooperation with the government and medical profession of the respective countries. The survey can result in recommendations made within the framework of a country's resources, designed to accelerate the necessary developments to improve the care of patients with advanced cancer. The impartial and respected humanitarian purposes of the U.I.C.C. will support the efforts of concerned physicians, public health officials and interested laymen within each country."

Panel 22

The Role of Medical Education in Cancer Control

Chairman:

Roald N. Grant (U.S.A.)

Members:

I. M. Bush (U.S.A.), E. C. Easson (U.K.), U. P. Guimaraes (Brazil)
H. J. Tagnon (Belgium), K. Oota (Japan), N. I. Perevodchikova (U.S.S.R.)

The panel addressed itself primarily to discussing the problem of undergraduate medical school education in cancer and agreed that the rapid proliferation of medical knowledge in recent years has made it increasingly difficult
for faculties to adequately cover the teaching of cancer. Dr. Roald N. Grant,
of the American Cancer Society in New York City, described the various
techniques which have been developed to increase the efficiency of teaching of
medical science. Among those which are being applied to the teaching of cancer
are the use of self-instructional audio-visual equipment utilizing 8 mm sound
motion picture cartridges, video-tape recordings, and computerized information
storage and retrieval machines which enable the student and the machine to
carry out a student-teacher dialogue.

In an effort to find ways of improving the undergraduate teaching of cancer,
a controlled study of a programmed learning technique was made by Dr.
Irving M. Bush, of Cook County Hospital in Chicago, Illinois, who compared
the results of teaching students with a programmed text on colon cancer with
using a standard monograph on "Cancer of the Colon and Rectum". The course
was given to students, interns and residents. He found that study by the use of
the traditional monograph resulted in a gain of 33 per cent in knowledge of
cancer of the colon and rectum compared to a 66 per cent gain in score by those
who utilized a programmed text.

In addition to the need for teaching numerous new basic science facts about
cancer, there is the more immediate need to provide the students with established
clinical information about the disease. That this is a problem was demonstrated
by Dr. Eric Easson, of the Christie Hospital and Holt Radium Institute in

Manchester, England, who gave a special test (see Appendix) on the prognosis of a variety of common forms of cancer to senior medical students, general practitioners and nurses. He found that all three groups greatly underestimated the curability of cancer. This reflected not only a lack of knowledge of how successful the treatment of favorable cases of cancer can be, but also a substantial degree of pessimism about cancer in general. That this pessimism was deeply rooted and wide-spread was demonstrated by the fact that there was no improvement in the scores of the students despite an intensive effort to concentrate on the teaching of the prognosis of cancer during the students' third and fourth years. The effect of this attitude on cancer treatment can be appreciated when one considers what will be the outcome of a consultation between a pessimistic patient and an equally pessimistic physician.

The panel discussed at length the various possible approaches to medical school curriculum-planning in cancer teaching. One of these is the establishment of a chair on oncology. It was agreed that medical school faculties, in general, were not receptive to this method of cancer teaching. However chairs of oncology have been established in several of the Egyptian medical schools and are apparently operating successfully. Dr. NATASHA PEREVODCHIKOVA, of the Institute of Experimental and Clinical Oncology of the U.S.S.R., reported that some institutions in her country were experimenting with chairs of oncology and modified similar approaches to the teaching of cancer in medical schools. The discussion brought out the fact that the United States' Cancer Coordinator system has been very successful in bringing improved cancer teaching to the medical schools and is a method which is highly acceptable to the faculty. The cancer coordinator is a member of the faculty who is given the assignment of assisting his fellow faculty members in bringing new information and techniques on cancer teaching to their attention, and helping in cancer teaching as requested. The cancer coordinator program is supported by a federal grant to each medical school. Another approach used by some medical schools is the appointment of a cancer committee which serves as a body to stimulate the faculty and promote improved cancer teaching. The panel was reminded by Dr. HENRI TAGNON, of the Institut Jules-Bordet in Brussels, Belgium, that cancer teaching and cancer care and research are inseparable, and that a team approach involving all three categories is desirable. He pointed out that individual oncologists were often missionaries whereas good teachers were needed.

Dr. KUNIO OOTA, of the University of Tokyo, Tokyo, Japan, brought out that medical students today have an overwhelming interest in research into the basic sciences as compared to a lesser interest in clinical medicine. This tendency seems to be fairly wide-spread in other countries and reflects the increasing emphasis on scientific practice of medicine. This trend makes it necessary for teachers to employ special efforts to capture the interest of students in the clinical aspects of cancer, and that special efforts should be made by the panel agreed that greater emphasis is needed in undergraduate education in the clinical aspects of cancer, and that special efforts should be made by the faculties of medical schools to provide for this in the curriculum, and that the UICC should make efforts to be helpful in that direction.

Appendix

Of 100 middle-aged people with the following diseases, how many would you expect to be alive and well five years after appropriate treatment? (Ring the number you think most likely in each case):

Early cancer of the breast	0	25	50	*75*	100
Early cancer of the vocal cord	0	25	50	*75*	100
Early cancer of the cervix uteri	0	25	50	*75*	100
Early seminoma testis	0	25	50	*75*	100
Early Hodgkin's disease	0	25	*50*	75	100

(italic figures are correct answers to questions)

Panel 23

International Cancer Organizations
— UICC, WHO, and IARC —

Chairman:

A. V. Chaklin (U.S.S.R)

Members:

E. von Haam (U.S.A.), J. Higginson (I.A.R.C.), M. J. Shear (U.I.C.C.),
H. L. Stewart (U.S.A.), H. Torloni (W.H.O.), A. J. Tuyns (W.H.O.),
J. Vikol (W.H.O.)

UICC Publications

Kaposi's Sarcoma. S. Karger AG., Basle (Switzerland) — New York (1963).

Cancer of the urinary bladder. S. Karger AG., Basle (Switzerland) — New York (1963).

Prognosis of malignant tumours of the breast. S. Karger AG., Basle (Switzerland) — New York (1963).

The lymphoreticular tumours in Africa. S. Karger AG., Basle (Switzerland) — New York (1964).

Cellular control mechanisms and cancer. Elsevier Publishing Company, Amsterdam — London — New York (1964).

Illustrated Tumor Nomenclature. Springer-Verlag Berlin — Heidelberg — New York (1965).

Structure and control of the melanocyte. Springer-Verlag Berlin — Heidelberg — New York (1966).

Public education about cancer; cancer education programmes in various countries. UICC, Geneva (1966).

Cancer incidence in five continents. Springer-Verlag Berlin — Heidelberg — New York (1966).

Choriocarcinoma. Springer-Verlag Berlin — Heidelberg — New York (1967).

Cancer detection. Springer-Verlag Berlin — Heidelberg — New York (1967).

Public education about cancer; research findings and theoretical concepts. Springer-Verlag Berlin — Heidelberg — New York (1967).

Tumour specific antigens. Munksgaard, Copenhagen (1967).

Cancer of the nasopharynx. Munksgaard, Copenhagen (1967).

Potential Carcinogenic Hazards from Drugs. Springer-Verlag Berlin — Heidelberg — New York (1967).

Treatment of Burkitt's Tumor. Springer-Verlag Berlin — Heidelberg — New York (1967).

Mechanisms of Invasion in Cancer. Springer-Verlag Berlin — Heidelberg — New York (1967).

Proceedings of the Ninth International Cancer Congress — Congress Lectures and Official Speeches. Springer-Verlag, Berlin — Heidelberg — New York (1967).

Ovarian Cancer. Springer-Verlag Berlin — Heidelberg — New York (1967).

Reprint from

UICC Monograph Series
Volume 10: Ninth International Cancer Congress

Edited by R. J. C. HARRIS

Springer-Verlag Berlin · Heidelberg · New York 1967

Printed in Germany / Not for sale

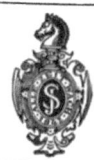

SPRINGER-VERLAG
BERLIN · HEIDELBERG · NEW YORK

Recent Results in Cancer Research
Fortschritte der Krebsforschung
Progrès dans les recherches sur le cancer

Edited by numerous experts. Editor in Chief: P. Rentchnick, Genève
Sponsored by the Swiss League Against Cancer

Volume 1: R. Schindler, Die tierische Zelle in Zellkultur
1965. Gebunden DM 16,—; US $ 4.00

Volume 2: Neuroblastomas · Biochemical Studies. Edited by C. Bohuon
1966. Cloth DM 16,—; US $ 4.00

Volume 3: W. C. Hueper, Occupational and Environmental Cancers of the Respiratory System. 1966. Cloth DM 34,—; US $ 8.50

Volume 4: L. Goldman, Laser Cancer Research. 1966. Cloth DM 16,—; US $ 4.00

Volume 5: D. Metcalf, The Thymus
Its Role in Immune Responses, Leukaemia Development and Carcinogenesis
1966. Cloth DM 24,—; US $ 6.00

Volume 6: Malignant Transformation by Viruses. Edited by W. H. Kirsten
1966. Cloth DM 32,—; US $ 8.00

Volume 7: Ch. G. Moertel, Multiple Primary Malignant Neoplasms
Their Incidence and Significance
1966. Cloth DM 18,—; US $ 4.50

■ Prospectus on request!

Volume 8: New Trends in the Treatment of Cancer
Edited by L. Manuila, S. Moles, P. Rentchnick
1967. Cloth DM 32,—; US $ 8.00

Volume 9: J. Lindenmann / P. A. Klein, Immunological Aspects of Viral Oncolysis
1967. Cloth DM 18,—; US $ 4.50

Volume 10: R. S. Nelson, Radioactive Phosphorus in the Diagnosis of Gastrointestinal Cancer
1967. Cloth DM 15,—; US $ 3.75

Volume 11: R. G. Freeman / J. M. Knox, Treatment of Skin Cancer
1967. Cloth DM 15,—; US $ 3.75

Volume 12: H. T. Lynch, Hereditary Factors in Carcinoma
1967. Cloth DM 24,—; US $ 6.00

Volume 13: Tumours in Children
Edited by J. K. Steward and H. B. Marsden
1967. In preparation

Special subscription rate at 20 % of list price applies when complete set is purchased.

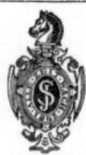